Sixth Edition

Essentials of
Equipment in Anaesthesia, Critical Care and Perioperative Medicine

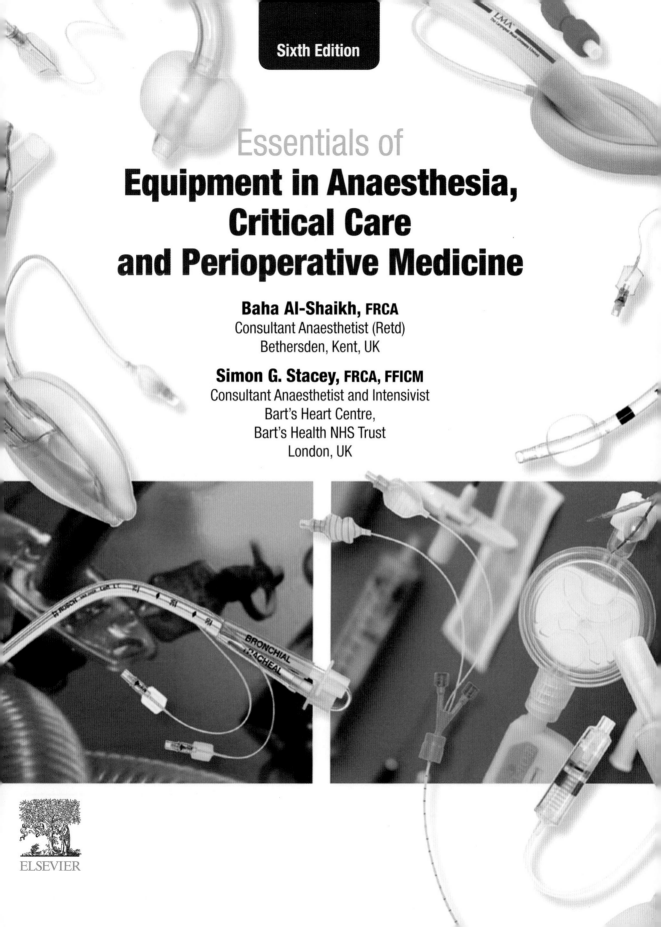

Sixth Edition

Essentials of
Equipment in Anaesthesia,
Critical Care
and Perioperative Medicine

Baha Al-Shaikh, FRCA
Consultant Anaesthetist (Retd)
Bethersden, Kent, UK

Simon G. Stacey, FRCA, FFICM
Consultant Anaesthetist and Intensivist
Bart's Heart Centre,
Bart's Health NHS Trust
London, UK

ELSEVIER

First edition 1995
Second edition 2002
Third edition 2007
Fourth edition 2013
Fifth edition 2019

The right of Baha Al-Shaikh and Simon G. Stacey to be identified as author of this work has been asserted by them in accordance with the Copyright, Designs and Patents Act 1988.

Notices

Practitioners and researchers must always rely on their own experience and knowledge in evaluating and using any information, methods, compounds or experiments described herein. Because of rapid advances in the medical sciences, in particular, independent verification of diagnoses and drug dosages should be made. To the fullest extent of the law, no responsibility is assumed by Elsevier, authors, editors or contributors for any injury and/or damage to persons or property as a matter of products liability, negligence or otherwise, or from any use or operation of any methods, products, instructions, or ideas contained in the material herein.

ISBN: 978-0-323-84845-9

Content Strategist: Trinity Hutton
Content Project Manager: Arindam Banerjee
Design: Miles Hitchen
Art Buyer: Nijantha Priyadharshini
Marketing Manager: Deborah Watkins

Printed in India

Last digit is the print number: 9 8 7 6 5 4 3 2 1

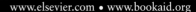

Working together
to grow libraries in
developing countries

www.elsevier.com • www.bookaid.org

Contents

Preface

In the last millennium, only Professors/Academics had access to the resources needed to publish a book. There was a very real disconnect at the time between the professorial authors and the exam-taking readership. So over 30 years after the novel idea of an abundantly illustrated equipment book, written by junior doctors who understood what the FRCA exam wanted them to know, here we are again.

This sixth edition holds true to the original format and philosophy of the trail blazing first edition: syllabus focused text, great illustration, and helpful questions, plus web links.

Ironically one of the authors was a Professor before retiring, but I trust the readers will not hold that against us!

We have maintained the high standards that have made this the equipment book of choice not only for trainees in Anaesthesia, but also for our Operating Department Practitioner and Nursing colleagues. We have extensively updated the text, images and illustrations.

Simplicity, Structure, Syllabus.

BA-S
SGS

Acknowledgements

We are extremely grateful to the manufacturers and suppliers for their help and assistance in the provision of the necessary images and information for this edition. Without their help, this sixth edition could not have gone ahead in its current format.

Below is the list of the people and their companies who helped us by providing images during the preparation of this book.

Staffan Ahlandsberg, Sylva Lindskog *(HemoCue AB)*

Kerrie Anson, Charlotte Green *(Diamedica)*

Joshua Ardon *(Haemonetics)*

Andrew Garnham *(Penlon)*

Louisa Giblin *(GE)*

Katrin Hueve *(Pajunk)*

Nicholas Jonassen, Irakli Jaliashvili *(Radiometer)*

Tannya Bagoban, Kevin Rowan *(Sonosite)*

James Bill, Jenine Sawyer, Alexandra Marheineke, Rosie McNamara *(Ambu)*

Vicki Brothers *(Rivanna Medical)*

Jennie Brownlie, Neil Manners *(Proact)*

Sean Duggan *(Intersurgical)*

Katie Figulla *(Philips)*

Michael Fox *(Getinge)*

Hollie Johnson *(Reliance Medical)*

Lynda Pedley *(Blue Box)*

Patricia Petit *(Smiths Medical)*

Charlotte Sowa *(Edwards Lifesciences)*

Ann Valerio *(Teleflex)*

Anton Yuzefovich *(Treaton)*

BA-S
SGS

Chapter 1

Medical gas supply

Gas supply

Medical gas supply takes the form of cylinders and/or a piped gas system, depending on the requirements of the hospital.

Cylinders

Components

1. Cylinders are made of thin-walled, seamless molybdenum steel in which gases and vapours are stored under pressure. They are designed to withstand considerable internal pressure.
2. The top end of the cylinder, the neck, ends in a tapered screw thread into which the valve is fitted. The thread is sealed with a material that melts if the cylinder is exposed to intense heat. This allows the gas to escape, thus reducing the risk of an explosion.
3. There is a plastic disc around the neck of the cylinder. The year when the cylinder was last examined and tested can be identified from the shape and colour of the disc.

4. Cylinders are manufactured in different sizes (sizes A–J) and contents (Table 1.1). Sizes A and H are not used for medical gases. Cylinders attached to the anaesthetic machine are usually size E (Figs. 1.1–1.4), while size J cylinders are commonly used for cylinder manifolds (see Fig. 1.19).
5. Lightweight cylinders can be made from aluminium alloy with a fibreglass covering in an epoxy resin matrix. These can be used to provide oxygen at home, during transport or in magnetic resonance scanners. They have a flat base for easy storage and handling.

Table 1.1 Contents of the commonly used cylinder sizes for oxygen, nitrous oxide and medical air			
Size	Oxygen	Nitrous oxide	Medical air
E (4.7 L H$_2$O capacity)	680 L	1,800 L	640 L
J (47.2 L H$_2$O capacity)	6,800 L	18,000 L	6,400 L
CD (2 L H$_2$O capacity)	460 L (23,000 kPa)		

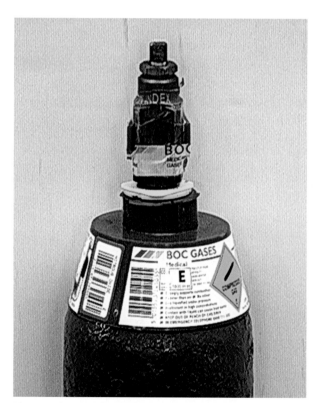

Fig. 1.1 Nitrous oxide cylinder (size E) with its wrapping and labels.

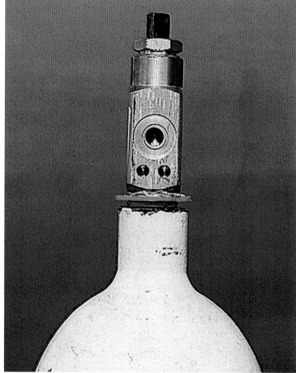

Fig. 1.2 Oxygen cylinder valve and pin index.

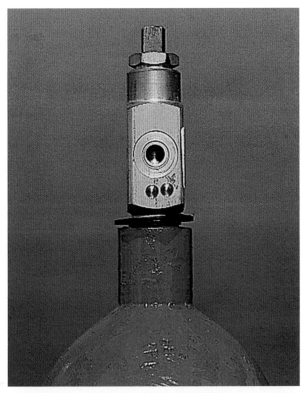

Fig. 1.3 Nitrous oxide cylinder valve and pin index.

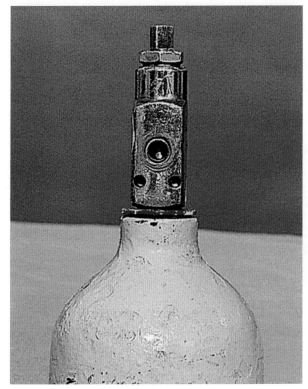

Fig. 1.4 Carbon dioxide cylinder valve and pin index.

- **Gas** exits in the gaseous state at room temperature. Its liquefaction at room temperature is impossible, since the room temperature is above its critical temperature.
- **Vapour** is the gaseous state of a substance below its critical temperature. At room temperature and atmospheric pressure, the substance is liquid.
- **Critical temperature** is the temperature above which a substance cannot be liquefied no matter how much pressure is applied. The critical temperatures for nitrous oxide and oxygen are 36.5°C and −118°C, respectively.

Gas laws
- Boyle's Law: at a constant temperature, pressure is inversely proportional to volume of a gas $(P \propto 1/V)$.
- Charles' Law: at a constant pressure, volume of a gas is directly proportional to its temperature $(V \propto T)$.
- Gay-Lussac's Law: at a fixed volume and mass of a gas, the pressure of that gas is directly proportional to its temperature $(P \propto T)$.
- Avogadro's Law: at a constant temperature and pressure, volume of gas is directly proportional to the amount of gas $(V \propto n)$.

At room temperature, oxygen is stored as a gas at a pressure of 13,700 kPa (above its critical temperature), whereas nitrous oxide is stored in a liquid phase with its vapour at equilibrium at a pressure of 4400 kPa (and usually below its critical temperature). As the liquid is less compressible than the gas, this means that the cylinder should only be partially filled. The amount of filling is called the *filling ratio*. Partially filling the cylinders with liquid minimizes the risk of dangerous increases in pressure due to increased vaporization of the liquid with increases in the ambient temperature. This scenario could lead to an explosion. In the United Kingdom, the filling ratio for nitrous oxide and carbon dioxide is 0.75. In hotter climates, the filling ratio is reduced to 0.67.

The filling ratio is the weight of the fluid in the cylinder divided by the weight of water required to fill the cylinder. However, it is important to remember that a filling ratio of 0.75 is not exactly the same as the cylinder being 75% filled. This is due to the differences in the physical properties of the contents, such as its density, and water content.

A full oxygen cylinder at atmospheric pressure can deliver 130 times its capacity of oxygen. A typical size E full oxygen cylinder delivering 4 L/min will last for 2 hours and 50 minutes but will last only 45 minutes when delivering 15 L/min.

At constant temperature, a gas-containing cylinder, e.g. oxygen, shows a linear and proportional reduction in cylinder pressure as it empties, obeying Boyle's law (first gas law).

For a cylinder that contains liquid and vapour, e.g. nitrous oxide, initially the pressure remains constant as more vapour is produced to replace that which was used. Once all the liquid has been used, the pressure in the cylinder starts to decrease. The temperature in such a cylinder can decrease because of the loss of the latent heat of vaporization leading to the formation of ice on the outside of the cylinder.

 Exam tip: In the exam, make sure you know the difference between gas and vapour. This difference causes the pressure changes in an oxygen cylinder compared to a nitrous oxide cylinder when used.

Cylinders in use are checked and tested by manufacturers at regular intervals, every 5–10 years. Test details are recorded on the plastic disc between the valve and the neck of the cylinder. They are also engraved on the cylinder:

1. An internal endoscopic examination is carried out.
2. Flattening, bend and impact tests are carried out on at least one cylinder in every 100.
3. A pressure test is conducted, whereby the cylinder is subjected to high pressures of about 22,000 kPa, which is more than 50% above their normal working pressure.
4. A tensile test is carried out on at least one cylinder in every 100, whereby strips of the cylinder are cut out and subjected to impact, stretching, flattening and other tests of strength.

The marks engraved on the cylinders are:

1. Test pressure.
2. Dates of test performed.
3. Chemical formula of the cylinder's content.
4. Tare weight (weight of nitrous oxide cylinder when empty).

Labelling

The cylinder label includes the following details:
- Name, chemical symbol, pharmaceutical form, specification of the product, its licence number and the proportion of the constituent gases in a gas mixture.
- Substance identification number and batch number.
- Hazard warnings and safety instructions.
- Cylinder size code.
- Nominal cylinder volume (litres).
- Maximum cylinder pressure (bars).
- Filling date, shelf life and expiry date.
- Directions for use.
- Storage and handling precautions.

Problems in practice and safety features

1. The gases and vapours should be free of water vapour when stored in cylinders. Water vapour freezes and blocks the exit port when the temperature of the cylinder decreases on opening.
2. The outlet valve uses the pin-index system to make it almost impossible to connect a cylinder to the wrong yoke (Fig. 1.5).
3. Cylinders are colour coded to reduce accidental use of the wrong gas or vapour. In the United Kingdom, the colour coding is a two-part colour, shoulder and body (Table 1.2). The Medicine and Healthcare Products Regulatory Agency in the United Kingdom has decided to bring it in line with the European Standard EN 1089-3 to aid cylinder identification and improve patient safety. All cylinders will have a white body but each gas/vapour will retain its

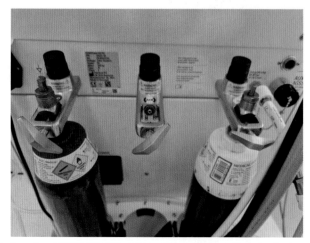

Fig. 1.5 Anaesthetic machine cylinder yokes. Note the Bodok seal in position in the medical air cylinder yoke.

Table 1.2 Colour-coding of medical gas cylinders (old and new system), their pressure when full and their physical state in cylinder

	Shoulder colour	Body colour (current/old system)	Body colour (new system)	Pressure at room temperature (kPa)	Physical state in cylinder
Oxygen	White	Black (green in USA)	White	13,700	Gas
Nitrous oxide	Blue	Blue	White	4400	Liquid/vapour
Carbon dioxide	Grey	Grey	White	5000	Liquid/vapour
Air	White/black quarters	Grey (yellow in USA)	White	13,700	Gas
Entonox	White/blue quarters	Blue	White	13,700	Gas
Oxygen/helium (Heliox)	White/brown quarters	Black	White	13,700	Gas

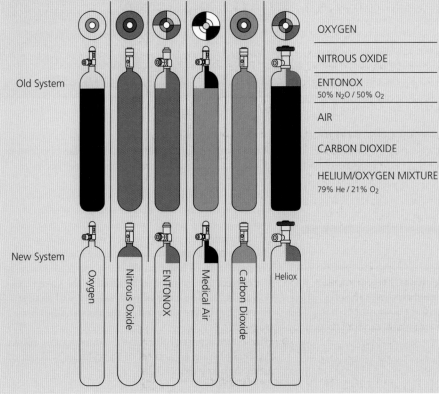

OXYGEN

NITROUS OXIDE

ENTONOX
50% N₂O / 50% O₂

AIR

CARBON DIOXIDE

HELIUM/OXYGEN MIXTURE
79% He / 21% O₂

current shoulder colour. It is hoped that these changes will take full effect by 2025. Already some oxygen and Entonox (BOC Healthcare, Manchester, UK) cylinders in the United Kingdom have started using the new scheme.

4. Cylinders should be checked regularly while in use to ensure that they have sufficient content and that leaks do not occur.
5. Cylinders should be stored in a purpose-built, dry, well-ventilated and fireproof room, preferably inside and

not subjected to extremes of heat. They should not be stored near flammable materials such as oil or grease or near any source of heat. They should not be exposed to continuous dampness, corrosive chemicals or fumes. This can lead to corrosion of cylinders and their valves.

6. To avoid accidents, full cylinders should be stored separately from empty ones. Size F, G and J cylinders are stored upright to avoid damage to the valves. Size C, D and E cylinders can be stored horizontally on shelves made of a material that does not damage the surface of the cylinders.

7. Overpressurized cylinders are hazardous and should be reported to the manufacturer.

Cylinders

- Cylinders are made of thin-walled molybdenum steel to withstand high pressures, e.g. 13,700 kPa and 4400 kPa for oxygen and nitrous oxide, respectively. Lightweight aluminium is also available.
- They are made in different sizes: size E cylinders are used on the anaesthetic machine; size J cylinders are used in cylinder banks.
- Oxygen cylinders contain gas, whereas nitrous oxide cylinders contain a mixture of liquid and vapour. In the United Kingdom, filling ratio for nitrous oxide cylinders is 0.75; in hotter climates, it is 0.67.
- At a constant temperature, the pressure in a gas cylinder decreases linearly and proportionally as it empties. This is not true in cylinders containing liquid/vapour.
- They are colour coded (shoulder and body). A new colour system is being introduced with white bodies but different coloured shoulders.

Cylinder valves

These valves seal the cylinder contents. The chemical formula of the particular gas is engraved on the valve (Fig. 1.6). Other types of valves (the bull nose, the hand wheel and the star) are used under special circumstances (Fig. 1.7).

Components

1. The valve is mounted on the top of the cylinder, screwed into the neck via a threaded connection. It is made of brass and is sometimes chromium plated.
2. An on/off spindle is used to open and close the valve by opposing a plastic facing against the valve seating.
3. The exit port is for supplying gas to the apparatus (e.g. anaesthetic machine).

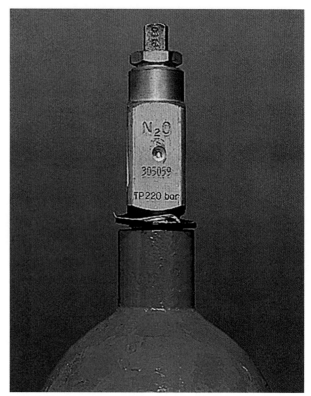

Fig. 1.6 Chemical formula (N_2O) engraved on a nitrous oxide cylinder valve.

4. A safety relief device allows the discharge of cylinder contents to the atmosphere if the cylinder becomes overpressurized.
5. The non-interchangeable safety system (pin-index system) is used on cylinders of size E or smaller as well as on size F and G Entonox cylinders. A specific pin configuration exists for each medical gas on the yoke of the anaesthetic machine. The matching configuration of holes on the valve block allows only the correct gas cylinder to be fitted in the yoke (Figs. 1.8 and 1.9). The gas exit port will not seal against the washer of the yoke unless the pins and holes are aligned.
6. The external part of the valve in some designs allows manual turning on and off of the cylinder without the need for a key (Fig. 1.10).

Mechanism of action

1. The cylinder valve acts as a mechanism for opening and closing the gas pathway.
2. A compressible yoke-sealing washer, Bodok seal (*bonded disk*), must be placed between the valve outlet and the apparatus to make a gas-tight joint (Fig. 1.11).

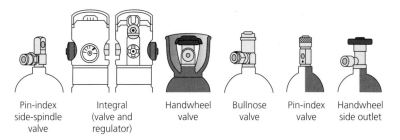

Pin-index side-spindle valve | Integral (valve and regulator) | Handwheel valve | Bullnose valve | Pin-index valve | Handwheel side outlet

Fig. 1.7 Cylinder valves.

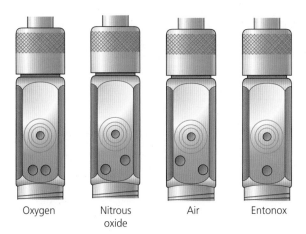

Oxygen   Nitrous   Air   Entonox
              oxide

Fig. 1.8 Pin-index system. Note the different configuration for each gas.

It is a gasket made of non-combustible material with a metal rim.

Problems in practice and safety features

1. The plastic wrapping of the valve should be removed just before use. The valve should be slightly opened and closed (cracked) before connecting the cylinder to the anaesthetic machine. This clears particles of dust, oil and grease from the exit port, which would otherwise enter the anaesthetic machine.
2. The valve should be opened slowly when attached to the anaesthetic machine or regulator. This prevents a rapid rise in pressure and an associated rise in temperature of the gas in the machine's pipelines. The cylinder valve should be fully open when in use (the valve must be turned two full revolutions).
3. During closure, overtightening of the valve should be avoided. This might lead to damage to the seal between the valve and the cylinder neck.
4. The Bodok seal should be inspected for damage prior to use. Having a spare seal readily available is advisable. This bonded non-combustible seal must be

kept clean and should never become contaminated with oil or grease. If a gas-tight seal cannot be achieved by moderate tightening of the screw clamp, it is recommended that the seal be renewed. Excessive force should never be used.

Cylinder valves
- They are mounted on the neck of the cylinder.
- Act as an on/off device for the discharge of cylinder contents.
- Pin-index system prevents cylinder identification errors.
- Bodok sealing washer must be placed between the valve and the yoke of the anaesthetic machine.
- Some designs allow manual (keyless) turning on and off.

Piped gas supply

Piped medical gas and vacuum (PMGV) is a system in which gases are delivered from central supply points to different sites in the hospital at a pressure of about 400 kPa. Special outlet valves supply the various needs throughout the hospital.

Oxygen, nitrous oxide, Entonox, compressed air and medical vacuum are commonly supplied through the pipeline system.

Components

1. Central supply points such as cylinder banks and/or liquid oxygen storage tank.
2. There is a labelled and colour-coded pipeline distribution network throughout the hospital.
3. Pipework is made of special high-quality copper alloy, which both prevents degradation of the gases it contains and has bacteriostatic properties. The fittings used are made from brass and are brazed rather than soldered.

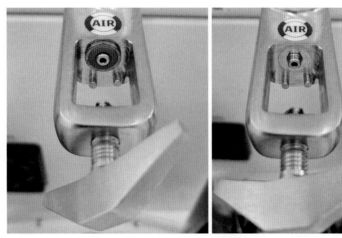

Fig. 1.9 A cylinder and pin-index system with Bodok seal in position *(left)* and with the Bodok seal removed *(right)*.

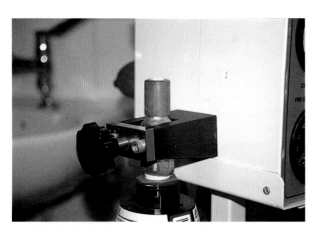

Fig. 1.10 A cylinder valve that allows manual opening and closing.

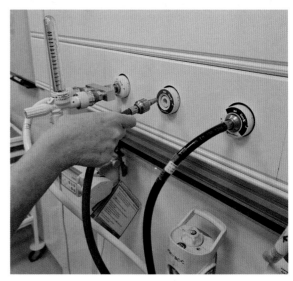

Fig. 1.12 Inserting a remote probe into its matching wall-mounted outlet socket.

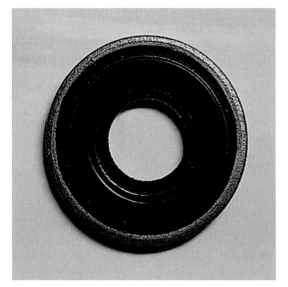

Fig. 1.11 A Bodok seal.

4. The size of the pipes differs according to the demand that they carry. Pipes with a 42-mm diameter are usually used for leaving the manifold. Smaller diameter tubes, such as 15 mm, are used after repeated branching.

5. Outlets are identified by gas colour coding, gas name and shape (Fig. 1.12). They accept matching quick connect/disconnect Schrader probes and sockets (Fig. 1.13), with an indexing collar specific for each gas (or gas mixture).

6. Outlets can be installed as flush-fitting units, surface-fitting units, on booms or pendants or suspended on a hose and gang mounted (Fig. 1.14).

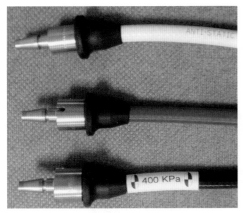

Fig. 1.13 Gas probes for oxygen *(top)*, nitrous oxide *(middle)* and air *(bottom)*. Note the locking groove on the probe to ensure connectivity.

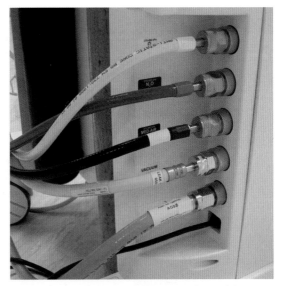

Fig. 1.15 Colour-coded hoses with non-interchangeable screw thread fittings attached to an anaesthetic machine.

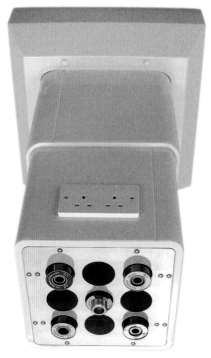

Fig. 1.14 Outlet sockets mounted in a retractable ceiling unit. (Courtesy Penlon Ltd, Abingdon, UK.)

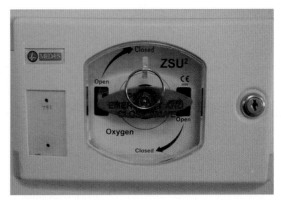

Fig. 1.16 An area valve service unit.

7. Flexible colour-coded hoses connect the outlets to the anaesthetic machine (Fig. 1.15). The anaesthetic machine end should be permanently fixed using a nut and liner union in which the thread is gas specific and non-interchangeable (a non-interchangeable screw thread [NIST] is the British Standard).
8. Isolating valves behind break-glass covers are positioned at strategic points throughout the pipeline network. They are also known as area valve service units (AVSUs)

(Fig. 1.16). They can be accessed to isolate the supply to an area in cases of fire or other emergency.

Problems in practice and safety features

1. A reserve bank of cylinders is available should the primary supply fail. Low-pressure alarms detect gas supply failure (Fig. 1.17).
2. A single-hose test is performed to detect cross-connection.
3. A tug test is performed to detect misconnection.
4. Regulations for PMGV installation, repair and modification are enforced.
5. Anaesthetists are responsible for the gases supplied from the terminal outlet through to the anaesthetic machine. Pharmacy, supplies and engineering departments share the responsibility for the gas pipelines 'behind the wall.'

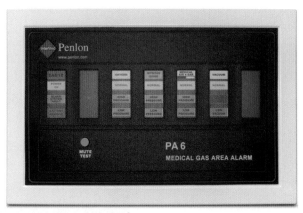

Fig. 1.17 Medical gas alarm panel. (Courtesy Penlon Ltd, Abingdon, UK.)

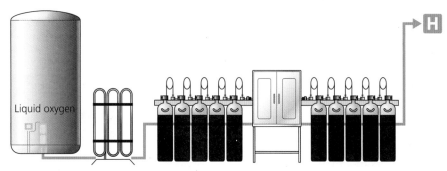

Fig. 1.18 Sources of oxygen supply in a hospital. A vacuum-insulated evaporator *(left)* and a cylinder manifold *(right)*.

6. There is a risk of fire from worn or damaged hoses that are designed to carry gases under pressure from a primary source such as a cylinder or wall-mounted terminal to medical devices such as ventilators and anaesthetic machines. Because of heavy wear and tear, the risk of rupture is greatest in oxygen hoses used with transport devices. Regular inspection and replacement, every 2–5 years, of all medical gas hoses is recommended.

Piped gas supply
- There is a network of labelled and colour-coded copper alloy pipelines throughout the hospital from central supply points.
- The outlets are colour- and shape-coded to accept matching 'Schrader' probes.
- Flexible and colour-coded pipelines run from the anaesthetic machine to the outlets.
- Single-hose and tug tests are performed to test for cross-connection and misconnection, respectively.
- There is a risk of fire from worn and damaged hoses.

Sources of gas supply

The source of supply can be cylinder manifold(s) and, in the case of oxygen, a liquid oxygen storage tank (vacuum-insulated evaporator [VIE]) or oxygen concentrator (Fig. 1.18).

Oxygen supplies are designed to meet the demand of the clinic/hospital. In a home or small institution, stand-alone cylinders or an oxygen concentrator would be sufficient. In a larger clinic, a cylinder manifold would be needed. In a large hospital with high oxygen demands, a VIE with an oxygen manifold backup would be usual.

CYLINDER MANIFOLD

Manifolds are used to supply nitrous oxide, Entonox and oxygen.

Components
1. Large cylinders (e.g. size J, each with 6800 L capacity) are usually divided into two equal groups, primary and secondary. The two groups alternate in supplying the

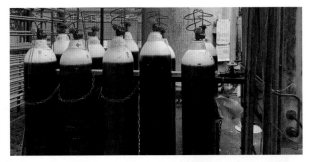

Fig. 1.19 An oxygen cylinder manifold.

pipelines (Fig. 1.19). The number of cylinders depends on the expected demand; usually to supply a typical day's demand so allowing one group of cylinders to change each day.
2. All cylinders in each group are connected through non-return valves to a common pipe. This in turn is connected to the pipeline through pressure regulators.
3. Pressure regulators reduce gas/vapour pressure to 400 kPa, the standard pipeline pressure.
4. As nitrous oxide is only available in cylinders (in contrast to liquid oxygen), its manifold is larger than that of oxygen. The latter usually acts as a backup to the liquid oxygen supply (see later).

Mechanism of action

1. In either group, all the cylinders' valves are opened. This allows them to empty simultaneously.
2. The supply is automatically changed to the secondary group when the primary group is nearly empty. The changeover is achieved through a pressure-sensitive device that detects when the cylinders are nearly empty.
3. The changeover activates an electrical signalling system to alert staff to the need to change the cylinders.

Problems in practice and safety features

1. The manifold should be housed in a well-ventilated room built of fireproof material away from the main buildings of the hospital.
2. The manifold room should not be used as a general cylinder store.
3. All empty cylinders should be removed immediately from the manifold room.

LIQUID OXYGEN

A VIE (Fig. 1.20) is the most economical way to store and supply oxygen. Stored liquid oxygen expands to 860 times its volume when vaporized at 20°C.

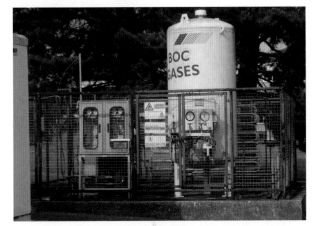

Fig. 1.20 A vacuum-insulated evaporator.

Components

1. A thermally insulated, double-walled steel tank with a layer of perlite in a vacuum is used as the insulation (Fig. 1.21). It can be described as a giant thermos flask, employing the same principles. They are built in different sizes depending on the need.
2. A pressure regulator allows gas to enter the hospital pipelines and maintains the pressure through the pipelines at about 400 kPa.
3. A safety valve opens at 1700 kPa, allowing the gas to escape when there is a build-up of pressure within the vessel. This can be caused by underdemand for oxygen.
4. An electronically controlled valve opens when there is an excessive demand on the system. This allows liquid oxygen to evaporate by passing through superheaters made of uninsulated coils of copper tubing. The 'superheaters' are not actively heated but rely on ambient temperature and heat from the air to warm the liquid oxygen.

Mechanism of action

1. Liquid oxygen is stored (up to 1500 L) at a temperature of –150°C to –170°C (lower than its critical temperature of –119°C) and at a pressure of 1000 kPa.

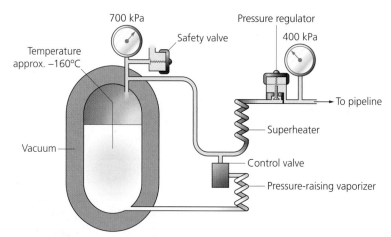

Fig. 1.21 Schematic diagram of a liquid oxygen supply system.

2. The VIE is not actively cooled. Instead, the temperature of the vessel is maintained by the high-vacuum shell insulation, thus minimizing conduction and convection of heat into the vessel. In addition, evaporation of the liquid oxygen requires heat (latent heat of vaporization). This heat is taken from the liquid oxygen, helping to maintain its low temperature.
3. The storage vessel rests on a weighing balance to measure the mass of the liquid using a tripod weighing scale. As the VIE's weight when empty (tare) is known, the weight of the liquid oxygen can be calculated. Instead of the weighing balance, a differential pressure gauge that measures the pressure difference between the bottom and top of the liquid oxygen can be used. This allows the height of the oxygen fluid column to be calculated. As the cross-sectional area of the VIE is constant, by measuring the difference in pressure, the volume of liquid oxygen can be calculated. As liquid oxygen evaporates, its mass decreases, reducing the pressure at the bottom. By measuring the difference in pressure, the contents of the VIE can be calculated. The information obtained is sent to the hospital alarm system. When required, fresh supplies of liquid oxygen are pumped from a tanker into the vessel.
4. The cold oxygen gas is warmed once outside the vessel in a coil of copper tubing. The increase in temperature causes an increase in pressure.
5. At a temperature of 15°C and atmospheric pressure, liquid oxygen can give 842 times its volume as gas.

Problems in practice and safety features

1. Reserve banks of cylinders are kept in case of supply failure.
2. A liquid oxygen storage vessel should be housed away from main buildings due to the fire hazard. The risk of fire is increased in cases of liquid spillage.
3. Spillage of cryogenic liquid can cause cold burns, frostbite and hypothermia.

 Exam tip: For the exam, make sure you understand how the VIE works. It is very important to memorize the relevant temperatures and pressures of liquid and gaseous oxygen.

You also need to be able to explain what happens when there is an overdemand or an underdemand for the oxygen supply.

Oxygen concentrators

Oxygen concentrators, also known as pressure swing adsorption systems, extract oxygen from air by differential adsorption. These devices may be small, are designed to supply oxygen to a single patient (Fig. 1.22) and supply oxygen to an anaesthetic machine (Fig. 1.23), or they can be large enough to supply oxygen for a medical gas pipeline system (Fig. 1.24).

Components

A zeolite molecular sieve is used. Zeolites are hydrated aluminium silicates of the alkaline earth metals in a powder or granular form in a lattice structure. Many zeolite columns are used.

Mechanism of action (Fig. 1.25)

1. Ambient air is filtered and pressurized to about 137 kPa by a compressor.
2. Air is exposed to a zeolite molecular sieve column, forming a very large surface area, at a certain pressure.
3. The sieve selectively retains nitrogen, water vapour and other unwanted components of air. These are released into the atmosphere after heating the column and applying a vacuum.

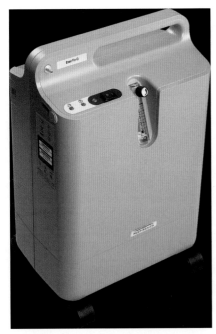

Fig. 1.22 The portable EverFlo Q home oxygen concentrator. (Courtesy of Philips RS North America LLC. All rights reserved.)

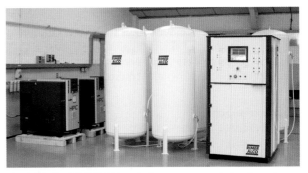

Fig. 1.24 The RA40/D/M hospital oxygen concentrator. It produces 80 L/min of oxygen. (Courtesy Rimer Alco Ltd, Thetford, UK.)

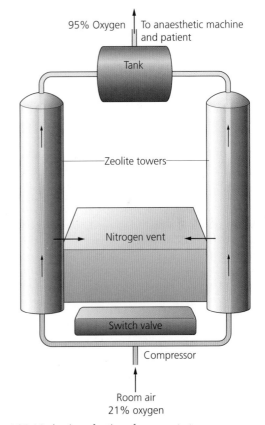

Fig. 1.25 Mechanism of action of a concentrator.

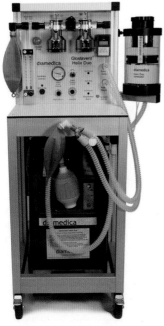

Fig. 1.23 The Glostavent Helix Duo, which has a built-in oxygen concentrator (see Chapter 2 for more details). (Courtesy of Diamedica, Barnstaple, Devon, UK.)

4. The sequential changeover between the columns is made by a time switch, typically cycles of around 20 seconds, allowing for a continuous supply of oxygen. When a column is not used, it is heated to release nitrogen and water vapour into the atmosphere.

5. The maximum oxygen concentration achieved is 95% by volume. Argon is the main remaining constituent with a concentration of approximately 5%. Argon is concentrated from air in a similar fashion to oxygen.

6. The life of the zeolite crystal can be expected to be at least 20,000 hours (which is about 10 years of use). Routine maintenance consists of changing filters at regular intervals.

Problems in practice and safety features

Although the oxygen concentration achieved is sufficient for the vast majority of clinical applications, its use with the circle system leads to argon accumulation. To avoid this, higher fresh gas flows are required.

> **Source of supply**
> - Cylinder manifold: banks of large cylinders, usually size J, are used.
> - Liquid oxygen: a thermally insulated vessel at a temperature of −150°C to −170°C and at a pressure of 500–1000 kPa is used.
> - Oxygen concentrator: a zeolite molecular sieve is used.

Entonox

This is a compressed gas mixture containing 50% oxygen and 50% nitrous oxide by volume. Gaseous oxygen is bubbled through liquid nitrous oxide, resulting in the vaporization of the liquid to form a gaseous O_2/N_2O mixture; **Poynting effect**. It is commonly used in the Accident and Emergency Department and in the labour ward and pre-hospital care settings to provide analgesia. A two-stage pressure demand regulator is attached to the Entonox cylinder when in use (Fig. 1.26). As the patient inspires through the mask or mouthpiece, gas flow is allowed to occur. Gas flow ceases at the end of an inspiratory effort. Entonox is compressed into cylinders to a pressure of 13,700 kPa. Entonox cylinders should be stored at 10°C for 24 hours before use.

If the temperature of the Entonox cylinder is decreased to below −5.5°C (the pseudo-critical temperature of Entonox in a cylinder), liquefaction and separation of the two components occurs, a process called *lamination*. This results in:
- a liquid mixture containing mostly nitrous oxide with about 20% oxygen dissolved in it, and
- above the liquid, a gas mixture of high oxygen concentration.

This means that, when used at a constant flow rate, a gas with a high concentration of oxygen is supplied first. This is followed by a gas of decreasing oxygen concentration as the liquid evaporates. This may lead to the supply of hypoxic mixtures, with less than 20% oxygen, as the cylinder is nearly empty.

Rewarming and mixing of both the cylinder and its contents reverses the separation and liquefaction.

Entonox pseudo-critical temperature when supplied via pipeline (400 kPa) is −30°C.

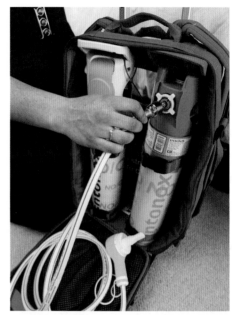

Fig. 1.26 Entonox cylinder showing the integrated valve, Schroder valve, hose and the patient's demand valve. (Courtesy BOC Healthcare, Manchester, UK.)

Problems in practice and safety features

- Liquefaction and separation of the components can be prevented by:
  1. Cylinders being stored horizontally for about 24 hours at temperatures of or above 5°C before use. The horizontal position increases the area for diffusion. If the contents are well mixed by repeated inversion, cylinders can be used earlier than 24 hours.
  2. Large cylinders are equipped with a dip tube with its tip ending in the liquid phase. This results in the liquid being used first, preventing the delivery of an oxygen concentration of less than 20%.
- Prolonged use of Entonox should be avoided because of the effect of nitrous oxide on the bone marrow, especially in critically ill patients. Adequate facilities for scavenging should be provided to protect hospital staff.

> **Entonox**
> - A compressed gas mixture with 50% oxygen and 50% nitrous oxide by volume (Poynting effect).
> - Supplied in cylinders at a pressure of 13,700 kPa and pipeline at a pressure of 400 kPa.
> - A two-stage pressure demand regulator is usually used.
> - Liquification and separation in a cylinder occurs at temperatures below −5.5°C. This can potentially lead to hypoxic mixtures. Large cylinders are designed to prevent this.

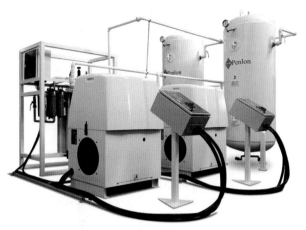

Fig. 1.27 Compressed medical air plant. (Courtesy Penlon Ltd, Abingdon, UK.)

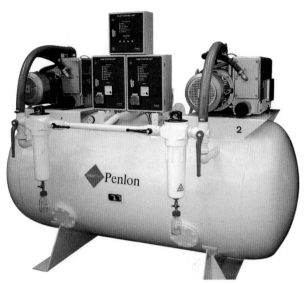

Fig. 1.28 Medical vacuum plant. (Courtesy Penlon Ltd, Abingdon, UK.)

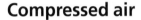

Compressed air

Medical air is supplied in a hospital for clinical uses or to drive power tools. The former is supplied at a pressure of 400 kPa and the latter at 700 kPa. The anaesthetic machines and most intensive care ventilator blenders accept a 400 kPa supply. The terminal outlets for the two pressures are different, each with its own Schrader valve, to prevent misconnection.

Air may be supplied from cylinder manifolds or more economically from a compressor plant with duty and backup compressors (Fig. 1.27). Each compressor is capable of meeting the hospital's expected demands. The temperature of air increases as it is compressed (Gay-Lussac's law, also known as the third gas law). The air is then cooled and the condensation is captured in special traps. Oil-free medical air is cleaned by filters and separators then dried and pressure regulated before use.

Compressor air intake should be carefully situated to prevent contamination with regular inspection.

Centralized vacuum or suction system (Fig. 1.28)

Suction devices play a crucial part in the care of patients in the operating theatre, intensive care unit and other parts of the hospital. It is recommended that one suction outlet is present in each anaesthetic room. It is also recommended that two suction outlets are present in each operating theatre, with one of them dedicated for anaesthetic use.

Components

1. A pump or a power source that is capable of continuously generating a negative pressure of –500 mmHg.
2. A suction controller with a filter.
3. A receiver or a collection vessel.
4. A suction tubing and suction nozzle (e.g. a Yankauer sucker) or catheter.

To determine the efficiency of central-piped vacuum systems
- A negative pressure of at least –53 kPa (–400 mmHg) should be maintained at the outlet.
- Each central-piped vacuum outlet should be able to withstand a flow of free air of at least 40 L/min.
- A unit should take no longer than 10 seconds to generate a vacuum (–500 mmHg) with a displacement of air of 25 L/min.

Mechanism of action

1. This is a high-pressure, low-flow system (compared with scavenging systems, which are low-pressure, high-flow systems; see Chapter 3).
2. Negative pressure is generated by an electric motor and pneumatic-driven pumps using the Venturi principle.
3. The amount of vacuum generated can be manually adjusted by the suction controller. This device has a variable orifice with a float assembly, a backup filter to

prevent liquid entering the system and ports to connect to a collection vessel or reservoir through flexible tubing.

4. The reservoir must have sufficient capacity to receive the aspirated material. Too large a capacity will make the system cumbersome and will take a long time to generate adequate negative pressure.

5. The suction tubing should be flexible and firm to prevent collapse. Also it should be transparent so that the contents aspirated can be visualized and of sufficient internal diameter and length for optimal suction.

6. The negative pressure (or degree of suctioning) can be adjusted to suit its use; e.g. a lesser degree of suctioning is required to clear oral secretions in a child than in an adult.

7. Bacterial filters are used to prevent the spread of infectious bacteria, with a removal of 99.999% of bacteria. Filters are also used to prevent fluids, condensate and smoke from contaminating the system.

8. It is recommended that there are at least two vacuum outlets in each operating theatre, one per anaesthetic room and one per post-anaesthesia recovery or intensive care unit bed.

Problems in practice and safety features

To prevent trauma to the tissues during suction, the nozzles should taper, be smooth and have multiple holes so that if one is blocked the others will continue suction.

Centralized vacuum or suction system

- Consists of a power source, a suction controller, a receiver, a suction tubing and a suction nozzle.
- Efficiency of the system should be tested before use.
- The amount of negative pressure should be adjusted according to its use.
- Trauma to tissues can be caused by the suction.

SUGGESTED FURTHER READING

Association of Anaesthetists, 2019. Safe handling of oxygen cylinders. Available from: https://anaesthetists.org/Home/Resources-publications/Safety-alerts/Safety-initiatives/Safe-handling-of-oxygen-cylinders.

BOC, 2016. Medical gas cylinder data chart. Available from: https://www.bochealthcare.co.uk/en/images/cylinder_data_med309965_2011_tcm409-54065.pdf.

Crombie, N., 2009. Confusing and ambiguous labelling of an oxygen cylinder. Anaesthesia 64 (1), 98.

Department of Health, 2006. Health Technical Memorandum 02-01. Medical gas pipeline systems. Part A: Design, Installation, Validation and Verification. The Stationery Office, London.

Department of Health, 2006. Health Technical Memorandum 02-01. Medical gas pipeline systems. Part B: Operational Management. The Stationery Office, London.

Department of Health, 2010. Unsecured medical gas cylinders, including cylinders on trolleys. Available from: https://www.gov.uk/government/publications/unsecured-medical-gas-cylinders-including-cylinders-on-trolleys.

Estates and Facilities Alert NHSE/I-2020/003, 19 November 2020 Covid-19 Response – Oxygen Supply and Fire Safety. Available from: https://www.cas.mhra.gov.uk/ViewandAcknowledgment/ViewAlert.aspx?AlertID=103024.

National Health Service (NHS), 2011. Airway suction equipment. Available from: http://www.nrls.npsa.nhs.uk/resources/?entryid45=94845.

National Health Service (NHS), 2018. Risk of death and severe harm from failure to obtain and continue flow from oxygen cylinders. Available from: https://www.england.nhs.uk/2018/01/failure-to-obtain-and-continue-flow-from-oxygen-cylinders/.

National Patient Safety Agency, 2009. Rapid Response Report, Oxygen safety in hospitals. Available from: https://www.sps.nhs.uk/wp-content/uploads/2011/08/RRR-Oxygen-safety-2009120092029_v1.pdf.

Poolacherla, R., Nickells, J., 2006. Suction devices. Anaesth. Intensive Care Med. 7 (10), 354–355.

Taylor, N.J., Davison, M., 2009. Inaccurate colour coding of medical gas cylinders. Anaesthesia 64 (6), 690.

SELF-ASSESSMENT QUESTIONS

Please check your eBook for additional self-assessment

MCQs

In the following lists, which of the statements (a) to (e) are true?

1. **Concerning cylinders**
   a. Oxygen is stored in cylinders as a gas.
   b. The pressure in a half-filled oxygen cylinder is 13,700 kPa.
   c. The pressure in a half-full nitrous oxide cylinder is 4400 kPa.
   d. Nitrous oxide is stored in the cylinder in the gas phase.
   e. Pressure in a full Entonox cylinder is 13,700 kPa.

2. **Entonox**
   a. Entonox is a 50:50 mixture by weight of O_2 and N_2O.
   b. Entonox has a pseudo-critical temperature of 5.5°C.
   c. Entonox cylinders should be stored upright.
   d. At room temperature, Entonox cylinders contain only gas.
   e. Entonox cylinders have blue bodies and white and blue quarters on the shoulders.

3. **Medical gas cylinders**
   a. They are made of manganese steel.
   b. They are engraved with the cylinder tare weight.
   c. They are tested every 5 years.
   d. Size E cylinders have an internal volume of 4.7 L.
   e. Grease should be applied to the valve to ensure a good seal with the anaesthetic machine.

4. **Oxygen**
   a. For medical use, oxygen is usually formed from fractional distillation of air.
   b. Long-term use can cause bone marrow depression.
   c. In hyperbaric concentrations, oxygen may cause convulsions.
   d. At constant volume, the absolute pressure of oxygen is directly proportional to its absolute temperature.
   e. The critical temperature of oxygen is −118°C.

5. **Oxygen concentrators**
   a. Oxygen concentrators concentrate O_2 that has been delivered from an oxygen cylinder manifold.
   b. Argon accumulation can occur when oxygen concentrators are used with the circle system.
   c. They are made of columns of a zeolite molecular sieve.
   d. They can achieve O_2 concentrations of up to 100%.
   e. They can only be used in home oxygen therapy.

6. **Concerning the safety features of medical gas cylinders**
   a. The valve is secured to the cylinder with a material that is resistant to heat so that it does not come loose in the event of a fire.
   b. At least one cylinder in every 100 manufactured is cut apart to test the strength of the cylinder.
   c. Valves are colour coded to aid identification.
   d. An oxygen cylinder can be fitted to the nitrous oxide yoke on an anaesthetic machine.
   e. A removable plastic seal is applied to the cylinder valve after filling to prevent ingress of dirt and to show if the cylinder has been tampered with.

7. **Oxygen**
   a. It is stored in cylinders at approximately 13,700 kPa.
   b. It has a critical temperature of 36.5°C.
   c. It is a liquid in its cylinder.
   d. It may form an inflammable mixture with oil.
   e. It obeys Boyle's law.

8. Concerning cylinders

   a. The filling ratio is equal to the weight of liquid in the cylinder divided by the weight of water required to fill the cylinder.

   b. The tare weight is the weight of the cylinder plus its contents.

   c. Nitrous oxide cylinders have a blue body and a blue and white top.

   d. A full oxygen cylinder has a pressure of approximately 137 bar.

   e. At 40°C, a nitrous oxide cylinder contains both liquid and vapour.

9. Concerning piped gas supply in the operating theatre

   a. Compressed air is supplied only under one pressure.

   b. The non-interchangeable screw thread system is the British Standard.

   c. Only oxygen and air are supplied.

   d. Size E cylinders are normally used in cylinder manifolds.

   e. Liquid oxygen is stored at temperatures above −100°C.

10. True or false

   a. There is no need for cylinders to undergo regular checks.

   b. The only agent identification on the cylinder is its colour.

   c. When attached to the anaesthetic machine, the cylinder valve should be opened slowly.

   d. When warmed, liquid oxygen can give 842 times its volume as gas.

   e. Cylinders are made of thick-walled steel to withstand the high internal pressure.

11. Regarding the pin-index system

   a. Cylinders do not engage with the pin-index system unless a Bodok seal is present.

   b. Nitrous oxide yokes have a single, central pin.

   c. The pin-index system is present on a size F oxygen cylinder.

   d. The system is used to identify the cylinder contents.

   e. A Bodok seal is made of non-combustible materials.

12. Regarding the piped medical vacuum system

   a. A negative pressure of −53 kPa is present at the outlet.

   b. The Venturi principle is used.

   c. A pressure of −500 kPa can be generated within 5 seconds.

   d. The medical vacuum supply does not require an area valve service unit (AVSU).

   e. The piped medical vacuum system cannot cause tissue damage at the pressures supplied.

Single best answer

13. Which of the following statements about Entonox is correct?

   a. When using a demand valve, gas is supplied to the patient at a fixed pressure.

   b. Entonox has a single pin in the pin-index system.

   c. Entonox is presented in a white cylinder with white and blue quartered shoulders.

   d. Entonox is stored as a liquid in cylinders.

   e. Entonox cylinders should be stored vertically.

14. Concerning piped medical gas and vacuum

   a. Outlets are only colour coded.

   b. Outlets are shape and colour coded.

   c. All the supplies can be interrupted using a single AVSU.

   d. Copper sulphate pipes are used to carry oxygen throughout the hospital.

   e. Backup cylinders for the oxygen supply are undesirable.

15. Entonox may laminate at temperatures less than

   a. 36.4°C.

   b. 23.5°C.

   c. 5°C.

   d. −5.5°C.

   e. −88°C.

Answers

1. *Concerning cylinders*
   a. *True. Oxygen is stored in the cylinder as a gas.*
   b. *False. Oxygen is stored in the cylinder as a gas where gas laws apply. The pressure gauge accurately reflects the contents of the cylinder. A full oxygen cylinder has a pressure of 13,700 kPa. Pressure in a half-full oxygen cylinder is therefore 6850 kPa.*
   c. *True. Nitrous oxide is stored in the cylinder in the liquid form. The pressure of a full nitrous oxide cylinder is about 4400 kPa. As the cylinder is used, the vapour above the liquid is used first. This vapour is replaced by new vapour from the liquid. Therefore the pressure is maintained. So the cylinder is nearly empty before the pressure starts to decrease. For this reason, the pressure gauge does not accurately reflect the contents of the cylinder.*
   d. *False. Nitrous oxide is stored in the cylinder as a liquid. The vapour above the liquid is delivered to the patient.*
   e. *True. Entonox is a compressed gas mixture containing 50% oxygen and 50% nitrous oxide by volume.*

2. *Entonox*
   a. *False. Entonox is a 50:50 mixture of O_2 and N_2O by volume and not by weight.*
   b. *False. The pseudo-critical temperature of Entonox is –5.5°C. At or below this temperature, liquefaction and separation of the two components occur.*
   c. *False. This increases the risk of liquefaction and separation of the components. To prevent this, Entonox cylinders should be stored horizontally for about 24 hours at temperatures at or above 5°C. This position increases the area for diffusion. With repeated inversion, Entonox cylinders can be used earlier than 24 hours.*
   d. *True. Liquefaction and separation of nitrous oxide and oxygen occur at or below –5.5°C.*
   e. *True.*

3. *Medical gas cylinders*
   a. *False. Standard medical gas cylinders are made of molybdenum steel. Lightweight cylinders can be made of an aluminium alloy or fibreglass.*
   b. *True.*
   c. *True.*
   d. *True.*
   e. *False. Grease should always be kept away from medical gas cylinders as it may enter the anaesthetic machine and contaminate the gas supply to the patient.*

4. *Oxygen*
   a. *True. Except for oxygen concentrators, which use zeolites.*
   b. *False. Long-term use of oxygen has no effect on the bone marrow. Long-term use of N_2O can cause bone marrow depression, especially with high concentrations in critically ill patients.*
   c. *True.*
   d. *True. This is Gay-Lussac's law where pressure = a constant × temperature. Oxygen also obeys the other gas laws (Dalton's law of partial pressures and Boyle's and Charles's laws).*
   e. *True. At or below –118°C, oxygen changes to the liquid phase. This is used in the design of the vacuum-insulated evaporator in which oxygen is stored in the liquid phase at temperatures of –150°C to –170°C.*

5. *Concerning the safety features of medical gas cylinders*
   a. *False. The valve is secured to the cylinder with a material that melts when exposed to extreme heat and releases the cylinder pressure in case of fire.*
   b. *True.*
   c. *False. Cylinders are colour coded to indicate contents.*
   d. *False. This would be prevented by the pin-index system.*
   e. *True.*

6. *Oxygen concentrators*
   a. *False. Oxygen concentrators extract oxygen from air using a zeolite molecular sieve. Many columns of zeolite are used. Zeolites are hydrated aluminium silicates of the alkaline earth metals.*
   b. *True. The maximum oxygen concentration achieved by oxygen concentrators is 95%. The rest is mainly argon. Using low flows with the circle breathing system can lead to the accumulation of argon. Higher fresh gas flows are required to avoid this.*

c. **True.** The zeolite molecular sieve selectively retains nitrogen and other unwanted gases in air. These are released into the atmosphere. The changeover between columns is made by a time switch.

d. **False.** Oxygen concentrators can deliver a maximum oxygen concentration of 95%.

e. **False.** Oxygen concentrators can be small, delivering oxygen to a single patient, or they can be large enough to supply oxygen to hospitals.

7. *Oxygen*

a. **True.** Molybdenum steel or aluminium alloy cylinders are used to store oxygen at pressures of approximately 13,700 kPa (137 bar).

b. **False.** The critical temperature of O_2 is –118°C. Above that temperature, oxygen cannot be liquefied however much pressure is applied.

c. **False.** Oxygen is a gas in the cylinder as its critical temperature is –118°C.

d. **True.** Oil is flammable while oxygen aids combustion. Oxygen cylinders should be stored away from oil.

e. **True.** At a constant temperature, the volume of a given mass of oxygen varies inversely with the absolute pressure (volume = a constant × 1/pressure). Oxygen obeys other gas laws.

8. *Concerning cylinders*

a. **True.** The filling ratio is used when filling cylinders with liquid, e.g. nitrous oxide. As the liquid is less compressible than the gas, the cylinder should be only partially filled. Depending on the ambient temperature, the filling ratio can be from 0.67 to 0.75.

b. **False.** The tare weight is the weight of the empty cylinder. This is used to estimate the amount of the contents of the cylinder. It is one of the marks engraved on the cylinders.

c. **False.** Nitrous oxide cylinders have a blue body and top. Entonox cylinders have a blue body and a blue and white top.

d. **True.**

e. **False.** At 40°C, nitrous oxide exists as a gas only. This is above its critical temperature, 36.5°C, so it cannot be liquefied above that.

9. *Concerning piped gas supply in the operating theatre*

a. **False.** Air is supplied at two different pressures; at 400 kPa when it is delivered to the patient and at 700 kPa when it is used to operate power tools in the operating theatre.

b. **True.** This stands for non-interchangeable screw thread. This is one of the safety features present in the piped gas supply system. Flexible colour-coded hoses connect the outlets to the anaesthetic machine. The connections to the anaesthetic machine should be permanently fixed using a nut and liner union where the thread is gas-specific and non-interchangeable.

c. **False.** Oxygen, nitrous oxide, air and vacuum can be supplied by the piped gas system.

d. **False.** Larger cylinders, e.g. size J, are normally used in a cylinder manifold. Size E cylinders are usually mounted on the anaesthetic machine.

e. **False.** Liquid oxygen has to be stored at temperatures below its critical temperature, –118°C. So oxygen stored at temperatures above –100°C (above its critical temperature) exists as a gas.

10. *True or false*

a. **False.** Cylinders should be checked regularly by the manufacturers. Internal endoscopic examination, pressure testing, flattening, bending and impact testing and tensile testing are done on a regular basis.

b. **False.** The name, chemical symbol, pharmaceutical form and specification of the agent, in addition to the colour of the cylinder, are used to identify the agent.

c. **True.** When attached to an anaesthetic machine, the cylinder valve should be opened slowly to prevent a rapid rise in pressure within the machine's pipelines.

d. **True.** It is more economical to store oxygen as a liquid before supplying it. At a temperature of 15°C and atmospheric pressure, liquid oxygen can give 842 times its volume as gas.

e. **False.** For ease of transport, cylinders are made of thin-walled, seamless molybdenum steel. They are designed to withstand considerable internal pressures and are tested up to pressures of about 22,000 kPa.

11. *Regarding the pin-index system*

a. **False.** Al though a Bodok seal should be present to ensure that the cylinder has a good seal with the yoke.

b. **False.** Entonox, not nitrous oxide, is marked by a single central pin.

c. **False.** The pin-index system is used on size E and smaller cylinders. Only Entonox cylinders have the pin-index system on size E cylinders.

d. **False.** The pin-index system is a safety system to ensure only the correct gas cylinder can be fitted to the yoke.

e. **True.**

12. *Regarding the piped medical vacuum system*
   a. **True.** *At least –53kPa is maintained at the outlet.*
   b. **True.**
   c. **False.** *A vacuum of –500 mmHg (not kPa) should be generated within 10 seconds (not 5 seconds).*
   d. **False.** *All of the piped medical gas supply and vacuum have AVSUs to allow isolation in emergencies and for maintenance.*
   e. **False.** *Depending on the intended use, vacuum pressure may need to be restricted to a lower pressure.*

13. *b.*

14. *b.*

15. *d.*

Chapter 2

The anaesthetic machine

The anaesthetic machine receives medical gases (oxygen, nitrous oxide, air) under pressure and provides a continuous and accurate flow of each gas individually. A gas mixture of the desired composition at a defined flow rate is created before a known concentration of an inhalational agent vapour is added. Gas and vapour mixtures are continuously delivered to the common gas outlet of the machine, as fresh gas flow (FGF), and to the breathing system and patient (Figs. 2.1 and 2.2). The anaesthetic machine consists of:

1. gas supplies (see Chapter 1)
2. pressure gauges
3. pressure regulators (reducing valves)
4. flowmeters
5. vaporizers
6. a common gas outlet
7. a variety of other features, e.g. high-flow oxygen flush, pressure relief valve and oxygen supply failure alarm and suction apparatus

Most modern anaesthetic machines or stations incorporate a circle breathing system (see Chapter 4) and a bag-in-bottle–type ventilator (see Chapter 8).

To ensure the delivery of a safe gas mixture, safety features of a modern anaesthetic machine should include the following:

- Colour-coded pressure gauges
- Colour-coded flowmeters
- An oxygen flowmeter controlled by a single touch-coded knob
- Oxygen is the last gas to be added to the mixture
- Oxygen concentration monitor or analyser
- Nitrous oxide is cut off when the oxygen pressure is low
- Oxygen:nitrous oxide ratio monitor and controller
- Pin-index safety system for cylinders and non-interchangeable screw thread for pipelines
- Alarm for failure of oxygen supply
- Ventilator disconnection alarm
- At least one reserve oxygen cylinder should be available on machines that use pipeline supply

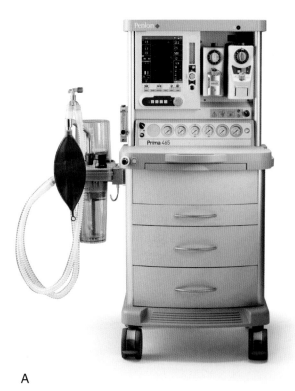

A

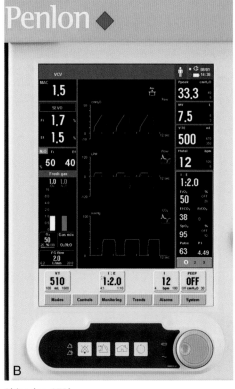

B

Fig. 2.1 (A, B) The Penlon Prima 465 with its control panel. (Courtesy Penlon, Abingdon, UK.)

Pressure gauge

This measures the pressure in the cylinder or pipeline. The pressure gauges for oxygen, nitrous oxide and medical air are mounted in a front-facing panel on the anaesthetic machine (Fig. 2.3).

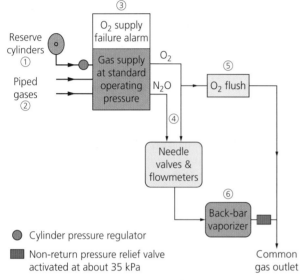

● Cylinder pressure regulator

▓ Non-return pressure relief valve
activated at about 35 kPa

Fig. 2.2 Diagrammatic representation of a continuous flow anaesthetic machine. Pressures throughout the system: *1*, O_2: 13,700 kPa, N_2O: 4400 kPa; *2*, pipeline: about 400 kPa; *3*, O_2 supply failure alarm activated at <250 kPa; *4*, regulated gas supply at about 400 kPa; *5*, O_2 flush: 45 L/min at a pressure of about 400 kPa; *6*, back-bar pressure 1–10 kPa (depending on flow rate and type of vaporizer).

Some anaesthetic machine designs have a digital display of the gas supply pressures (Fig. 2.4).

Components

1. A robust, flexible and coiled tube, which is oval in cross section (Fig. 2.5). It should be able to withstand the sudden high pressure when the cylinder is switched on.
2. The tube is sealed at its inner end and connected to a needle pointer that moves over a dial.
3. The other end of the tube is exposed to the gas supply.

Mechanism of action

1. The high-pressure gas causes the tube to uncoil (Bourdon gauge).
2. The movement of the tube causes the needle pointer to move on the calibrated dial, indicating the pressure.

Problems in practice and safety features

1. Each pressure gauge is colour-coded and calibrated for a particular gas or vapour. The pressure measured indicates the contents available in an oxygen cylinder. Oxygen is stored as a gas and obeys Boyle's law (pressure × volume = constant). This is not the case in a nitrous oxide cylinder since it is stored as a liquid and vapour.
2. A pressure gauge designed for pipelines should not be used to measure cylinder pressure and vice versa. This leads to inaccuracies and/or damage to the pressure gauge.
3. Should the coiled tube rupture, the gas vents from the back of the pressure gauge casing. The face of the pressure gauge is made of heavy glass as an additional safety feature.

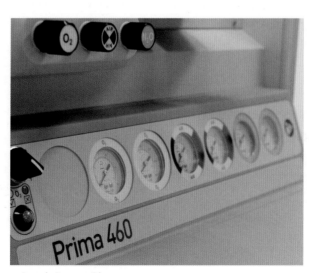

Fig. 2.3 Pressure gauges for oxygen, air and nitrous oxide.

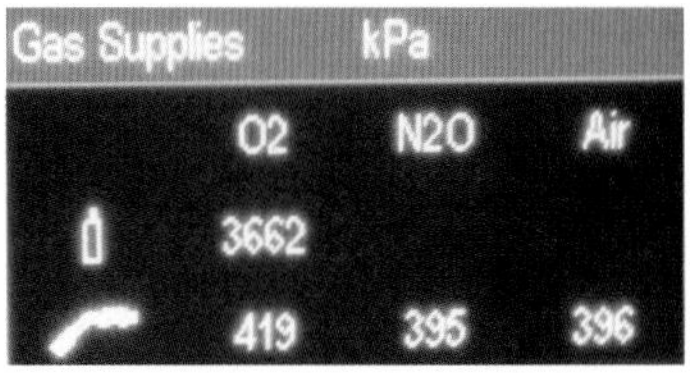

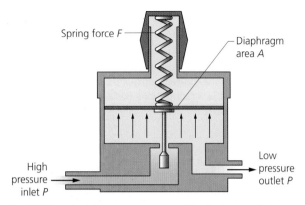

Fig. 2.4 Digital display of pressure gauges for oxygen (cylinder and pipeline), nitrous oxide (pipeline) and air (pipeline).

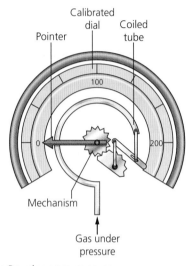

Fig. 2.5 The Bourdon pressure gauge.

Fig. 2.6 The principles of a pressure regulator (reducing valve).

Pressure gauge
- Measures pressure in cylinder or pipeline.
- Pressure acts to straighten a coiled tube.
- Colour-coded and calibrated for a particular gas or vapour.

Pressure regulator (reducing valve)

Pressure regulators are used because:
- Gas and vapour are stored under high pressure in cylinders. A regulator reduces the variable cylinder pressure to a constant safer operating pressure of about 400 kPa (just below the pipeline pressure) (Fig. 2.6).

- The temperature and pressure of the cylinder contents decrease with use. In order to maintain flow, constant adjustment is required in the absence of regulators.
- Regulators protect the components of the anaesthetic machine against pressure surges.
- The use of pressure regulators allows low-pressure piping and connectors to be used in the machine. This makes the consequences of any gas leak much less serious.

They are positioned between the cylinders and the rest of the anaesthetic machine (Figs. 2.7 and 2.8).

Components
1. An inlet, with a filter, leading to a high-pressure chamber with a valve.
2. This valve leads to a low-pressure chamber and outlet.
3. A diaphragm attached to a spring is situated in the low-pressure chamber.

Mechanism of action
1. Gas enters the high-pressure chamber and passes into the low-pressure chamber via the valve.
2. The force exerted by the high-pressure gas tries to close the valve. The opposing force of the diaphragm and spring tries to open the valve. A balance is reached between the two opposing forces. This maintains a gas flow under a constant pressure of about 400 kPa.

Problems in practice and safety features
1. Formation of ice inside the regulator can occur. If the cylinder contains water vapour, this may condense and freeze as a result of the heat lost when gas expands on entry into the low-pressure chamber.
2. The diaphragm can rupture.

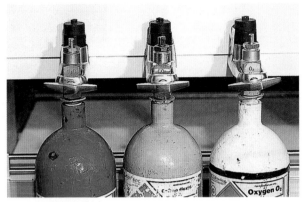

Fig. 2.7 Cylinder pressure regulators (black domes) positioned above the cylinder yokes in the Datex-Ohmeda Flexima anaesthetic machine.

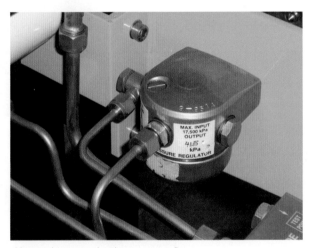

Fig. 2.8 Cylinder pressure regulator (the machine's tray has been removed).

3. Relief valves (usually set at 700 kPa) are fitted downstream of the regulators and allow the escape of gas should the regulators fail.
4. A one-way valve is positioned within the cylinder supply line. This prevents backflow and loss of gas from the pipeline supplies should a cylinder not be connected. This one-way valve may be incorporated into the design of the pressure regulator.

Pressure regulator
- Reduces pressure of gases from cylinders to about 400 kPa (similar to pipeline pressure).
- Allows fine control of gas flow and protects the anaesthetic machine from high pressures.
- A balance between two opposing forces maintains a constant operating pressure.

Second-stage regulators and flow restrictors

The control of pipeline pressure surges can be achieved either by using a second-stage pressure regulator or a flow restrictor (Fig. 2.9)—a constriction—between the pipeline supply and the rest of the anaesthetic machine. A lower pressure (100–200 kPa) is achieved. If there are only flow restrictors and no regulators in the pipeline supply, adjustment of the flowmeter controls is usually necessary whenever there is change in pipeline pressure.

Flow restrictors may also be used downstream of vaporizers to prevent a back pressure effect (see later).

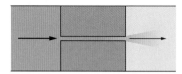

Fig. 2.9 A flow restrictor. The constriction causes a significant pressure drop when there is a high gas flow rate.

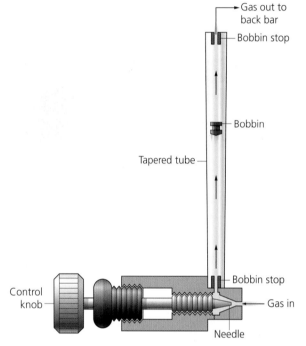

Fig. 2.10 A flow control (needle) valve and flowmeter.

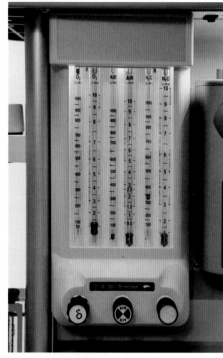

Fig. 2.11 A flowmeter panel.

One-way valve or backflow check valves

These valves are usually placed next to the inlet yoke. Their function is to prevent loss or leakage of gas from an empty yoke. They also prevent accidental cross-filling between paired cylinders.

Flow control (needle) valves

These valves control the flow through the flowmeters by manual adjustment. As the valve is opened, the orifice around the needle becomes larger and flow increases. They are positioned at the base of the associated flowmeter tube (Fig. 2.10). Increasing the flow of a gas is achieved by turning the valve in an anticlockwise direction. These valves reduce the gas pressure from around 44 kPa to just above atmospheric pressure before entry to the flowmeter block.

Components

1. The body, made of brass, screws into the base of the flowmeter.
2. The stem screws into the body and ends in a needle. It has screw threads allowing fine adjustment.
3. The flow control knobs are labelled and colour-coded.
4. A touch-coded knob controls the oxygen flowmeter.
5. A flow control knob guard is fitted to protect against accidental adjustment in the flowmeters.

Flowmeters

Flowmeters measure the flow rate of a gas passing through them. They are individually calibrated for each gas. Calibration occurs at room temperature and atmospheric pressure (sea level). They have an accuracy of about ±2.5%. For flows above 1 L/min, the units are L/min, and for flows below that, the units are 100 mL/min (Fig. 2.11).

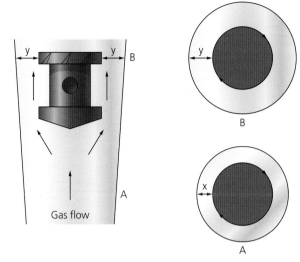

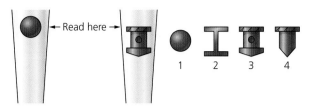

Fig. 2.13 Reading a flowmeter (top). Different types of bobbins: 1, ball; 2, non-rotating H float; 3, skirted; 4, non-skirted.

Fig. 2.12 Mechanism of action of the flowmeter. As the bobbin rises from A to B, the clearance increases (from x to y).

Components

1. A flow control (needle) valve.
2. A tapered (wider at the top), transparent plastic or glass tube.
3. A lightweight rotating bobbin or ball. Bobbin stops at either end of the tube ensure that it is always visible to the operator at extremes of flow.

Mechanism of action

1. When the needle valve is opened, gas is free to enter the tapered tube.
2. The bobbin is held floating within the tube by the gas flow passing around it. The higher the flow rate, the higher the bobbin rises within the tube.
3. The effect of gravity on the bobbin is counteracted by the gas flow. The pressure difference across the bobbin remains constant as it floats.
4. The clearance between the bobbin and the tube wall widens as the gas flow increases (Fig. 2.12).
5. At low flow rates, the clearance is longer and narrower, thus acting as a tube. Under these circumstances, the flow is laminar and a function of gas viscosity (Poiseuille's law).
6. At high flow rates, the clearance is shorter and wider, thus acting as an orifice. Here, the flow is turbulent and a function of gas density.
7. The top of the bobbin has slits (flutes) cut into its side. As gas flows past it, the slits cause the bobbin to rotate. A dot on the bobbin indicates to the operator that the bobbin is rotating and not stuck.

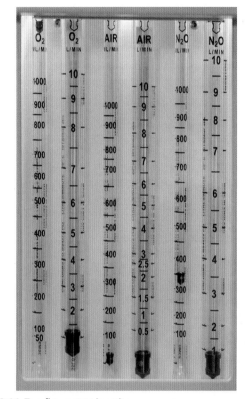

Fig. 2.14 Two flowmeters in series.

8. The reading of the flowmeter is taken from the top of the bobbin (Fig. 2.13). When a ball is used, the reading is generally taken from the midpoint of the ball.
9. When very low flows are required, e.g. in the circle breathing system, an arrangement of two flowmeters in series is used. One flowmeter reads a maximum of 1 L/min, allowing fine adjustment of the flow. One flow control per gas is needed for both flowmeters (Fig. 2.14).
10. There is a stop on the oxygen flow control valve to ensure a minimum oxygen flow of 200–300 mL/min past the needle valve. This ensures that the oxygen flow cannot be discontinued completely.

 Exam tip: Make sure you understand how the flow-meter works and the effects of viscosity and density on the function of the flowmeter.

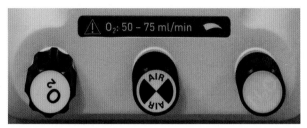

Fig. 2.15 Flow control knobs. Note the colour-coding and the distinctive-shape of oxygen control knob.

Problems in practice and safety features

1. The flow control knobs are colour-coded for their respective gases. The oxygen control knob is situated to the left (in the United Kingdom) and, in some designs, is larger with larger ridges and has a longer stem than the other control knobs, so sticking out farthest, making it easily recognizable (Fig. 2.15). In the United States and Canada, the oxygen control knob is situated to the right.

2. The European Standard for anaesthetic machines (EN 740) requires them to have the means to prevent the delivery of a gas mixture with an oxygen concentration below 25%. Current designs make it impossible for nitrous oxide to be delivered without the addition of a fixed percentage of oxygen. This is achieved by using interactive oxygen and nitrous oxide controls. This helps to prevent the possibility of delivering a hypoxic mixture to the patient. In the mechanical system, two gears are connected together by a precision stainless steel link chain. One gear with 14 teeth is fixed on the nitrous oxide flow control valve spindle. The other gear has 29 teeth and can rotate the oxygen flow control valve spindle, rather like a nut rotating on a bolt. For every 2.07 revolutions of the nitrous oxide flow control knob, the oxygen knob and spindle set to the lowest oxygen flow will rotate once. Because the gear on the oxygen flow control is mounted like a nut on a bolt, oxygen flow can be adjusted independently of nitrous oxide flow.

3. They are leak-proof due to the neoprene O-ring washers at both ends of the flowmeter block.

4. A crack in a flowmeter may result in a hypoxic mixture (Fig. 2.16). To avoid this, oxygen is the last gas to be added to the mixture that is delivered to the back bar.

5. Flow measurements can become inaccurate if the bobbin sticks to the inside wall of the flowmeter. The commonest causes are:
   a. dirt: this is a problem at low flow rates when the clearance is narrow. The source of the dirt is usually

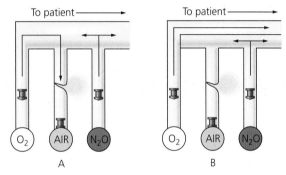

Fig. 2.16 (A) A broken air flowmeter allows oxygen to escape and a hypoxic mixture to be delivered from the back bar. (B) A possible design measure to prevent this.

   a contaminated gas supply. Filters, acting before gas enters the flowmeters, will remove the dirt.
   b. static electricity: the charge usually builds up over a period of time, leading to inaccuracies of up to 35%. Using antistatic materials in flowmeter construction helps to eliminate any build-up of charge. Application of antistatic spray removes any charge present.

5. Flowmeters are designed to be read in a vertical position, so any change in the position of the machine can affect the accuracy.

6. Pressure rises at the common gas outlet are transmitted back to the gas above the bobbin. This results in a drop in the level of the bobbin with an inaccurate reading. This can happen with minute volume divider ventilators as back pressure is exerted as they cycle with inaccuracies of up to 10%. A flow restrictor is fitted downstream of the flowmeters to prevent this from occurring.

7. Accidents have resulted from failure to see the bobbin clearly at the extreme ends of the tube. This can be prevented by illuminating the flowmeter bank and installing a wire stop at the top to prevent the bobbin from reaching the top of the tube.

8. Highly accurate computer-controlled gas mixers are available (see later).

Flowmeter

- Both laminar and turbulent flows are encountered, making both the viscosity and density of the gas relevant.
- The bobbin should not stick to the tapered tube.
- Oxygen is the last gas to be added to the mixture.
- It is very accurate with an error margin of ±2.5%.

Vaporizers

A vaporizer is designed to add a controlled amount of an inhalational agent, after changing it from liquid to vapour, to the FGF. This is normally expressed as a percentage of saturated vapour added to the gas flow. Vaporizers are positioned downstream of the flowmeters.

Characteristics of the ideal vaporizer

- Its performance is not affected by changes in FGF, volume of the liquid agent, ambient temperature and pressure, decrease in temperature due to vaporization and pressure fluctuation due to the mode of respiration.
- Low resistance to flow.
- Lightweight with small liquid requirement.
- Economy and safety in use with minimal servicing requirements.
- Corrosion- and solvent-resistant construction.

Vaporizers can be classified according to location:
1. Inside the breathing system. Gases pass through a very low-resistance, draw-over vaporizer due to the patient's respiratory efforts (e.g. Goldman, Oxford Miniature Vaporizer [OMV]). Such vaporizers are simple in design, lightweight, agent non-specific, i.e. allowing the use of any volatile agent, small and inexpensive. For these reasons, they are used in the 'field' or in otherwise difficult environments. However, they are not as efficient as the plenum vaporizers as their performance is affected as the temperature of the anaesthetic agent decreases due to loss of latent heat during vaporization. The Diamedica vaporizer (Fig. 2.17) has a low resistance and is thermally stable. It can be used with halothane/isoflurane and sevoflurane. It can also be used as a plenum vaporizer.
2. Outside the breathing system. Gases are driven through a plenum (high-resistance, unidirectional and agent-specific) vaporizer due to gas supply pressure. These vaporizers are reliable and easy to use.

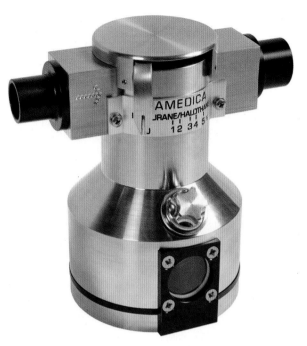

Fig. 2.17 Diamedica draw-over vaporizer. (Courtesy Diamedica, Barnstaple, Devon, UK.)

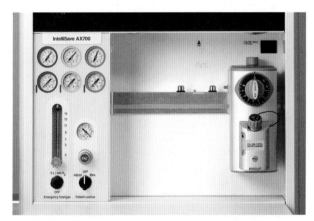

Fig. 2.18 A plenum vaporizer mounted on the back bar of an anaesthetic machine. (Courtesy Philips Healthcare, Guildford, UK.)

PLENUM VAPORIZER (Fig. 2.18)

Components

1. The case with the filling level indicator and a port for the filling device.
2. Percentage control dial on top/face of the case. The control dial opens in an anticlockwise direction.
3. The bypass channel and the vaporization chamber. The latter has Teflon wicks or baffles, cowls or nebulizers to increase the surface area available for vaporization (Fig. 2.19).

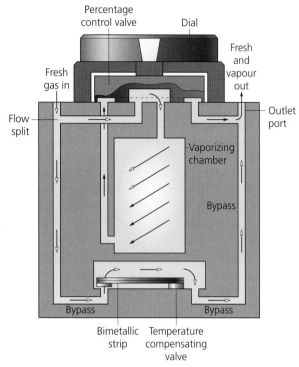

Fig. 2.19 A schematic diagram of the Tec Mk 5, an example of a plenum vaporizer.

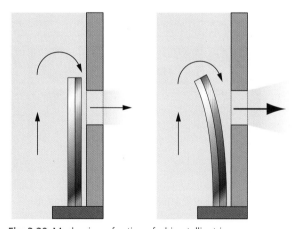

Fig. 2.20 Mechanism of action of a bimetallic strip.

4. The splitting ratio is controlled by a temperature-sensitive valve utilizing a bimetallic strip (Fig. 2.20). The latter is made of two strips of metal with different coefficients of thermal expansion bonded together. It is positioned inside the vaporization chamber in the older designs (Tec Mk 2). In modern designs (Tec Mk 3, 4, 5 and 7 and the Sigma Delta series), it is outside the vaporization chamber.

5. The vaporizers are mounted on the back bar (Fig. 2.21) using the interlocking Selectatec™ Vaporizer

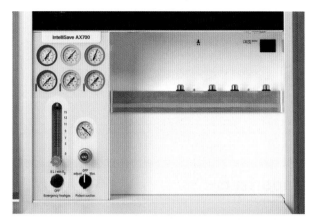

Fig. 2.21 An empty Selectatec back bar of an anaesthetic machine showing the O-rings. (Courtesy Philips Healthcare, Guildford, UK.)

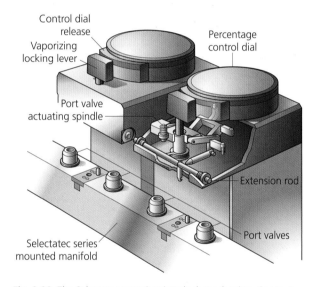

Fig. 2.22 The Selectatec vaporizer interlock mechanism. See text for details. (Courtesy GE Healthcare, Hatfield, UK.)

Manifold system (Fig. 2.22) with two male valve ports, each with an O-ring for a gas-tight fit, to take the vaporizer's two female ports.

6. The percentage control dial cannot be moved unless the locking lever of the system is engaged (in Mk 4–7 and Sigma Delta). The interlocking extension rods prevent more than one vaporizer from being used at any one time, preventing contamination of the one downstream (in Mk 4–7 and Sigma Delta). The FGF only enters the vaporizer when it is switched on (Fig. 2.23).

Mechanism of action

1. The calibration of each vaporizer is agent-specific.
2. FGF is split into two streams on entering the vaporizer. One stream flows through the bypass

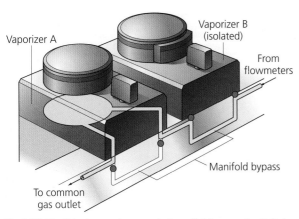

Vaporizer A

Vaporizer B (isolated)

From flowmeters

Manifold bypass

To common gas outlet

Fig. 2.23 The Selectatec series mounted manifold bypass circuit. Only when a vaporizer is locked in position and turned on can fresh gas enter. Vaporizer B is turned off and is isolated from the fresh gas, which only enters vaporizer A, which is turned on. If no vaporizer is fitted, the port valves are closed. (Courtesy GE Healthcare, Hatfield, UK.)

channel and the other smaller stream (typically less than 20% of total) flows through the vaporizing chamber. The two gas streams reunite as the gas leaves the vaporizer.

3. The vaporization chamber is designed so that the gas leaving it is always fully saturated with vapour before it rejoins the bypass gas stream. This should be achieved despite changes in the FGF.

4. Full saturation with vapour is achieved by increasing the surface area of contact between the carrier gas and the anaesthetic agent. This is achieved by having wicks saturated by the inhalational agent, a series of baffles or by bubbling the gas through the liquid. The presence of wicks and baffles significantly increases the internal resistance of the vaporizer.

5. The desired concentration is obtained by adjusting the percentage control dial. This alters the amount of gas flowing through the bypass channel to that flowing through the vaporization chamber.

6. In the modern designs, the vapour concentration supplied by the vaporizer is virtually independent of the FGFs between 0.25 and 15 L/min.

7. During vaporization, cooling occurs due to the loss of latent heat of vaporization. Lowering the temperature of the agent decreases its saturated vapour pressure (SVP) and makes it less volatile. In order to stabilize the temperature and compensate for temperature changes:
   a. the vaporizer is made of a material with high density and high specific heat capacity with a very high thermal conductivity, e.g. copper. As a temperature stabilizer, copper acts as a heat sink, readily giving heat to the anaesthetic agent and maintaining its temperature

   b. a temperature-sensitive valve (e.g. bimetallic strip or bellows) within the body of the vaporizer automatically adjusts the splitting ratio according to the temperature. It allows more flow into the vaporizing chamber as the temperature decreases.

8. The amount of vapour carried by the FGF is a function of both the SVP of the agent and the atmospheric pressure. At high altitudes, the atmospheric pressure is reduced, whereas the SVP remains the same. This leads to an increased amount of vapour, whereas the saturation of the agent remains the same. The opposite occurs in hyperbaric chambers. This is of no clinical relevance as it is the partial pressure of the agent in the alveoli that determines the clinical effect of the agent.

Problems in practice and safety features

1. In modern vaporizers (e.g. Tec Mk 5 onwards), the liquid anaesthetic agent does not enter the bypass channel even if the vaporizer is tipped upside down due to internal valves acting as an antispill mechanism. In earlier designs, dangerously high concentrations of anaesthetic agent could be delivered to the patient in cases of agent spillage into the bypass channel. Despite that, it is recommended that the vaporizer is purged with an FGF of 5 L/min for 30 minutes with the percentage control dial set at 5%.

2. The Selectatec system increases the potential for leaks. This is due to the risk of accidental removal of the O-rings with changes of vaporizers (see Fig. 2.21).

3. Minute volume divider ventilators exert back pressure as they cycle. This pressure forces some of the gas exiting the outlet port back into the vaporizing chamber, where more vapour is added. Retrograde flow may also contaminate the bypass channel. These effects cause an increase in the inspired concentration of the agent, which may be toxic. These pressure fluctuations can be compensated for by:
   a. long inlet port into the vaporizing chamber as in Tec Mk 3. This ensures that the bypass channel is not contaminated by retrograde flow from the vaporizing chamber
   b. downstream flow restrictors used to maintain the vaporizer at a pressure greater than any pressure required to operate commonly used ventilators
   c. both the bypass channel and the vaporizing chamber are of equal volumes, so gas expansion and compression are equal.

4. Preservatives, such as thymol in halothane, accumulate on the wicks of vaporizers with time. Large quantities may interfere with the function of the vaporizer. Thymol can also cause the bimetallic strip in the Tec Mk 2 to stick. Modern inhalational agents do not contain preservatives.

5. A pressure relief valve downstream of the vaporizer opens at about 35 kPa. This prevents damage to flowmeters or vaporizers if the common gas outlet is blocked.
6. The bimetallic strip has been situated in the bypass channel since the Tec Mk 3. It is possible for the chemically active strip to corrode in a mixture of oxygen and the inhalational agent within the vaporizing chamber (Tec Mk 2).
7. The vaporizer needs regular servicing to ensure accurate calibration.
8. Despite its temperature-compensation properties, the vaporizer can deliver unreliable inhalational agent concentrations in extreme ambient temperatures.

Vaporizers
- The case is made of copper, which is a good heat sink.
- Consists of a bypass channel and vaporization chamber. The latter has wicks to increase the surface area available for vaporization.
- A temperature-sensitive valve controls the splitting ratio. It is positioned outside the vaporizing chamber in modern vaporizers (Tec Mk 3, 4, 5 and 7 and Sigma Delta series).
- The gas leaving the vaporizing chamber is fully saturated.
- The effect of temperature changes and back pressure are compensated for.

Vaporizer-filling devices

These are agent-specific, being geometrically coded (keyed) to fit the safety filling port of the correct vaporizer and anaesthetic agent supply bottle (Fig. 2.24). They prevent the risk of adding the wrong agent to the wrong vaporizer and decrease the extent of spillage. The safety filling system, in addition, ensures that the vaporizer cannot overflow. Fillers used for desflurane and sevoflurane have valves that are only opened when fully inserted into their ports. This prevents spillage.

The fillers are colour-coded:
- Red: halothane
- Orange: enflurane
- Purple: isoflurane
- Yellow: sevoflurane
- Blue: desflurane

A more recent design feature is the antipollution cap, allowing the filler to be left fitted to the bottle between uses to prevent the agent from vaporizing. It also eliminates

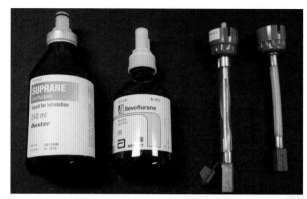

Fig. 2.24 Agent-specific, colour-coded filling devices; *(left to right)* desflurane, sevoflurane, isoflurane and enflurane.

airlocks, speeding up vaporizer filling, and ensures that the bottle is completely emptied, reducing wastage.

Non-return pressure relief safety valve

1. This is situated downstream of the vaporizers either on the back bar itself or near the common gas outlet (Fig. 2.25). Its non-return design helps to prevent back pressure effects commonly encountered using minute volume divider ventilators.
2. It opens when the pressure in the back bar exceeds about 35 kPa. Flowmeter and vaporizer components can be damaged at higher pressures.

Emergency oxygen flush

This is usually activated by a non-locking button (Fig. 2.26). When pressed, pure oxygen is supplied from the outlet of the anaesthetic machine. The flow bypasses the flowmeters and the vaporizers. A flow of about 35–75 L/min at a pressure of about 400 kPa is expected. The emergency oxygen flush is usually activated by a non-locking button and using a self-closing valve. It is designed to minimize unintended and accidental operation by staff or other equipment. The button is recessed in a housing to prevent accidental depression.

Problems in practice and safety features

1. The high operating pressure and flow of the oxygen flush puts the patient at a higher risk of barotrauma.
2. When the emergency oxygen flush is used inappropriately, it leads to dilution of the anaesthetic gases and possible awareness.

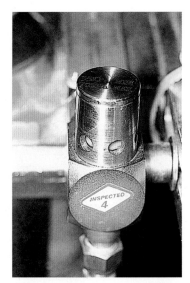

Fig. 2.25 A non-return pressure relief valve situated at the end of the back bar.

3. It should not be activated while ventilating a patient using a minute volume divider ventilator.

Compressed oxygen outlet(s)

One or more compressed oxygen outlets are used to provide oxygen at about 400 kPa (Fig. 2.27). It can be used to drive ventilators or a manually controlled jet injector.

Oxygen supply failure alarm

Many designs are available (Fig. 2.28), but the characteristics of the ideal warning device are as follows:
1. Activation depends on the pressure of oxygen itself.
2. It requires no batteries or mains power.
3. It gives an audible signal of a special character and of sufficient duration and volume to attract attention.
4. It should give a warning of impending failure and a further alarm that failure has occurred.
5. It should have pressure-linked controls that interrupt the flow of all other gases when it comes into operation. Atmospheric air is allowed to be delivered to the patient without carbon dioxide accumulation. It should be impossible to resume anaesthesia until the oxygen supply has been restored.

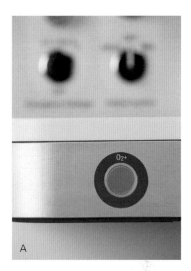

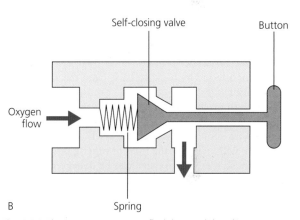

Fig. 2.26 The emergency oxygen flush button (A) and its mechanism of action (B). (A, Courtesy Philips Healthcare, Guildford, UK.)

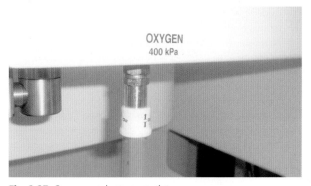

Fig. 2.27 Compressed oxygen outlet.

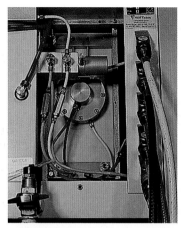

Fig. 2.28 The oxygen supply failure alarm in the Datex-Ohmeda Flexima anaesthetic machine.

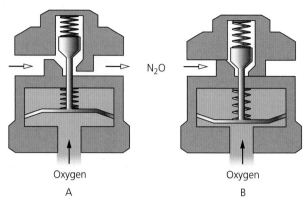

Fig. 2.29 Oxygen supply failure alarm mechanism of action. (A) O_2 pressure is higher than 200 kPa, so allowing N_2O flow *(blue)*. (B) O_2 pressure is lower than 200 kPa, so cutting off N_2O flow.

6. The alarm should be positioned on the reduced pressure side of the oxygen supply line.
7. It should be tamper-proof.
8. It is not affected by back pressure from the anaesthetic ventilator.

In modern machines, if the oxygen supply pressure falls below 200 kPa, the low-pressure supply alarm sounds. With supply pressures below 137 kPa, the 'fail-safe' valve will interrupt the flow of other gases to their flowmeters so that only oxygen can be delivered (Fig. 2.29). The oxygen flow set on the oxygen flowmeter will not decrease until the oxygen supply pressure falls below 100 kPa.

Anti-hypoxic safety features

These features are designed to prevent the delivery of gaseous mixtures with oxygen concentrations of less than 25%. This can be achieved by:

- Mechanical means: a chain links the oxygen and nitrous oxide flow control valves. Increasing the flow rate of nitrous oxide leads to a proportional increase in oxygen flow rate. The oxygen flowmeter control valve has a stop to ensure a minimum flow of oxygen at 175–250 mL/min, even with the valve apparently closed.
- Pneumatic means: a pressure-sensitive diaphragm measuring the changes in oxygen and nitrous oxide concentrations. The diaphragm is designed to ensure an increase in oxygen flow rate by a ratio of 25% of any increase in the nitrous oxide flow rate.
- A paramagnetic oxygen analyser continuously measuring the oxygen concentration. Nitrous oxide flow is switched off automatically when oxygen concentration falls under 25%.

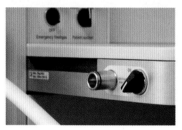

Fig. 2.30 Common gas outlet. (Courtesy Philips Healthcare, Guildford, UK.)

Common gas outlet (Fig. 2.30)

The common gas outlet is where the anaesthetic machine 'ends'. At the common gas outlet, the gas mixture made at the flowmeters plus any inhaled anaesthetic agent added by the vaporizer exit the machine and enter the fresh gas tubing that conducts it to the breathing system. The common gas outlet is a conically tapered pipe with a 22-mm male/15-mm female connector fitting. It can be fixed or on a swivelling connector. The connector of the common gas outlet should be strong enough to withstand a torque of up to 10 Nm because of the heavy equipment that may be attached.

 Exam tip: Pay attention to the order in which you check the anaesthetic machine. You need to follow the gas flow.

Other modifications and designs

1. **Desflurane vaporizer** (Figs. 2.31 and 2.32). Desflurane is an inhalational agent with unique physical properties, making it extremely volatile. Its SVP is 664 mmHg at 20°C and, with a boiling point of 23.5°C at

atmospheric pressure, which is only slightly above normal room temperature, precludes the use of a normal variable-bypass type vaporizer. Due to its low boiling point, changes in ambient temperature can lead to large and unpredictable changes in vapour pressure and its delivered concentration. In order to overcome these physical properties, vaporizers with a completely different design are used despite the similar appearance. They are mounted on the Selectatec system.

a. An electrically heated desflurane vaporization chamber (sump) with a capacity of 450 mL requires a warm-up period of 5–10 minutes to reach its operating temperature of 39°C (i.e. above its boiling point) and an SVP of more than 1550 mmHg (about two atmospheric pressures). The vaporizer will not function below this temperature and pressure. Due to the previously mentioned circumstances, temperature compensation is not required.

b. A fixed restriction/orifice is positioned in the FGF path. The FGF does not enter the vaporization chamber. Instead, the FGF enters the path of the regulated concentration of desflurane vapour before the resulting gas mixture is delivered to the patient.

c. A differential pressure transducer adjusts a pressure-regulating valve at the outlet of the vaporization chamber. The transducer senses pressure at the fixed restriction on one side and the pressure of desflurane vapour upstream to the pressure-regulating valve on the other side. This transducer ensures that the pressure of desflurane vapour upstream of the control valve equals the pressure of FGF at the fixed restriction.

d. A percentage control dial with a rotary valve adjusts a second resistor, which controls the flow of desflurane vapour into the FGF and thus the output concentration. The dial calibration is from 0% to 18%.

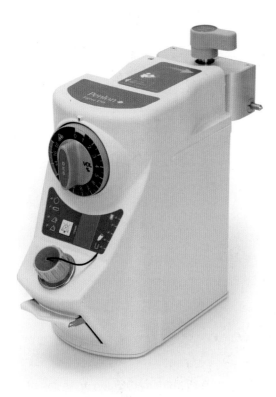

Fig. 2.31 Penlon Sigma EVA desflurane vaporizer. (Courtesy Penlon, Abingdon, UK.)

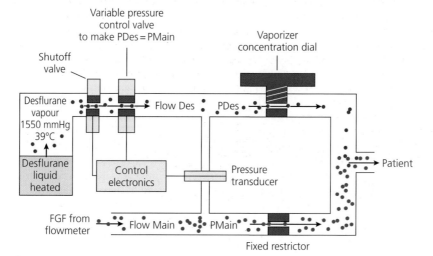

Fig. 2.32 A schematic diagram of the desflurane vaporizer.

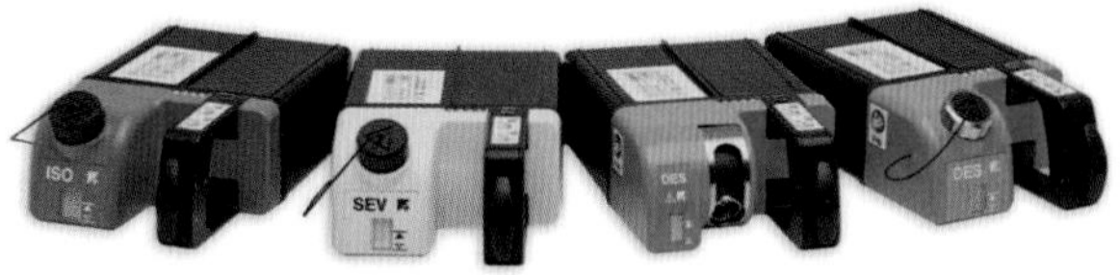

Fig. 2.33 Aladin₂™ cassettes. (Courtesy GE, Hatfield, Hertfordshire, UK.)

e. The fixed restriction/orifice ensures that the pressure of the carrier gas within the vaporizer is proportional to gas flow. The transducer ensures that the pressure of desflurane vapour upstream of the resistor equals the pressure of FGF at the orifice. This means that the flow of desflurane out of the vaporizing chamber is proportional to the FGF, so enabling the output concentration to be made independent of FGF rate.

f. The vaporizer incorporates malfunction alarms (auditory and visual). There is a backup 9-V battery should there be a main power system failure.

2. **Newly designed anaesthetic machines** are more sophisticated than that described previously. Many important components have become electrically or electronically controlled as an integrated system. Thermistors can be used to measure the flow of gases. Gas flow causes changes in temperature, which are measured by the thermistors. Changes in temperature are calibrated to measure flows of gases. Other designs measure flows using electronic flow sensors based on the principle of the pneumotachograph. Pressure difference is measured across a laminar flow resistor through which the gas flows. Using a differential pressure transducer, flow is measured and displayed on a screen in the form of a virtual graduated flowmeter, together with a digital display.

a. Aladin₂™ cassettes (Fig. 2.33) are refillable vaporizers that are designed by GE for use with the *Aisys™ CS² anesthesia delivery system* (Fig. 2.34), replacing the conventional vaporizers. They are agent-specific, very accurate and lightweight (less than 3.5 kg). They have electronic controls, allowing automatic record keeping, gas usage calculation, FGF and temperature/pressure compensation, self-check and diagnostics with electronic level sensing and agent identification. They are service-free with no handling or tilting restrictions.

They are functionally similar to conventional vaporizers, with a bypass channel and a vaporizing chamber. However, the bypass channel is positioned in the vaporizer housing in the anaesthetic machine rather than the cassette itself. A proportional valve regulates the amount of fresh gas flowing through the cassette, so adjusting the agent

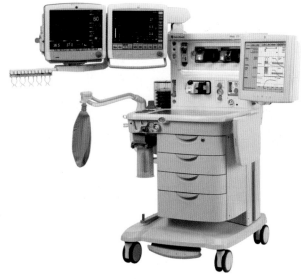

Fig. 2.34 The GE Aisys™ CS² anesthesia delivery system with Alladin₂™ cassette. (Courtesy GE, Hatfield, Hertfordshire, UK.)

concentration. The more fresh gas allowed to pass through the cassette, so getting fully saturated with the agent, the greater the concentration with part of the fresh gas bypassing the cassette.

Each cassette is magnetically coded allowing the *Aisys™ CS² anesthesia delivery system* to recognize which type of agent cassette is inserted.

In the GE *Aisys™ CS² anesthesia delivery system*, the fractional inspired oxygen concentration (FiO₂) and end-tidal anaesthetic agent concentration can be set by the anaesthetist with the workstation working to achieve these targets in the quickest and safest way.

b. The Dräger Zeus IE workstation (Dräger, Hemel Hempstead, UK) (Fig. 2.35) uses direct injectors instead of the traditional vaporizers. This allows direct injection of the inhalational agent into the breathing system. This in turn allows for rapid changes in the inhalational agent concentration independent of the FGF. The FiO₂ and end-tidal anaesthetic agent concentration are set by the

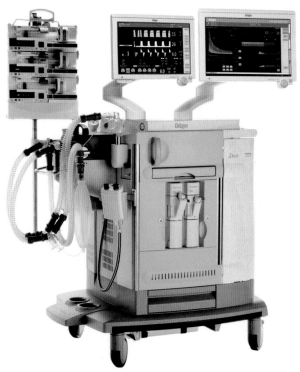

Fig. 2.35 Dräger Zeus IE anaesthetic workstation. (Courtesy Dräger, Hemel Hempstead, UK.)

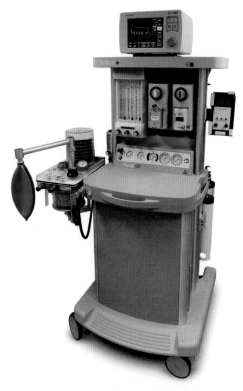

Fig. 2.36 Penlon non-ferrous Prima 451 magnetic resonance imaging anaesthetic machine with AV-S monitor. (Courtesy Penlon, Abingdon, UK.)

anaesthetist. The system achieves these targets in the safest and quickest way. The workstation also has a number of pumps, allowing intravenous infusion when required.

3. **MRI compatible anaesthetic machines.** Since most of the anaesthetic machine is made from metal, it should not be used close to a magnetic resonance imaging (MRI) scanner. Distorted readings and physical damage to the scanner are possible because of the attraction of the strong magnetic fields. Newly designed anaesthetic machines made of totally non-ferrous material solve this problem (Fig. 2.36).

4. **Small and compact anaesthetic machines** are available (Fig. 2.37). Such machines can be used in restricted space areas.

5. **Quantiflex Anaesthetic Machine** (Fig. 2.38). This machine has the following features:
   a. Two flowmeters, one for oxygen and one for nitrous oxide, with one control knob for both flowmeters.
   b. The oxygen flowmeter is situated to the right, whereas the nitrous oxide flowmeter is situated to the left.
   c. The relative concentrations of oxygen and nitrous oxide are adjusted by a mixture control wheel. The oxygen concentration can be adjusted in 10% increments from 30% to 100%.

d. This design prevents the delivery of hypoxic mixtures.
e. It is mainly used in dental anaesthesia.

6. Some **newly designed anaesthetic machines** have an extra outlet with its own flowmeter to deliver oxygen to conscious or lightly sedated patients via a face mask. This can be used in patients undergoing surgery under regional anaesthesia with sedation.

7. The **Glostavent Helix Duo** (Figs 1.23). This was developed to enable the provision of anaesthesia in low-resource environments where compressed gases and electricity supplies are unreliable.

   The machine has two low-resistance, draw-over vaporizers allowing the delivery of gaseous induction using sevoflurane for induction then isoflurane for maintenance. The switching mechanism between vaporizers has a unique vaporizer select design with a 'break before make' safety feature (see Fig. 2.39), permitting easy and controlled changeover with no possibility of having both vaporizers in use at the same time.

   The machine is mains and battery powered and uses its own integral oxygen concentrator to supply the oxygen at a flow of 10 L/min. The machine

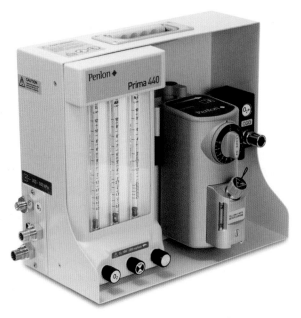

Fig. 2.37 Penlon compact Prima 440 anaesthetic machine. (Courtesy Penlon, Abingdon, UK.)

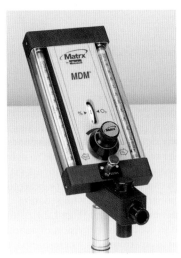

Fig. 2.38 Matrx MDM Anaesthetic Machine. (Courtesy Porter Instrument, Parker Hannifin Corporation, Hatfield, PA, USA.)

has its own built ventilator (pressure and volume controlled) and a fuel cell as an inspired oxygen concentration analyser. A built-in uninterruptable power supply allows the machine to fully function for 30 minutes. It can be used for adults, paediatrics and neonates.

 Exam tip: Make sure you know the safety features of a modern anaesthetic machine in delivering a safe gas mixture.

Anaesthesia in remote areas

The apparatus used must be compact, portable and robust. The Triservice apparatus is suitable for use in remote areas where supply of compressed gases and vapours is difficult (Figs. 2.40 and 2.41). The Triservice anaesthetic apparatus name derives from the three branches of military services: Army, Navy and Air Force.

Components

1. A face mask with a non-rebreathing valve fitted.
2. A short length of tubing leading to a self-inflating bag.
3. A second length of tubing leading from the self-inflating bag to two OMVs.
4. An oxygen cylinder can be connected upstream of the vaporizers. A third length of tubing acts as an oxygen reservoir during expiration.

Mechanism of action

1. The Triservice apparatus can be used for both spontaneous and controlled ventilation.
   a. The patient can draw air through the vaporizers. The exhaled gases are vented out via the non-rebreathing valve.
   b. The self-inflating bag can be used for controlled or assisted ventilation.

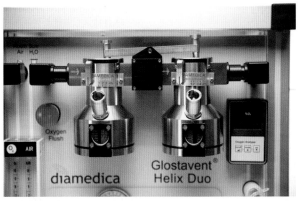

Fig. 2.39 The selection mechanism between the two vaporizers in the Glostavent Helix Duo. (Courtesy Diamedica, Barnstaple, Devon, UK.)

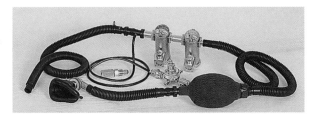

Fig. 2.40 The Triservice apparatus.

2. The OMV is a variable bypass, low-resistance draw-over vaporizer with a capacity for 50 mL of anaesthetic agent. The wick is made of metal with no temperature-compensation features. However, there is an ethylene glycol jacket acting as a heat sink to help to stabilize the vaporizer temperature. The calibration scale on the vaporizer can be detached, allowing the use of different inhalational agents. A different inhalational agent can be used after blowing air for 10 minutes and rinsing the wicks with the new agent. The vaporizer casing has extendable feet fitted.
3. The downstream vaporizer is traditionally filled with trichloroethylene to compensate for the absence of the analgesic effect of nitrous oxide.

Problems in practice and safety features

1. The vaporizers' heat sink (ethylene glycol jacket) is not suitable for prolonged use at high gas flows. The vapour concentration decreases as the temperature decreases.

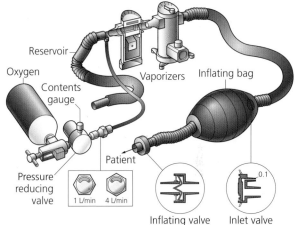

Fig. 2.41 Mechanism of action of the Triservice apparatus.

2. During use, accidental tipping of the vaporizer can spill liquid agent into the breathing system. The vaporizer is spill proof when turned off.

Triservice apparatus
- Consists of two OMVs, a self-inflating bag and a non-rebreathing valve.
- The apparatus is suitable for both spontaneous and controlled breathing.
- The OMV is a draw-over vaporizer with no temperature compensation. It has a heat sink. It can be used with different inhalational agents.

SUGGESTED FURTHER READING

Auxiliary Common Gas Outlet (ACGO) for Anaesthetic Machine – no FGF to Patient With Wrong Setting. Available from: https://www.gov.uk/drug-device-alerts/medical-device-alert-auxiliary-common-gas-outlet-acgo-for-anaesthetic-machine-no-fresh-gas-flow-to-patient-with-wrong-setting.

Medicines and Healthcare products Regulatory Agency (MHRA), 2014. All anaesthetic breathing systems, anaesthetic machines and anaesthetic ventilators - inadequate ventilation. Available from: https://www.gov.uk/drug-device-alert-all-anaesthetic-breathing-systems-anaesthetic-machines-and-anaesthetic-ventilators-inadequate-ventilation.

Medicines and Healthcare products Regulatory Agency (MHRA), 2014. Anaesthetic machines: off-label use during the COVID-19 pandemic. (MDA/2020/012). Available from: https://www.gov.uk/drug-device-alerts/anaesthetic-machines-off-label-use-during-the-covid-19-pandemic-mda-2020-012.

National Institute for Health and Care Excellence (NICE), 2014. End-tidal control software for use with aisys closed circuit anaesthesia systems for automated gas control during general anaesthesia. Available from: http://www.nice.org.uk/advice/mib10.

University of Bristol, 2017. The Anaesthetic Machine Anatomy. Available from: https://www.bristol.ac.uk/media-library/sites/vetscience/documents/clinical-skills/Anaesthetic%20Machine%20Anatomy.pdf.

SELF-ASSESSMENT QUESTIONS

Please check your eBook for additional self-assessment

MCQs

In the following lists, which of the following statements (a) to (e) are true?

1. **Flowmeters in an anaesthetic machine**
   a. N_2O may be used in an O_2 flowmeter without a change in calibration.
   b. Flowmeters use a tube and bobbin.
   c. They are an example of a variable orifice device.
   d. They have a linear scale.
   e. Both laminar and turbulent flows are encountered.

2. **Vaporizers**
   a. Manual ventilation using a vaporizer in circle (VIC) causes a reduction in the inspired concentration of the inhalational agent.
   b. A Tec Mk 3 vaporizer can be used as a VIC.
   c. Gas flow emerging from the vaporizing chamber should be fully saturated with the inhalational agent.
   d. The bimetallic strip valve in Tec Mk 5 is in the vaporizing chamber.
   e. In modern vaporizers, the inhalational agent concentration delivered to the patient gradually decreases the longer the vaporizer is used due to cooling of the agent.

3. **Pressure gauges on an anaesthetic machine**
   a. Use the Bourdon pressure gauge principle.
   b. The pressure reflects accurately the cylinders' contents for both oxygen and nitrous oxide.
   c. Can be interchangeable between oxygen and nitrous oxide.
   d. The same pressure gauge can be used for both cylinder and pipeline gas supply.
   e. They are colour-coded for a particular gas or vapour.

4. **Regarding safety features on modern anaesthetic machines**
   a. The nitrous oxide flow control knob can be rotated 2.07 times for each revolution of the oxygen flow control knob.
   b. The nitrous oxide control knob has distinctive knurling to reduce accidental activation.
   c. The oxygen failure alarm activates when supply pressure falls below 200 kPa.
   d. European standard EN740 requires anaesthetic machines to have a mechanism to prevent delivery of gas mixtures of less than 25% oxygen.
   e. A fail-safe valve prevents air supply to the patient when oxygen supply pressure drops below 137 kPa.

5. **Laminar flow**
   a. It is directly proportional to the square root of pressure.
   b. Halving the radius results in a flow equivalent to a 16th of the original laminar flow.
   c. It is related to the density of the fluid.
   d. The flow is greatest in the centre.
   e. Laminar flow changes to turbulent when Reynold's number exceeds 2000.

6. **Flowmeters on an anaesthetic machine**
   a. They have an accuracy of ±2.5%.
   b. They have a tapered tube with a narrow top.
   c. Oxygen is the first gas to be added to the mixture at the back bar.
   d. At high flows, the density of the gas is important in measuring the flow.
   e. The reading of the flow is from the top of the bobbin.

7. Concerning the Triservice apparatus
   a. Two plenum vaporizers are used.
   b. It can be used for both spontaneous and controlled ventilation.
   c. An inflating bag and a one-way valve are used.
   d. The Oxford Miniature Vaporizer (OMV) has a metal wick and a heat sink.
   e. Supplementary oxygen can be added to the system.

8. Pressure regulators
   a. They are only used to reduce the pressure of gases.
   b. They maintain a gas flow at a constant pressure of about 400 kPa.
   c. Their main purpose is to protect the patient.
   d. Relief valves open at 700 kPa in case of failure.
   e. Flow restrictors can additionally be used in pipeline supply.

9. The safety features found in an anaesthetic machine include
   a. Oxygen supply failure alarm.
   b. Colour-coded flowmeters.
   c. Vaporizer level alarm.
   d. Ventilator disconnection alarm.
   e. Two vaporizers can be safely used at the same time.

10. The non-return valve on the back bar of an anaesthetic machine between the vaporizer and common gas outlet
    a. Decreases the pumping effect.
    b. Often is incorporated with a pressure relief valve on modern machines.
    c. Is designed to protect the patient.
    d. Is designed to protect the machine.
    e. Opens at a pressure of 70 kPa.

11. The oxygen emergency flush on an anaesthetic machine
    a. Operates at 20 L/min.
    b. Is always safe to use during anaesthesia.
    c. Operates at 40 L/min.
    d. Increases risk of awareness during anaesthesia.
    e. Can be safely used with a minute volume divider ventilator.

12. Regarding the Glostavent Helix Duo
    a. Uses a draw-over vaporizer.
    b. Oxygen is supplied from cylinders only.
    c. Incorporates an uninterruptable power supply unit.
    d. Can be used to deliver sevoflurane.
    e. Incorporates a paramagnetic oxygen analyser.

Single best answer

13. Concerning a desflurane vaporizer
    a. Is ready for use immediately.
    b. Can be used with other inhalational agents.
    c. Needs an electrical supply to function.
    d. Fresh gas flow (FGF) enters the vaporization chamber.
    e. Is colour-coded red.

14. The pressure supplied by activating the emergency oxygen flush button is
    a. 13,700 kPa.
    b. 4400 kPa.
    c. 400 kPa.
    d. 250 kPa.
    e. 10 kPa.

15. Which of the following will not affect the reading on a flowmeter
    a. Temperature
    b. Atmospheric pressure
    c. Angle of flowmeter
    d. Setting of a vaporizer
    e. Use of a ventilator

16. Which of the following features of vaporizers are designed to protect against the effects of back pressure
    a. Having bypass and vaporizing chambers of the same volume
    b. Bimetallic strips
    c. Wicks
    d. Selectatec system
    e. Low resistance to flow

Answers

1. *Flowmeters in an anaesthetic machine*
   a. *False. The flowmeters in an anaesthetic machine are calibrated for the particular gas(es) used, taking into consideration the viscosity and density of the gas(es). N_2O and O_2 have different viscosities and densities so unless the flowmeters are recalibrated, false readings will result.*
   b. *True. They are constant pressure, variable orifice flowmeters. A tapered transparent tube with a lightweight rotating bobbin. The bobbin is held floating in the tube by the gas flow. The clearance between the bobbin and the tube wall widens as the flow increases. The pressure across the bobbin remains constant as the effect of gravity on the bobbin is countered by the gas flow.*
   c. *True. See above.*
   d. *False. The flowmeters do not have a linear scale. There are different scales for low and high flow rates.*
   e. *True. At low flows, the flowmeter acts as a tube, as the clearance between the bobbin and the wall of the tube is longer and narrower. This leads to laminar flow, which is dependent on the viscosity (Poiseuille's law). At high flows, the flowmeter acts as an orifice. The clearance is shorter and wider. This leads to turbulent flow, which is dependent on density.*

2. *Vaporizers*
   a. *False. During manual (or controlled) ventilation using a VIC vaporizer, the inspired concentration of the inhalational agent is increased. It can increase to dangerous concentrations. Unless the concentration of the inhalational agent(s) is measured continuously, this technique is not recommended.*
   b. *False. As the patient is breathing through a VIC vaporizer, it should have very low internal resistance. The Tec Mk 3 has a high internal resistance because of the wicks in the vaporizing chamber.*
   c. *True. This can be achieved by increasing the surface area of contact between the carrier gas and the anaesthetic agent. Full saturation should be achieved despite changes in FGF. The final concentration is delivered to the patient after mixing with the FGF from the bypass channel.*
   d. *False. The bimetallic strip valve in the Tec Mk 5 is in the bypass chamber. The bimetallic strip has been positioned in the bypass chamber since the Tec Mk 3. This was done to avoid corrosion of the strip in a mixture of oxygen and inhalational agent when positioned in the vaporizing chamber.*
   e. *False. The concentration delivered to the patient stays constant because of temperature-compensating mechanisms. This can be achieved by:*
      • using a material with high density and high specific thermal conductivity (e.g. copper) that acts as a heat sink, readily giving heat to the agent and maintaining its temperature
      • a temperature-sensitive valve within the vaporizer that automatically adjusts the splitting ratio according to the temperature, so if the temperature decreases due to loss of latent heat of vaporization, it allows more flow into the vaporizing chamber.

3. *Pressure gauges on an anaesthetic machine*
   a. *True. A pressure gauge consists of a coiled tube that is subjected to pressure from the inside. The high-pressure gas causes the tube to uncoil. The movement of the tube causes a needle pointer to move on a calibrated dial, indicating the pressure.*
   b. *False. Oxygen is stored as a gas in the cylinder hence it obeys the gas laws. The pressure changes in an oxygen cylinder accurately reflect the contents. Nitrous oxide is stored as a liquid and vapour so it does not obey Boyle's law. This means that the pressure changes in a nitrous oxide cylinder do not accurately reflect the contents of the cylinder.*
   c. *False. The pressure gauges are calibrated for a particular gas or vapour. Oxygen and nitrous oxide pressure gauges are not interchangeable.*
   d. *False. Cylinders are kept under much higher pressures (13,700 kPa for oxygen and 5400 kPa for nitrous oxide) than the pipeline gas supply (about 400 kPa). Using the same pressure gauges for both cylinders and pipeline gas supply can lead to inaccuracies and/or damage to pressure gauges.*
   e. *True. Colour-coding is one of the safety features used in the use and delivery of gases in medical practice. In the United Kingdom, white is for*

oxygen, blue for nitrous oxide and black for medical air.

4. *Regarding safety features on modern anaesthetic machines*
   a. **True.**
   b. **False.** The oxygen flow control knob has distinctive knurling to aid identification.
   c. **True.**
   d. **True.**
   e. **False.** The fail-safe valve prevents nitrous oxide supply when the oxygen supply pressure falls below 137 kPa.

5. *Laminar flow*
   a. **False.** Laminar flow is directly proportional to pressure. Hagen–Poiseuille equation: Flow $\propto$ pressure × radius^4/viscosity × length.
   b. **True.** From the above equation, the flow $\propto$ radius^4.
   c. **False.** Laminar flow is related to viscosity. Turbulent flow is related to density.
   d. **True.** Laminar flow is greatest in the centre at about twice the mean flow rate. The flow is slower nearer to the wall of the tube. At the wall the flow is almost zero.
   e. **True.** Reynold's number is the index used to predict the type of flow, laminar or turbulent. Reynold's number = velocity of fluid × density × radius of tube/viscosity. In laminar flow, Reynold's number is <2000. In turbulent flow, Reynold's number is >2000.

6. *Flowmeters on an anaesthetic machine*
   a. **True.** The flowmeters on the anaesthetic machine are very accurate with an accuracy of ±2.5%.
   b. **False.** The flowmeters on an anaesthetic machine are tapered tubes; however, the top is wider than the bottom.
   c. **False.** Oxygen is the last gas to be added to the mixture at the back bar. This is a safety feature in the design of the anaesthetic machine. If there is a crack in a flowmeter, a hypoxic mixture may result if oxygen is added first to the mixture.
   d. **True.** At high flows, the flow is turbulent, which is dependent on density. At low flows, the flow is laminar, which is dependent on viscosity.
   e. **True.** When a ball is used, the reading is taken from the midpoint.

7. *Concerning the Triservice apparatus*
   a. **False.** In the Triservice apparatus, two draw-over OMVs are used. Plenum vaporizers are not used due to their high internal resistance. The OMV is lightweight, and, by changing its calibration scale, different inhalational agents can be used easily.
   b. **True.** The system allows both spontaneous and controlled ventilation. The resistance to breathing is low, allowing spontaneous ventilation. The self-inflating bag provides the means to control ventilation.
   c. **True.** As above.
   d. **True.** The OMV has a metal wick to increase area of vaporization within the vaporization chamber. The heat sink consists of an ethylene glycol jacket to stabilize the vaporizer temperature.
   e. **True.** Supplementary oxygen can be added to the system from an oxygen cylinder. The oxygen is added to the reservoir proximal to the vaporizer(s).

8. *Pressure regulators*
   a. **False.** Pressure regulators are used to reduce pressure of gases and to maintain a constant flow. In the absence of pressure regulators, the flowmeters need to be adjusted regularly to maintain constant flows as the contents of the cylinders are used up. The temperature and pressure of the cylinder contents decrease with use.
   b. **True.** Pressure regulators are designed to maintain a gas flow at a constant pressure of about 400 kPa irrespective of the pressure and temperature of the contents of the cylinder.
   c. **False.** Pressure regulators offer no protection to the patient. Their main function is to protect the anaesthetic machine from the high pressure of the cylinder and to maintain a constant flow of gas.
   d. **True.** In situations in which the pressure regulator fails, a relief valve that opens at 700 kPa prevents the build-up of excessive pressure.
   e. **True.** Flow restrictors can be used in a pipeline supply. They are designed to protect the anaesthetic machine from pressure surges in the system. They consist of a constriction between the pipeline supply and the anaesthetic machine.

9. *The safety features found in an anaesthetic machine include*
   a. **True.** This is an essential safety feature in the anaesthetic machine. The ideal design should operate under the pressure of oxygen itself, give a characteristic audible signal, be capable of warning of impending failure and give a further alarm when failure has occurred, be capable of interrupting the flow of other gases and not require batteries or mains power to operate.
   b. **True.** The flowmeters are colour-coded, and the shape and size of the oxygen flowmeter knob is different from that of the nitrous oxide knob. This allows the identification of the oxygen knob even in a dark environment.

c. False. The vaporizer level can be monitored by the anaesthetist. This is part of the anaesthetic machine checklist. There is no alarm system. However, some of desflurane vaporizers have a level alarm.

d. True. A ventilator disconnection alarm is essential when a ventilator is used. They are also used to monitor leaks, obstruction and malfunction. They can be pressure- and/or volume-monitoring alarms. In addition, clinical observation, end-tidal carbon dioxide concentration and airway pressure are 'disconnection alarms'.

e. False. Only one vaporizer can be used at any one time. This is due to the interlocking Selectatec system in which interlocking extension rods prevent more than one vaporizer being used at any one time. These rods prevent the percentage control dial from moving, preventing contamination of the downstream vaporizer.

10. The non-return valve on the back bar of an anaesthetic machine between the vaporizer and common gas outlet

a. True. Minute volume divider ventilators exert back pressure as they cycle. This causes reversal of the FGF through the vaporizer. This leads to an uncontrolled increase in the concentration of the inhalational agent. Also the back pressure causes the fluctuation of the bobbins in the flowmeters as the ventilator cycles. The non-return valve on the back bar prevents these events from happening.

b. True. The non-return valve on the back bar opens when the pressure in the back bar exceeds 35 kPa. Flowmeters and vaporizer components can be damaged at higher pressures.

c. True. By preventing the effects of back pressure on the flowmeters and vaporizer as the minute volume divider ventilator cycles, the non-return

valve on the back bar provides some protection to the patient. The flows on the flowmeters and the desired concentration of the inhalational agent can be accurately delivered to the patient.

d. True. See b.

e. False. The non-return valve on the back bar of the anaesthetic machine opens at a pressure of 35 kPa.

11. The oxygen emergency flush on an anaesthetic machine:

a. False. 35–75 L/min can be delivered by activating the oxygen emergency flush on the anaesthetic machine.

b. False. The inappropriate use of the oxygen flush during anaesthesia increases risk of awareness (a 100% oxygen can be delivered) and barotrauma to the patient (because of the high flows delivered).

c. True. See a.

d. True. This can happen by diluting the anaesthetic mixture (see b).

e. False. Because of the high FGF (35–70 L/min), the minute volume divider ventilator does not function appropriately.

12. Regarding the Glostavent Helix Duo

a. True.

b. False. Uses its own oxygen concentrator as its source of oxygen.

c. True.

d. True.

e. False. A fuel cell oxygen analyser is used.

13. c.

14. c.

15. d.

16. a.

Chapter 3

Pollution in theatre and scavenging

Since the late 1960s there has been speculation that trace anaesthetic gases/vapours may have a harmful effect on operating theatre personnel. It has been concluded from currently available studies that there is no association between occupational exposure to trace levels of waste anaesthetic vapours in scavenged operating theatres and adverse health effects. However, it is desirable to vent out the exhaled anaesthetic vapours and maintain a vapour-free theatre environment. A prudent plan for minimizing exposure includes maintaining equipment, training personnel and monitoring exposure routinely. Although not universally agreed upon, the recommended maximum accepted concentrations in the United Kingdom (issued in 1996), over an (see Table 3.1 for main causes) 8-hour time-weighted average, are as follows:

- 100 particles per million (ppm) for nitrous oxide
- 50 ppm for enflurane
- 50 ppm for isoflurane
- 10 ppm for halothane
- 20 ppm for sevoflurane (recommended by Abbot Laboratories)
- no limit is set for desflurane, although a 50-ppm target is advisable due to its similarity to enflurane.

These levels were chosen because they are well below the levels at which any significant adverse effects occurred in animals and represent levels at which there is no evidence to suggest human health would be affected.

Table 3.1 Causes of operating theatre pollution

Anaesthetic techniques	Incomplete scavenging of the gases from ventilator and/or APL valve
	Poorly fitting face mask
	Paediatric breathing systems, e.g. T-piece
	Failure to turn off fresh gas and/or vaporizer at the end of an anaesthetic
	Uncuffed tracheal tubes
	Filling of the vaporizers
	Exhalation of the gases/vapours during recovery
Anaesthetic machine	Leaks from the various connections used, e.g. O-rings, soda lime canister
Others	Cryosurgery units and cardiopulmonary bypass circuit if a vapour is used

In the United States, the maximum accepted concentrations of any halogenated agent should be less than 2 ppm. When such agents are used in combination with nitrous oxide, levels of less than 0.5 ppm should be achieved. Nitrous oxide, when used as the sole anaesthetic agent, at 8-hour time-weighted average concentrations should be less than 25 ppm during the administration of an anaesthetic.

The Netherlands has a limit of 25 ppm for nitrous oxide, whereas Italy, Sweden, Norway and Denmark set 100 ppm as their limit for exposure to nitrous oxide. The differences illustrate the difficulty in setting standards without adequate data.

Methods used to decrease theatre pollution are listed as follows.

1. The facility should have adequate theatre ventilation and air conditioning, with frequent and rapid changing of the circulating air (15–20 times/h). This is one of the most important factors in reducing pollution. Unventilated theatres are four times as contaminated with anaesthetic gases and vapours compared to those with proper ventilation. A non-recirculating ventilation system is usually used. A recirculating ventilation system is not recommended. In labour wards where anaesthetic agents including Entonox are used, rooms should be well ventilated with a minimum of 5 air changes/h.
2. The circle breathing system recycles the exhaled anaesthetic vapours, absorbing CO_2. It requires a very low fresh gas flow, so reducing the amount of inhalational agents used. This decreases the level of theatre environment contamination.
3. The use of total intravenous anaesthesia.
4. Regional anaesthesia is another option.
5. Avoid spillage and use fume cupboards during vaporizer filling. This used to be a significant contributor to the hazard of pollution in the operating theatre. Modern vaporizers use special agent-specific filling devices as a safety feature and to reduce spillage and pollution.
6. Scavenging.

Sampling procedures for evaluating waste anaesthetic vapour concentrations in air should be conducted for nitrous oxide and halogenated agents on a yearly basis in the United Kingdom and on a quarterly basis in the United States in each location where anaesthesia is administered. Monitoring should include:

- leak testing of equipment and
- sampling air in the theatre personnel breathing zone.

Anaesthetic equipment, gas scavenging, gas supply, flowmeters and ventilation systems must be subject to a planned preventative maintenance (PPM) programme. At least once annually, the general ventilation system and the scavenging equipment should be examined and tested by a responsible person.

It is important to remember that the inhalational anaesthetic agents—chlorofluorocarbons (isoflurane), hydro-fluorocarbons (sevoflurane and desflurane) and nitrous oxide—are greenhouse gases and have an effect on the climate.

Pollution in the operating theatre
- In scavenged areas, there is no association between occupational exposure to anaesthetic agents trace levels and adverse health effects.
- There are no agreed international standards of the maximum accepted concentrations of agents in the theatre environment.
- Routine monitoring and testing (PPM) are mandatory.

 Exam tip: It is important to know the causes of pollution in the operating theatre, the methods used to reduce the pollution and the acceptable maximum concentrations (in ppm) of vapours in the operating theatre.

Anaesthetic Gas Scavenging Systems (AGSS)

In any location where inhalation anaesthetics are administered, an adequate and reliable system should be used for scavenging waste anaesthetic gases. A scavenging system is capable of collecting the waste anaesthetic gases from the breathing system and discarding them safely.

Unscavenged operating theatres can show N_2O levels of 400–3000 ppm.

The ideal scavenging system
- Should not affect the ventilation and oxygenation of the patient.
- Should not affect the dynamics of the breathing system.

A well-designed scavenging system should consist of a collecting device for gases from the breathing system/ventilator at the site of overflow, a ventilation system to carry waste anaesthetic gases from the operating theatre and a method for limiting both positive and negative pressure variations in the breathing system.

The performance of the scavenging system should be part of the anaesthetic machine check.

Scavenging systems can be divided into passive and active systems.

Passive system

The passive system is simple to construct with zero running cost.

Components

1. The collecting and transfer system consists of a shroud connected to the adjustable pressure limiting (APL) valve (or expiratory valve of the ventilator). A 30-mm connector attached to transfer tubing leads to a receiving system (Fig. 3.1). The 30-mm wide-bore connector is designed as a safety measure in order to

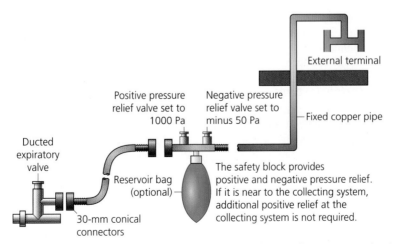

Fig. 3.1 Diagram of a passive scavenging system. (With permission from Aitkenhead, R., Smith, G., 1996. Textbook of Anaesthesia, 3rd ed. Churchill Livingstone.)

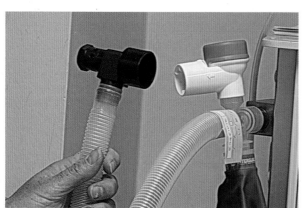

Fig. 3.2 Attaching a 30-mm connector to the adjustable pressure limiting valve of the breathing system. The 30-mm wide bore is designed as a safety measure.

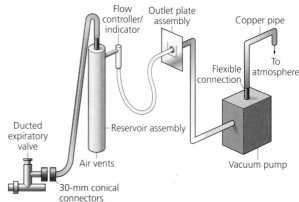

Fig. 3.3 Diagram of an active scavenging system. (With permission from Aitkenhead, R., Smith, G., 1996. Textbook of Anaesthesia, 3rd ed. Churchill Livingstone.)

prevent accidental misconnection to other ports of the breathing system (Fig. 3.2).

2. A receiving system (reservoir bag) can be used. Two spring-loaded valves guard against excessive positive (1000 Pa) in case of a distal obstruction or negative (−50 Pa) pressures in case of increased demand in the scavenging system. Without these valves, excessive positive pressure increases the risk of barotrauma should there be an obstruction beyond the receiving system. Excessive negative pressure could lead to the collapse of the reservoir bag of the breathing system and the risk of rebreathing.

3. The disposal system is a wide-bore copper pipe leading to the atmosphere directly or via the theatre ventilation system.

Mechanism of action

1. The exhaled gases are driven by either the patient's respiratory efforts or the ventilator.

2. The receiving system should be mounted on the anaesthetic machine to minimize the length of transfer tubing, therefore minimizing resistance to flow.

Problems in practice and safety features

1. Connecting the scavenging system to the exit grille of the theatre ventilation is possible. Recirculation or reversing of the flow is a problem in this situation.

2. Excess positive or negative pressures caused by the wind at the outlet might affect the performance and even reverse the flow.

3. The outlet should be fitted with a wire mesh to protect against insects.

4. Compressing or occluding the passive hose may lead to the escape of gases/vapours into the operating

theatre, thereby polluting it. The disposal hose should be made of non-compressible materials and not placed on the floor.

Active system

Components

1. The collecting and transfer system is similar to that of the passive system (Fig. 3.3).

2. The receiving system (Fig. 3.4) is usually a valveless, open-ended reservoir positioned between the receiving and disposal components. A bacterial filter situated downstream and a visual flow indicator positioned between the receiving and disposal systems can be used. A reservoir bag with two spring-loaded safety valves can also be used as a receiving system.

3. The active disposal system consists of a fan or a pump used to generate a vacuum (Fig. 3.5).

Mechanism of action

1. The low-pressure vacuum system drives the gases through the system. Active scavenging systems are able to deal with a wide range of expiratory flow rates (30–130 L/min).

2. A motorized fan, a pump or a venturi system is used to generate the vacuum or negative pressure that is transmitted through pipes.

3. The receiving system is capable of coping with changes in gas flow rates. Increased demand (or excessive negative pressure) allows ambient air to be entrained, thereby maintaining the pressure. The opposite occurs

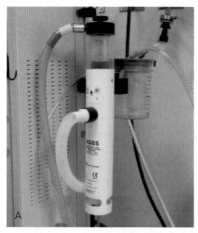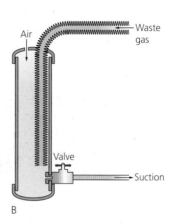

Fig. 3.4 Anaesthetic gases receiving system (A). Its mechanism of action (B).

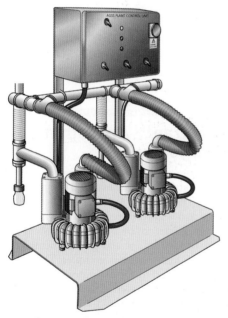

Fig. 3.5 Anaesthetic Gas Scavenging Systems *(AGSS)* vacuum pumps used in an active scavenging system. (Courtesy Penlon Ltd, Abingdon, UK [http://www.penlon.com].)

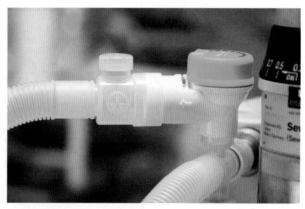

Fig. 3.6 Anaesthesia gas scavenging pressure relief valve. (Courtesy Intersurgical, Wokingham, UK.)

during excessive positive pressure. As a result, a uniform gas flow is passed to the disposal system.

Problems in practice and safety features

1. The reservoir is designed to prevent excessive negative or positive pressures being applied to the patient. Excessive negative pressure leads to the collapse of the reservoir bag of the breathing system and the risk of rebreathing. Excessive positive pressure increases the risk of barotrauma should an obstruction occur beyond the receiving system.
2. An independent vacuum pump should be used for scavenging purposes.
3. The ISO standard 80601-2-13 Anaesthetic Workstation states, 'under single fault conditions, the pressure at the inlet to the anaesthetic gas scavenging system shall not exceed 20 cm H_2O with an exhaust flow rate of 75 L/min.' A safety valve (Fig. 3.6) prevents the build-up of pressure in the breathing system in case the transfer system/tubing is occluded, causing back pressure to the patient. Gases are released into the atmosphere.

Exam tip: All the safety features in both the passive and active scavenging systems need to be understood. How is the patient protected against excessive positive or negative pressures within the breathing system?

Charcoal canisters (Cardiff Aldasorber)

The canister is a compact passive scavenging system (Fig. 3.7).

Components
1. A canister.
2. Charcoal particles.
3. Transfer tubing connecting the canister to the APL valve of the breathing system or the expiratory valve of the ventilator.

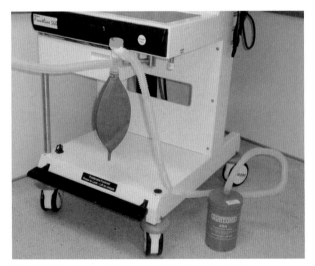

Fig. 3.7 Charcoal canister connected to the adjustable pressure limiting valve of the breathing system.

Mechanism of action
1. The charcoal particles absorb the halogenated inhalational agents (halothane, enflurane and isoflurane).
2. The increasing weight of the canister is the only indication that it is exhausted.
3. It is usually replaced after every 12 hours of use.

Problems in practice and safety features
1. It cannot absorb nitrous oxide.
2. Heating the canister causes the release of the inhalational agents.

Contrafluran™ Anaesthetic Gas Capture System

Modern inhalational agents undergo minimal metabolism. They are mainly exhaled unchanged. This system is designed to reduce their effect on the environment. Pioneered by Baxter, the system allows the capture of sevoflurane and desflurane in special canisters using highly porous granules. The compact canister is connected to the expiratory limb of the breathing system and attached to the anaesthetic machine. One canister can hold about 240 mL of desflurane, equivalent to one bottle. Separate canisters for sevoflurane and desflurane should be used. A visual indicator and an audible alarm signal a full canister. Once full, the manufacturers collect the canisters to extract, separate and sterilize the captured vapours that could be reused as active ingredients for new anaesthetic vapours. Licence approval for the use of the recycled vapours is still pending in the United Kingdom at the time of publication.

SUGGESTED FURTHER READING

Boiano, J.M., Steege, A.L., 2016. Precautionary practices for administering anesthetic gases: a survey of physician anesthesiologists, nurse anesthetists and anesthesiologist assistants. J. Occup. Environ. Hyg. 13 (10), 782–793.

Controlling Waste Anaesthetic Gases in Healthcare Settings, Information Sheet (HSA) 2014. Available from: https://www.hsa.ie/eng/Publications_and_Forms/Publications/Healthcare_Sector/Waste_Anaesthetic_Gases_Information_Sheet.pdf.

Herzog-Niescery, J., Gude, P., Gahlen, F., et al., 2016. Surgeons' exposure to sevoflurane during paediatric adenoidectomy: a comparison of three airway devices. Anaesthesia 71, 915–920.

Hiller, K.N., Altamirano, A.V., Cai, C.Y., Tran, S.F., Williams, G.W., 2015. Evaluation of waste anesthetic gas in the postanesthesia care unit within the patient breathing zone. Anesthesiol. Res. Pract. 354184.

Medicines and Healthcare products Regulatory Agency (MHRA), 2010. Anaesthetic gas scavenging systems (AGSS) – all manufacturers. MDA/2010/021). Available from: https://assets.publishing.service.gov.uk/media/5485ac3c40f0b602440002a5/con076137.pdf.

Molina Aragonés J.M., Ayora, A., Barbara Ribalta, A., et al., 2016. Occupational exposure to volatile anaesthetics: a systematic review. Occupational Medicine 66, 202–207.

Tallent, R., Corcoran, J., Sebastian, J., 2018. Evaluation of a novel waste anaesthetic gas scavenger device for use during recovery from anaesthesia. Anaesthesia 73, 59–64.

Waste Anesthetic Gases, 2007. Occupational Hazards in Hospitals (NIOSH). Available from: https://www.cdc.gov/niosh/docs/2007-151/pdfs/2007-51.pdf?id=10.26616/NIOSHPUB2007151.

SELF-ASSESSMENT QUESTIONS

Please check your eBook for additional self-assessment

MCQs

In the following lists, which of the statements (a) to (e) are true?

1. **Pollution in theatre**
   a. The Cardiff Aldasorber can absorb N_2O and the inhalational agents.
   b. The circulating air in theatre should be changed 15–20 times/h.
   c. In the scavenging system, excessive positive and negative pressures should be prevented from being applied to the patient.
   d. In the active scavenging system, an ordinary vacuum pump can be utilized.
   e. The maximum accepted concentration of nitrous oxide is 100 ppm.

2. **Important factors in reducing pollution in the operating theatre**
   a. Scavenging.
   b. Low-flow anaesthesia using the circle system.
   c. Adequate theatre ventilation.
   d. The use of fume cupboards when filling vaporizers.
   e. Cardiff Aldasorber.

3. **Passive scavenging system**
   a. Is easy to build and maintain.
   b. Is efficient.
   c. There is no need to have positive or negative relief valves in the collecting system.
   d. The exhaled gases are driven by the patient's respiratory effort or the ventilator.
   e. Commonly uses 15-mm connectors in the United Kingdom.

4. **Concerning anaesthetic agents pollution**
   a. There is an international standard for the concentrations of trace inhalational agents in the operating theatre environment.
   b. In the United Kingdom, monitoring of inhalational agents concentration in the operating theatre is done annually.
   c. PPM stands for particles per million.
   d. An unscavenged operating theatre would have less than 100 ppm of nitrous oxide.
   e. A T-piece paediatric breathing system can cause theatre pollution.

5. **Regarding the maximum permitted concentrations of anaesthetic gases in the UK theatre environment**
   a. The limits are based on international guidelines.
   b. The limits are based on a 24-hour time-weighted average.
   c. The limit for halothane is 50 ppm.
   d. The limit for sevoflurane is specified in the Control of Substances Hazardous to Health regulations.
   e. The limit for isoflurane is the same as the limit for enflurane.

6. **Which of the following limits for anaesthetic vapour concentrations in the theatre environment are correct?**
   a. A limit of 20 ppm of sevoflurane is recommended by the manufacturer.
   b. A limit of 10 ppm is set for enflurane.
   c. A limit of 50 ppm is set for halothane.
   d. A limit of 50 ppm is set for isoflurane.
   e. A limit of 200 ppm is set for nitrous oxide.

Single best answer

7. Operating theatre pollution
a. Does not exist.
b. Only occurs in anaesthetic rooms.
c. Can be detected by analysing a sample from theatre's atmosphere.
d. Can be eliminated by regular monitoring alone.
e. Can be eliminated by using the laryngeal mask more often.

8. What is the limit for isoflurane vapour concentration in the theatre environment?
a. 100 ppm.
b. 75 ppm.
c. 50 ppm.
d. 20 ppm.
e. 10 ppm.

9. Use of which of the following can reduce theatre pollution?
a. The T-piece anaesthesia circuit for paediatric cases.
b. Cardiopulmonary bypass.
c. Uncuffed endotracheal tubes.
d. High (>10 L/min) fresh gas flows.
e. Agent-specific vaporizer filling devices.

10. Which of the following statements regarding scavenging devices is true?
a. The reservoir in an active scavenging system is open to air.
b. An ideal scavenging system increases the circuit dead space.
c. The Cardiff Aldasorber is an example of an active scavenging system.
d. Scavenging can only be fitted to circle breathing circuits.
e. Passive scavenging systems require a one-way valve at the external terminal.

Answers

1. *Pollution in theatre*
   a. *False. Cardiff Aldasorber can only absorb the inhalational agents but not nitrous oxide. This limits its use in reducing pollution in the operating theatre.*
   b. *True. Changing the circulating air in the operating theatre 15–20 times/h is one of the most effective methods of reducing pollution. An unventilated theatre is about four times more polluted compared to a properly ventilated one.*
   c. *True. The patient should be protected against excessive positive and negative pressures being applied by the scavenging system. Excessive positive pressure puts the patient under the risk of barotrauma. Excessive negative pressure causes the reservoir in the breathing system to collapse, thus leading to incorrect performance of the breathing system.*
   d. *False. Because of the nature of the flow of the exhaled gases, the scavenging system should be capable of tolerating high and variable gas flows. The flow of exhaled gases is very variable during both spontaneous and controlled ventilation. An ordinary vacuum pump might not be capable of coping with such variable flows, from 30 to 120 L/min. The active scavenging system is a high flow, low-pressure system. A pressure of –0.5 cm H_2O to the patient breathing system is needed. This cannot be achieved with an ordinary vacuum pump (low-flow, high-pressure system).*
   e. *True. In the United Kingdom, the maximum accepted concentration of nitrous oxide is 100 ppm over an 8-hour time-weighted average.*

2. *Important factors in reducing pollution in the operating theatre*
   a. **True.** In any location in which inhalation anaesthetics are administered, there should be an adequate and reliable system for scavenging waste anaesthetic gases. Unscavenged operating theatres can show 400–3000 ppm of N_2O, which is much higher than the maximum acceptable concentration.
   b. **True.**
   c. **True.** One of the most important factors in reducing pollution is adequate theatre ventilation. The circulating air is changed 15–20 times/h. Unventilated theatres are four times more contaminated than properly ventilated theatres.
   d. **False.** Modern vaporizers use agent-specific filling keys, which limit spillage.
   e. **False.** Cardiff Aldasorber absorbs the inhalational agents but not nitrous oxide.

3. *Passive scavenging system*
   a. **True.** A passive scavenging system is easy and cheap to build and costs nothing to maintain. There is no need for a purpose-built vacuum pump system with the necessary maintenance required.
   b. **False.** The passive system is not an efficient system. Its efficiency depends on the direction of the wind blowing at the outlet. Negative or positive pressure might affect the performance and even reverse the flow.
   c. **False.** The positive pressure relief valve protects the patient against excessive pressure build-up in the breathing system and barotrauma. The negative pressure relief valve prevents the breathing system reservoir from being exhausted, ensuring correct performance of the breathing system.
   d. **True.** The driving forces for gases in the passive system are the patient's respiratory effort or the ventilator. For this reason the transfer tubing should be made as short as possible to reduce resistance to flow.
   e. **False.** 30-mm connectors are used in the United Kingdom as a safety feature to prevent misconnection.

4. *Concerning anaesthetic agents pollution*
   a. **False.** There is no international standard for the concentrations of trace inhalational agents in the operating theatre environment. This is mainly because of the unavailability of adequate data. Different countries set their own standards, but there is an agreement on the importance of maintaining a vapour-free environment in the operating theatre.
   b. **True.** Monitoring of inhalational agents concentration in the operating theatre is done annually in the United Kingdom and on a quarterly basis in the United States in each location where anaesthesia is administered.
   c. **False.** PPM (capitals) stands for planned preventative maintenance, whereas ppm (lowercase letters) stands for particles per million.
   d. **False.** An unscavenged operating theatre would have 400–3000 ppm of nitrous oxide. In the United Kingdom, the recommended maximum accepted concentration over an 8-hour time-weighted average is 100 ppm of nitrous oxide.
   e. **True.** A T-piece paediatric breathing system can cause theatre pollution because of the open-ended reservoir. A modified version has an APL valve, allowing scavenging of the anaesthetic vapours (see Chapter 4).

5. *Regarding the maximum permitted concentrations of anaesthetic gases in the UK theatre environment*
   a. **False.** There are no international regulations on occupational exposure to anaesthetic gases, and countries differ in their legislation.
   b. **False.** An 8-hour time-weighted average is used.
   c. **False.** The halothane concentration must be kept below 10 ppm.
   d. **False.** The limit of 20 ppm for sevoflurane is a manufacturer's recommendation; the limits for the other gases were set in 1996, before sevoflurane was in common use.
   e. **True.** It is 50 ppm.

6. *Which of the following limits for anaesthetic vapour concentrations in the theatre environment are correct*
   a. **True.**
   b. **False.** It is 50 ppm.
   c. **False.** It is 10 ppm.
   d. **True.**
   e. **False.** It is 100 ppm.

7. *c.*

8. *c.*

9. *e.*

10. *a.*

Chapter 4

Breathing systems

Breathing systems must fulfil three objectives:

1. delivery of oxygen,
2. removal of carbon dioxide (CO_2) from the patient and
3. delivery of inhaled anaesthetic agents. These agents are predominantly eliminated by the lungs also, so the breathing system must be able to expel them as necessary.

Several breathing systems are used in anaesthesia. Mapleson classified them into A, B, C, D and E. After further revision of the classification, a Mapleson F breathing system was added. Currently, only A, D, E and F systems and their modifications are commonly used during anaesthesia. Mapleson B and C systems are used more frequently in post-anaesthesia recovery units and in emergency situations.

The fresh gas flow (FGF) rate required to prevent rebreathing of alveolar gas is a measure of the efficiency of a breathing system.

Properties of the ideal breathing system

1. Simple and safe to use.
2. Delivers the intended inspired gas mixture.
3. Permits spontaneous, manual and controlled ventilation in all age groups.
4. Efficient, requiring low FGF rates.
5. Protects the patient from barotrauma.
6. Sturdy, compact, portable and lightweight in design.
7. Permits the easy removal of waste exhaled gases and is effective in eliminating CO_2.
8. Has a low resistance and minimal dead space.
9. Ability to conserve heat and moisture.
10. Easy to maintain with minimal running costs.

Components of the breathing systems

ADJUSTABLE PRESSURE LIMITING VALVE

The adjustable pressure limiting (APL) valve is a valve that allows the exhaled gases and excess FGF to leave the breathing system (Fig. 4.1). It does not allow room air to enter the breathing system. It allows control of the pressure within the breathing system and the patient's airway. The APL valve is an essential component of most breathing systems, except Mapleson E or F (see later).

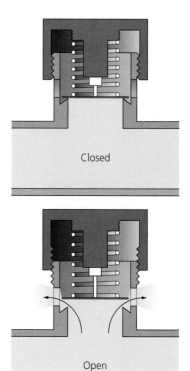

Closed

Open

Fig. 4.1 Diagram of an adjustable pressure limiting valve.

Synonymous terms for the APL valve are *expiratory valve, spill valve* and *relief valve*.

Components

1. The APL valve has three ports: the inlet, the patient and the exhaust. The latter can be opened to the atmosphere or connected to the scavenging system using a shroud.
2. A lightweight disc rests on a knife-edge seating. The disc is held onto its seating by a spring. The tension in the spring, and therefore the valve's opening pressure, is controlled by the valve dial.

Mechanism of action

1. This is a one-way, adjustable, spring-loaded valve. The spring is used to adjust the pressure required to open the valve. The disc rests on a knife-edge seating in order to minimize its area of contact.
2. The valve allows gases to escape when the pressure in the breathing system exceeds the valve's opening pressure.
3. During spontaneous ventilation, the patient generates a positive pressure in the system during expiration, causing the valve to open. A pressure of less than 1 cm

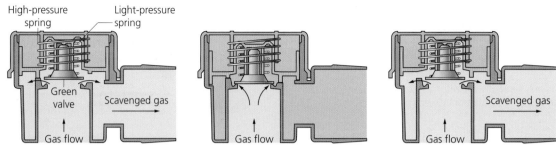

Fig. 4.2 Intersurgical adjustable pressure limiting valve. In the open position *(left)*, the valve is actuated by pressures of less than 0.1 kPa (1 cm H_2O) with minimal resistance to flow. A 3/4 clockwise turn of the dial takes the valve through a range of pressure limiting positions to the closed position *(centre)*. In the closed position, the breathing system pressure, and therefore the intrapulmonary pressure, is protected by a pressure relief mechanism *(right)* actuated at 6 kPa (60 cm H_2O). This safety relief mechanism cannot be overridden.

H_2O (0.1 kPa) is needed to actuate the valve when it is in the open position.

4. During positive pressure ventilation, a controlled leak is produced by adjusting the valve dial during inspiration. This allows control of the patient's airway pressure.

Problems in practice and safety features

1. Malfunction of the scavenging system may cause excessive negative pressure. This can lead to the APL valve remaining open throughout respiration. This leads to an unwanted enormous increase in the breathing system's dead space.
2. The patient may be exposed to excessive positive pressure if the valve is closed during assisted ventilation. A pressure relief safety mechanism actuated at a pressure of about 60 cm H_2O is present in modern designs (Fig. 4.2), even when the cap is screwed down and the valve is fully closed.
3. Water vapour in exhaled gas may condense on the valve. The surface tension of the condensed water may cause the valve to stick. The disc is usually made of a hydrophobic (water repelling) material, which prevents water from condensing on the disc.
4. The valve can add bulk to the breathing system.

Adjustable pressure limiting valve
- One-way spring-loaded valve with three ports.
- The spring adjusts the pressure required to open the valve.
- When fully open, a pressure of less than 1 cm H_2O (0.1 kPa) is needed to actuate it.
- A pressure relief safety mechanism is actuated at 60 cm H_2O (6 kPa) even when closed.

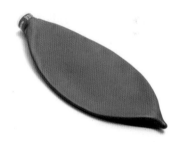

Fig. 4.3 Intersurgical standard 2-L adult size reservoir bag.

RESERVOIR BAG

The reservoir bag is an important component of most breathing systems, improving efficiency and allowing manual ventilation.

Components

1. It is made of plastic (latex-free) or antistatic rubber. Designs tend to be ellipsoidal in shape.
2. The standard adult size is 2 L (Fig. 4.3). The smallest size for paediatric use is 0.5 L. Volumes from 0.5 to 6 L exist. Bigger size reservoir bags are useful during inhalational induction, e.g. adult induction with sevoflurane.

Mechanism of action

1. The reservoir bag accommodates the FGF during expiration, acting as a reservoir available for the following inspiration. Otherwise, the FGF must be at least the patient's peak inspiratory flow to prevent rebreathing. As this peak inspiratory flow may exceed 30 L/min in adults, breathing directly from the FGF will be insufficient.
2. It acts as a monitor of the patient's ventilatory pattern during spontaneous breathing. It serves as a very inaccurate guide to the patient's tidal volume.

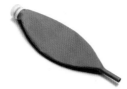

Fig. 4.4 Intersurgical 0.5-L double-ended reservoir.

3. It can be used to assist or control ventilation.
4. When employed in conjunction with the T-piece (Mapleson F system), a 0.5-L double-ended bag is used. The distal hole acts as an expiratory port (Fig. 4.4).

Problems in practice and safety features

1. Because of its compliance, the reservoir bag can accommodate rises in pressure in the breathing system better than other parts. When grossly overinflated, the rubber reservoir bag can limit the pressure in the breathing system to about 40 cm H_2O. This is due to Laplace's law dictating that the pressure (P) will fall as the bag's radius (r) increases: $P = 2$ (tension)/r.
2. The size of the bag depends on the breathing system and the patient. A small bag may not be large enough to provide a sufficient reservoir for a large tidal volume.
3. Too large a reservoir bag makes it difficult for it to act as a respiratory monitor.

> **Reservoir bag**
> - Made of rubber or plastic.
> - 2-L size commonly used for adults. Bigger sizes can be used for inhalational induction in adults.
> - Accommodates FGF.
> - Can assist or control ventilation.
> - Limits pressure build-up in the breathing system.

TUBINGS

These connect one part of a breathing system to another. They also act as a reservoir for gases in certain systems. They tend to be made of plastic, but other materials such as silicone rubber and silver-impregnated bactericidal plastics are available.

The length of the breathing tubing is variable depending on the configuration of the breathing system used. They must promote laminar flow wherever possible, and this is achieved by their being of a uniform and large diameter. The size for adults is 22-mm wide. However, paediatric tubing is 15-mm wide to reduce bulk. The

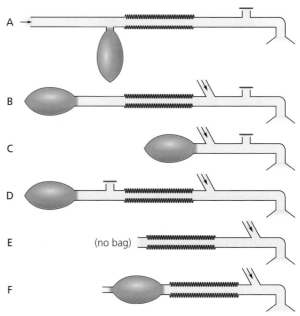

Fig. 4.5 Mapleson classification of anaesthetic breathing systems. The *arrow* indicates entry of fresh gas to the system. See text for details.

corrugations resist kinking and increase flexibility, but they produce greater turbulence than smooth-bore tubes.

Specific configurations are described as follows.

Mapleson classification

In 1954, Mapleson classified the breathing systems into five configurations (A to E) and a sixth (F) was added later (Fig. 4.5). The classification is according to the relative positions of the APL valve, reservoir bag and FGF. Mapleson systems need significantly higher FGF to prevent rebreathing compared to the circle breathing system and therefore the expensive use of volatile agents. Their use in modern anaesthesia is very limited with the widespread use of the circle breathing system.

Magill system (Mapleson A)

This breathing system was popular and widely used in the United Kingdom.

Components

1. Corrugated rubber or plastic tubing (usually 110–180 cm in length) and an internal volume of at least 550 mL.

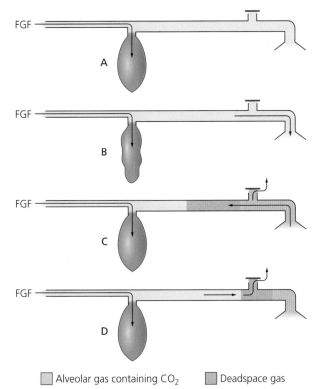

FGF

A

FGF

B

FGF

C

FGF

D

◻ Alveolar gas containing CO_2 ◻ Deadspace gas

Fig. 4.6 Mechanism of action of the Magill breathing system during spontaneous ventilation; see text for details. *FGF,* Fresh gas flow.

2. A reservoir bag mounted at the machine end.
3. APL valve situated at the patient's end.

Mechanism of action

1. During the first inspiration, all the gases are fresh and consist of oxygen and anaesthetic gases from the anaesthetic machine (Fig. 4.6A and B).
2. As the patient exhales (Fig. 4.6C), the gases coming from the anatomical dead space (i.e. they have not undergone gas exchange so contain no CO_2) are exhaled first and enter the tubing and are channelled back toward the reservoir bag, which is being filled continuously with FGF.
3. The alveolar gases follow the anatomical dead space gases and enter the tubing.
4. During the expiratory pause, pressure build-up within the system allows the FGF to expel the alveolar gases first out through the APL valve (Fig. 4.6D).
5. By that time the patient inspires again (Fig. 4.6B), getting a mixture of FGF and the rebreathed anatomical dead space gases.
6. It is a very efficient system for spontaneous breathing. Because there is no gas exchange in the anatomical dead space, the FGF requirements to prevent

rebreathing of alveolar gases are theoretically equal to the patient's alveolar minute volume (about 70 mL/kg/min).
7. The Magill system is not an efficient system for controlled ventilation. An FGF rate of three times the alveolar minute volume is required to prevent rebreathing.

Problems in practice and safety features

The Magill system is not suitable for use with children of less than 25–30 kg body weight. This is because of the increased dead space caused by the system's geometry at the patient's end. Dead space is further increased by the angle piece and face mask.

One of its disadvantages is the heaviness of the APL valve at the patient's end, especially if connected to a scavenging system. This places a lot of drag on the connections at the patient's end.

Magill (Mapleson A) breathing system

● Efficient for spontaneous ventilation. FGF required is equal to alveolar minute volume (about 70 mL/kg/min).
● Inefficient for controlled ventilation. FGF three times alveolar minute volume.
● APL valve is at the patient's end.
● Not suitable for paediatric practice.

Lack system (Mapleson A)

This is a coaxial modification of the Magill Mapleson A system.

Components

1. 1.8-m length coaxial tubing (tube inside a tube). The FGF is through the outside tube, and the exhaled gases flow through the inside tube (Fig. 4.7A).
2. The inside tube is wide in diameter (14 mm) to reduce resistance to expiration. The outer tube's diameter is 30 mm.
3. The reservoir bag is mounted at the machine end.
4. The APL valve is mounted at the machine end, eliminating the drag on the connections at the patient's end, which is a problem with the Magill system.

Mechanism of action

1. It has a similar mechanism to the Magill system except the Lack system is a coaxial version. The fresh gas flows through the outside tube, whereas the exhaled gases flow through the inside tube.

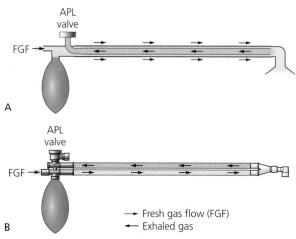

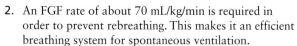

Fig. 4.7 (A) The coaxial Lack breathing system. (B) The parallel Lack breathing system. *APL,* Adjustable pressure limiting.

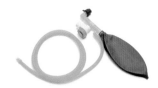

Fig. 4.8 Intersurgical adult Mapleson C system.

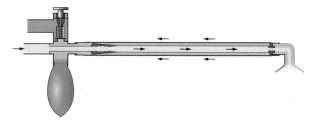

Fig. 4.9 The Bain breathing system.

2. An FGF rate of about 70 mL/kg/min is required in order to prevent rebreathing. This makes it an efficient breathing system for spontaneous ventilation.
3. Since it is based on the Magill system, it is not suitable for controlled ventilation.

Instead of the coaxial design, a parallel tubing version of the system exists (Fig. 4.7B). This has separate inspiratory and expiratory tubing and retains the same flow characteristics as the coaxial version.

> **Lack breathing system**
> - Coaxial version of Mapleson A, making it efficient for spontaneous ventilation. FGF rate of about 70 mL/kg/min is required.
> - FGF is delivered along the outside tube and the exhaled gases flow along the inner tube.
> - APL valve is at the machine end.
> - Not suitable for controlled ventilation.

Mapleson B and C systems
(Figs. 4.5 and 4.8)

Components
1. A reservoir bag. In the B system, corrugated tubing is attached to the bag and both act as a reservoir.
2. An APL valve at the patient's end.
3. FGF is added just proximal to the APL.

Mechanism of action
Both systems are not efficient during spontaneous or controlled ventilation. An FGF of more than 1.5–2 times the minute volume is required to prevent rebreathing.

During controlled ventilation, the B system is slightly more efficient due to the corrugated tubing acting as a reservoir. An FGF of more than 50% of the minute ventilation is still required to prevent rebreathing.

Mapleson C (also known as the Waters circuit) is lightweight and compact. It is used in resuscitation situations as an alternative to a self-inflating bag. By adjusting the APL valve, it allows positive end-expiratory pressure (PEEP) with a visual and tactile ventilation monitor.

> **Mapleson B and C breathing systems**
> - B system has a tubing and bag reservoir.
> - Both B and C systems are not efficient for spontaneous and controlled ventilation.
> - B system is more efficient than the A system during controlled ventilation.
> - C system is lightweight and used in resuscitation situations.

Bain system (Mapleson D)

The Bain system is a coaxial version of the Mapleson D system (Fig. 4.9). It is lightweight and compact at the patient's end. It is useful where access to the patient is limited, such as during head and neck surgery.

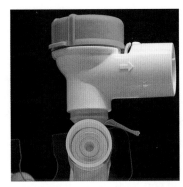

Fig. 4.10 The proximal (machine's) end of coaxial Bain's breathing system. The fresh gas flow flows through the narrow inner tube.

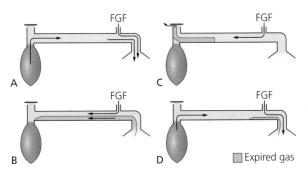

Fig. 4.11 Mechanism of action of the Mapleson D breathing system during spontaneous ventilation; see text for details. *FGF,* Fresh gas flow.

The Manley ventilator, which has been switched to a spontaneous ventilation mode, is an example of a non-coaxial Mapleson D system.

Components

1. A length of coaxial tubing (tube inside a tube). The usual length is 180 cm, but it can be supplied at 270 cm (for dental or ophthalmic surgery) and 540 cm (for magnetic resonance imaging [MRI] scans for which the anaesthetic machine needs to be kept outside the scanner's magnetic field). Increasing the length of the tubing does not affect the physical properties of the breathing system.
2. The fresh gas flows through the narrow inner tube (6 mm) while the exhaled gases flow through the outside tube (22 mm) (Fig. 4.10). The internal lumen has a swivel mount at the patient's end. This ensures that the internal tube cannot kink, thereby ensuring delivery of fresh gas to the patient.
3. The reservoir bag is mounted at the machine end.
4. The APL valve is mounted at the machine end.

Mechanism of action

1. During spontaneous ventilation, the patient's exhaled gases are channelled back to the reservoir bag and become mixed with fresh gas (Fig. 4.11B). Pressure build-up within the system will open the APL valve, allowing the venting of the mixture of the exhaled gases and fresh gas (Fig. 4.11C).
2. The FGF required to prevent rebreathing (as seen in Fig. 4.11D) during spontaneous ventilation is about 1.5–2 times the alveolar minute volume. A flow rate of 150–200 mL/kg/min is required. This makes it an

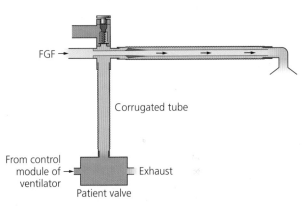

Fig. 4.12 The Bain breathing system connected to a ventilator (e.g. Penlon Nuffield 200) via tubing connected to the bag mount. *FGF,* Fresh gas flow.

inefficient and uneconomical system for use during spontaneous ventilation.
3. It is a more efficient system for controlled ventilation. A flow of 70–100 mL/kg/min will maintain normocapnia. A flow of 100 mL/kg/min will cause moderate hypocapnia during controlled ventilation.
4. Connection to a ventilator is possible (Fig. 4.12). By removing the reservoir bag, a ventilator such as the Penlon Nuffield 200 can be connected to the bag mount using a 1-m length of corrugated tubing (the volume of tubing must exceed 500 mL if the driving gas from the ventilator is not to enter the breathing system). The APL valve must be fully closed. In this situation it acts as a T-piece.
5. A parallel version of the D system is available.

Problems in practice and safety features

1. The internal tube can kink, preventing fresh gas from being delivered to the patient.
2. The internal tube can become disconnected at the machine end, causing a large increase in the dead space and resulting in hypoxaemia and hypercapnia. Movement of the reservoir bag during spontaneous ventilation is not therefore an indication that the fresh gas is being delivered to the patient.

Bain breathing system

- Coaxial version of Mapleson D. A parallel version exits.
- Fresh gas flows along the inner tube, and the exhaled gases flow along the outer tube.
- Not efficient for spontaneous ventilation. Fresh gas flow (FGF) rate required is 150–200 mL/kg/min.
- Efficient during controlled ventilation. FGF rate required is 70–100 mL/kg/min.

Exam tip: A common question is how to safety test the Bain breathing system to ensure that there is no kinking, obstruction or dislodgment of the inner tube delivering the FGF.

Exam tip: It is important to know the differences between Lack and Bain breathing systems; both are coaxial but differ in which tube is used for FGF and exhaled gases. Also, the reasons for the different diameters of the outside tubing.

T-piece system (Mapleson E and F)

This is a valveless breathing system used in anaesthesia for children up to 25–30 kg body weight (Fig. 4.13). It is suitable for both spontaneous and controlled ventilation.

Components

1. A T-shaped tubing with three open ports (Fig. 4.14).
2. Fresh gas from the anaesthetic machine is delivered via a tube to one port.
3. The second port leads to the patient's mask or tracheal tube/supraglottic airway device. The connection should be as short as possible to reduce dead space.
4. The third port leads to reservoir tubing. Jackson-Rees added a double-ended bag to the end of the reservoir tubing (making it Mapleson F).
5. A modification exists where an APL valve is included before a closed-ended 500-mL reservoir bag. A pressure relief safety mechanism in the APL valve is actuated at a pressure of 30 cm H_2O (Fig. 4.15). This design allows effective scavenging.

Mechanism of action

1. The system requires an FGF of 2.5–3 times the minute volume to prevent rebreathing with a minimal flow of 4 L/min. This makes the system inefficient.
2. The double-ended bag acts as a visual monitor during spontaneous ventilation. In addition, the bag can be used for assisted or controlled ventilation.

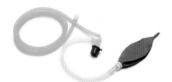

Fig. 4.13 Intersurgical paediatric T-piece breathing system.

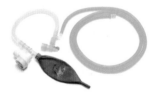

Fig. 4.15 Intersurgical T-piece incorporating an adjustable pressure limiting valve and closed reservoir bag to enable effective scavenging.

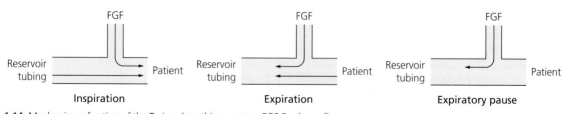

Fig. 4.14 Mechanism of action of the T-piece breathing system. *FGF*, Fresh gas flow.

3. The bag can provide a degree of continuous positive airway pressure (CPAP) during spontaneous ventilation.
4. Controlled ventilation is performed either by manual squeezing of the double-ended bag (intermittent occlusion of the reservoir tubing in the Mapleson E) or by removing the bag and connecting the reservoir tubing to a ventilator such as the Penlon Nuffield 200.
5. The volume of the reservoir tubing determines the degree of rebreathing (too large a tube) or entrainment of ambient air (too small a tube). The volume of the reservoir tubing should approximate the patient's tidal volume.

Problems in practice and safety features

1. Since there is no APL valve used in this breathing system, scavenging is a problem.
2. Patients younger than 6 years of age have a low functional residual capacity (FRC). Mapleson E was designed before the advantages of CPAP were recognized for increasing the FRC. This problem can be partially overcome in the Mapleson F with the addition of the double-ended bag.

T-piece E and F breathing systems
- Used in paediatric practice up to 25–30 kg body weight.
- Requires a high FGF during spontaneous ventilation, making it inefficient.
- Offers minimal resistance to expiration.
- Valveless breathing system.
- Scavenging is difficult.
- A modified design with an APL valve and a closed-ended reservoir allows effective scavenging.

 Exam tip: Make sure you can talk about and reassemble the separate components of a breathing system (tubing, reservoir, APL valve and face mask).

The Humphrey ADE breathing system

This is a very versatile breathing system that combines the advantages of the Mapleson A, D and E systems. It can therefore be used efficiently for spontaneous and controlled ventilation in both adults and children. The mode of use is determined by the position of a lever that is mounted on the Humphrey block. Both parallel and coaxial versions exist with similar efficiency. The parallel version will be considered here.

Components

1. Two lengths of 15-mm smooth-bore tubing (corrugated on outside but smooth on inside). One delivers the fresh gas and the other carries away the exhaled gas. Distally they are connected to a Y-connection leading to the patient. Proximally they are connected to the Humphrey block.
2. The Humphrey block is at the machine end and consists of
   a. an APL valve featuring a visible indicator of valve performance,
   b. a 2-L reservoir bag,
   c. a lever to select either spontaneous or controlled ventilation,
   d. a port to which a ventilator can be connected, e.g. Penlon Nuffield 200,
   e. a safety pressure relief valve that opens at pressure in excess of 60 cm H_2O and
   f. a modified design incorporating a soda lime canister.

Mechanism of action

1. With the lever up in the spontaneous mode, the reservoir bag and APL valve are connected to the breathing system as in the Magill system (Fig. 4.16A).
2. With the lever down in the ventilator mode, the reservoir bag and the APL valve are isolated from the breathing system as in the Mapleson E system (Fig. 4.16B). The expiratory tubing channels the exhaled gas via the ventilator port. Scavenging occurs at the ventilator's expiratory valve.
3. The system is suitable for paediatric and adult use. The tubing is rather narrow, with a low internal volume. Because of its smooth bore, there is no significant increase in resistance to flow compared to the 22-mm corrugated tubing used in other systems. Small tidal volumes are possible during controlled ventilation, and less energy is needed to overcome the inertia of gases during spontaneous ventilation.
4. The presence of an APL valve in the breathing system offers a physiological advantage during paediatric anaesthesia, since it is designed to offer a small amount of PEEP (1 cm H_2O).
5. During spontaneous ventilation
   a. an FGF of about 50–60 mL/kg/min is needed in adults
   b. the recommended initial FGF for children weighing less than 25 kg body weight is 3 L/min. This offers a considerable margin for safety.
6. During controlled ventilation
   a. an FGF of 70 mL/kg is needed in adults
   b. the recommended initial FGF for children weighing less than 25 kg body weight is 3 L/min.

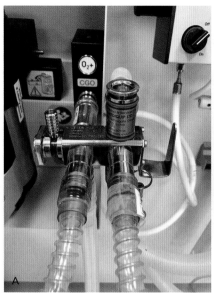 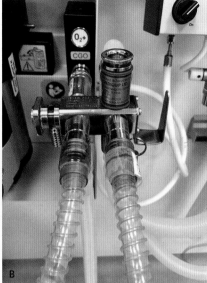

Fig. 4.16 Humphry block with (A) lever up in the spontaneous mode; (B) lever down in ventilator mode.

However, adjustment may be necessary to maintain normocarbia.

Humphrey ADE breathing system
- Can be used efficiently for spontaneous and controlled ventilation.
- Can be used in both adult and paediatric anaesthetic practice.
- Both parallel and coaxial versions exist.
- A ventilator can be connected.

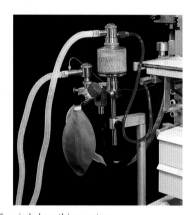

Fig. 4.17 The circle breathing system.

The circle breathing system and soda lime

Over 80% of the anaesthetic gases/vapours are wasted when FGF of 5.0 L/min is used. Typically, the reduction of FGF from 3.0 L/min to 1.0 L/min results in a saving of about 50% of the total consumption of any volatile anaesthetic agent.

In this breathing system, soda lime is used to absorb the patient's exhaled CO_2 (Fig. 4.17). FGF requirements are low, making the circle system very efficient and causing minimal pollution. As a result, there has been an increasing interest in low-flow anaesthesia due to the cost of expensive inhalational agents, together with the increased awareness of the pollution caused by the inhalational agents themselves (see Table 3.1).

Depending on the FGF, the system can be one of the following:

- **Closed-circle anaesthesia.** The FGF is just sufficient to replace the volume of gas and vapour taken up by the patient. No gas leaves via the APL valve, and the exhaled gases are rebreathed after CO_2 is absorbed. Leaks from the breathing system should be eliminated. In practice, this is possible only if the gases sampled by the gas analyser are returned back to the system.
- **Minimal-flow anaesthesia.** The FGF is reduced to 0.5 L/min.

- **Low-flow anaesthesia.** The FGF used is less than the patient's alveolar ventilation (usually below 1.5 L/min). Excess gases leave the system via the APL valve.

Components

1. A vertically positioned canister contains soda lime. The canister has two ports: one to deliver inspired gases to the patient and the other to receive exhaled gases from the patient.
2. Inspiratory and expiratory tubings are connected to the canister. Each port incorporates a unidirectional valve. Corrugated tubings are used to prevent kinking.
3. FGF from the anaesthetic machine is positioned distal to the soda lime canister but proximal to the unidirectional inspiratory valve, i.e. on the inspiratory limb.
4. An APL valve is positioned between the unidirectional expiratory valve and canister, i.e. on the expiratory limb. It is connected to a 2-L reservoir bag.
5. A vaporizer is mounted on the anaesthetic machine back bar (*vaporizer out*side circle [VOC]) or a vaporizer positioned on the expiratory limb within the system (*vaporizer in*side circle [VIC]).
6. Soda lime consists of 94% calcium hydroxide ($Ca(OH)_2$) and 5% sodium hydroxide (NaOH) with a small amount (less than 0.1%) of potassium hydroxide (KOH). It has a pH of 13.5 and a moisture content of 14%–19%. Some modern types of soda lime have no KOH. Soda lime granules are prone to powder formation, especially during transport. Disintegrated granules increase resistance to breathing. Because of this, silica (0.2%) is added to harden the absorbents and reduce powder formation. A dye or colour indicator is added to change the granules' colour when the soda lime is exhausted. Colour changes can be from white to violet/purple (ethyl violet dye), from pink to white (titan yellow dye) or from green to violet. Colour changes occur when the pH is less than 10. Some types of soda lime have a low concentration of a zeolite added. This helps to maintain the pH at a high level for longer and retains moisture, so improving CO_2 absorption and reducing the formation of carbon monoxide (CO) and compound A.
7. The size of soda lime granules is 4–8 mesh. Strainers with 4–8 mesh have four and eight openings/in, respectively. Therefore, the higher the mesh number, the smaller the particles are. Recently produced soda lime made to a uniform shape of 3- to 4-mm spheres allows a more even flow of gases and a reduction in channelling. This results in a longer life with lower dust content and lower resistance to flow: 1 kg can absorb more than 120 L of CO_2.

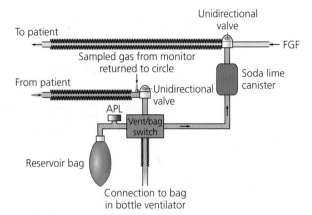

Fig. 4.18 Mechanism of action of the circle breathing system. *APL,* Adjustable pressure limiting; *FGF,* fresh gas flow.

8. Baralyme (or Baralime), consists of 80% barium hydroxide ($Ba(OH)_2$) and 20% $Ca(OH)_2$. It is widely used in the United States. Another absorber is 'Amsorb Plus,' which consists of calcium chloride and $Ca(OH)_2$. Being free of strong alkali, this absorber offers environmental advantages.

Mechanism of action

1. High FGF of several litres per minute is needed in the initial period to denitrogenate the circle system and the FRC. This is important to avoid the build-up of unacceptable levels of nitrogen in the system. In closed-circle anaesthesia, a high FGF is needed for up to 15 minutes. In low-flow anaesthesia, a high FGF of up to 6 minutes is required. The FGF can be later reduced to 0.5–1 L/min. If no N_2O is used during anaesthesia (i.e. an oxygen/air mix is used), it is not necessary to eliminate nitrogen because air contains nitrogen. A short period of high flow is needed to prime the system and the patient with the inhalational agent.
2. Exhaled gases are circled back to the canister, where CO_2 absorption takes place and water and heat (exothermic reaction) are produced. The warmed and humidified gas joins the FGF to be delivered to the patient (Fig. 4.18).
3. Chemical sequences for the absorption of CO_2 by soda lime:
    a. Note how both NaOH and KOH are regenerated at the expense of $Ca(OH)_2$. This explains soda lime's mix—only a little NaOH and KOH and a lot of $Ca(OH)_2$:

    $$H_2O + CO_2 \rightarrow H_2CO_3$$

    then

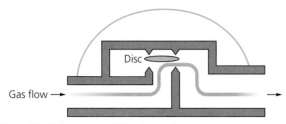

Fig. 4.19 Circle system unidirectional valve.

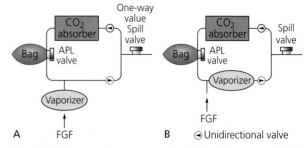

Fig. 4.20 Diagrammatic representation of the circle system with (A) vaporizer outside the circle and (B) vaporizer inside the circle. *APL*, Adjustable pressure limiting; *FGF*, fresh gas flow.

$$H_2CO_3 + 2KOH \rightarrow K_2CO_3 + 2H_2O$$

then

$$K_2CO_3 + Ca(OH)_2 \rightarrow CaCO_3 + 2KOH$$

or

$$CO_2 + 2NaOH \rightarrow Na_2CO_3 + H_2O + heat$$

then

$$Na_2CO_3 + Ca(OH)_2 \rightarrow 2NaOH + CaCO_3$$

b. As can be seen in the previous equations, this is an exothermic reaction that alters the pH of the whole system. The reaction also produces water. One mole of water is produced for each mole of CO_2 absorbed.

c. The direction of gas flow is controlled via the unidirectional valves made of discs that rest on a 'knife-edge' (Fig. 4.19). They allow gas to flow in one direction only and prevent the mixing of inspired and expired gases, thus preventing rebreathing. These are mounted in see-through plastic domes so that they can be seen to be working satisfactorily.

4. The canister is positioned vertically to prevent exhaled gas channelling through unfilled portions. Larger canisters are more efficient than smaller ones because of the higher litres of CO_2/kg weight capacity.

5. The lower the FGF used, the more rapidly soda lime granules are consumed. This is because most of the exhaled gases pass through the absorber with very little being discarded through the APL valve. For a 70- to 80-kg patient with a tidal volume of 500 mL, respiratory rate of 12 breaths/min and CO_2 production of 250 mL/min, using an FGF of 1 L/min, the soda lime will be exhausted after 5–7 hours of use. For the same patient but using an FGF of 3 L/min, the soda lime will be exhausted after 6–8 hours of use.

6. The circle system can be used for both spontaneous and controlled ventilation.

7. Disposable circle breathing systems exist. They feature coaxial inspiratory tubing. The inner tubing delivers the FGF from the anaesthetic machine, and the outer tubing delivers the recirculated gas flow. Both gas flows mix distally. This allows a more rapid change in the inhalational gas and vapour concentration at the patient's end.

Use of vaporizers in the circle breathing system

VOC vaporizers (Fig. 4.20A) are positioned on the back bar of the anaesthetic machine. They are high-efficiency vaporizers that can deliver high-output concentrations at low flows. They have high internal resistance.

1. The vaporizer should be able to deliver accurate concentrations of inhalational agent with both high and low FGFs. This is easily achieved by most modern vaporizers, e.g. the Tec and Sigma Delta series.

2. The volume of the circle system is large in relation to the low FGF used. Rapid changes in the concentration of the inspired vapour can be achieved by increasing the FGF to the circle system. Delivering the FGF distally, using a coaxial inspiratory tubing design, allows faster changes in inspired vapour concentration compared to conventional circle systems at low flows.

VIC vaporizers (see Fig. 4.20B) are designed to offer minimal resistance to gas flow and have no wicks on which water vapour might condense (e.g. Goldman vaporizer). The VIC vaporizer is a low-efficiency vaporizer adding only small amounts of vapour to the gas recirculating through it. Such a configuration is rarely used in current practice.

1. FGF will be vapour free and thus dilutes the inspired vapour concentration.

2. During spontaneous ventilation, respiration is depressed with deepening of anaesthesia. Uptake of the anaesthetic agent is therefore reduced. This

is an example of a feedback safety mechanism. The safety mechanism is lost during controlled ventilation.

Problems in practice and safety features

1. Adequate monitoring of inspired oxygen, end-tidal CO_2 and inhalational agent concentrations is essential and mandatory. Expired gas has lower concentrations of oxygen and inhalational agent than the inspired gas due to the uptake by patients. At low FGF flows, due to the progressive dilution by the recycled expired gases, the inspired concentration drifts downward. This can be prevented by setting high concentrations of oxygen (at flowmeter) and agent (at vaporizer).

2. The unidirectional valves may stick and fail to close because of water vapour condensation. This leads to an enormous increase in dead space and/or resistance.

3. The resistance to breathing is increased especially during spontaneous ventilation. The main cause of resistance to breathing is due to the unidirectional valves. Dust formation can increase resistance to breathing further. It can also lead to clogging and channelling, so reducing efficiency. Current soda lime designs claim less dust formation.

4. Compound A (a pentafluoroisopropenyl fluoromethyl ether, which is nephrotoxic in rats) is produced when sevoflurane is used in conjunction with soda lime. This is due to the degradation of sevoflurane (dehydrohalogenation) as a result of the alkali metal hydroxide present in soda lime.

   Factors that increase the production of compound A are:
   a. increasing temperature,
   b. high sevoflurane concentrations,
   c. use of Baralyme rather than soda lime,
   d. low FGF and
   e. newer designs of soda lime, being non-caustic (no KOH and only very low levels of NaOH), claim less or no production of compound A. For substance A production, baralyme is worse than soda lime. Amsorb is the safest.

5. CO production can occur when volatile agents containing the CHF_2 moiety (enflurane, isoflurane and desflurane) are used with very dry granules when the water content is less than 1.5% in soda lime or less than 5% in baralyme. This can occur when the system is left unused for a long period of time, e.g. overnight or during weekends, or when a small basal flow from the anaesthetic machine occurs. CO accumulation and subsequent carboxyhaemoglobin formation are said to occur

at less than 0.1%/h and, so may become significant in smokers when ultra-low flows are used; oxygen flushes of the system (e.g. once per hour) will prevent this.

   More recent designs of soda lime claim less or no production of CO. The association of strong alkalis such as KOH and NaOH with the production of CO has led to the subsequent removal of KOH and reduction in amounts of NaOH used. Some absorbers (e.g. Amsorb) do not use strong alkalis at all.

6. Other substances can accumulate such as methane, acetone, ethanol and hydrogen. However, they do not generally become clinically significant.

7. Uneven filling of the canister with soda lime leads to channelling of gases and decreased efficiency.

8. The circle system is bulkier, less portable and more difficult to clean.

9. Soda lime is corrosive. Protective clothing, gloves and eye/face protection can be used.

10. Because of the many connections, there is an increased potential for leaks and disconnection.

The circle breathing system

- Soda lime canister with two unidirectional valves attached to inspiratory and expiratory tubings. An APL valve and a reservoir bag are connected to the system.
- Soda lime consists of 94% $Ca(OH)_2$, 5% NaOH and a small amount of KOH. More recent versions have no KOH and a much lower percentage of NaOH.
- Soda lime absorbs the exhaled CO_2 and produces water and heat (so it humidifies and warms inspired gases).
- Very efficient breathing system using low FGF and reducing pollution.
- A high initial flow is required.
- Vaporizers can be VIC or VOC.

Waters canister ('to-and-fro') bidirectional flow breathing system

Currently, this system is not widely used in anaesthetic practice. It consists of a Mapleson C system with a soda lime canister positioned between the APL valve and the reservoir. A filter is positioned in the canister to prevent

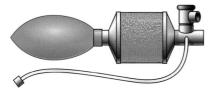

Fig. 4.21 The Waters canister breathing system.

the soda lime granules from 'entering' the breathing system and the risk of inhaling them. It is not an efficient system as the granules nearest to the patient are exhausted first, so increasing the dead space. It is also a cumbersome system, since the canister has to be positioned horizontally and packed tightly with the soda lime granules to prevent channelling of the gases (Fig. 4.21).

Table 4.1 Summary of advantages and disadvantages of the various breathing systems

System	Advantages	Disadvantages
Mapleson A	Efficient in spontaneous ventilation	Inefficient in controlled ventilation
Mapleson B		Inefficient in both spontaneous and controlled ventilation
Mapleson C	Lightweight and compact	Inefficient in both spontaneous and controlled ventilation
Mapleson D	Efficient in ventilated ventilation The inspiratory limb can be very long (suitable for head/neck surgery and for use in an MRI setting)	Inefficient in spontaneous ventilation
Mapleson E	Useful for patients under 30 kg as low resistance due to the lack of a valve	Difficult to scavenge waste gas High FGF is needed
Mapleson F	Useful for patients under 30 kg as low resistance due to the lack of a valve Reservoir bag allows ventilation.	Difficult to scavenge waste gas. A specially designed APL valve can be used allowing scavenging High FGF is needed
Circle	Very efficient when used at minimal flows	FGF must match patient demands at all times.
Humphrey's ADE	Used efficiently in adults and children Efficient in spontaneous and controlled ventilation	Large and cumbersome valve block

APL, Adjustable pressure limiting; *FGF,* fresh gas flow; *MRI,* magnetic resonance imaging.

SUGGESTED FURTHER READING

Department of Health, 2004. Protecting the Breathing Circuit in Anaesthesia. DoH, London. Available from: http://www.frca.co.uk/documents/Protecting%20the%20PBC.pdf.

Gott, K., Dolling, S., 2016. Anaesthetic breathing systems. Anaesth. Intens. Care. Med. 17 (3), 137–140.

Mapleson, W.W., 2004. Fifty years after – reflections on 'The elimination of rebreathing in various semi-closed anaesthetic systems'. Editorial. I Br. J. Anaesth. 93 (3), 319–321.

Tsim, P., Howatson, A., 2016. Breathing systems in anaesthesia. Available from: http://anaesthesiology.gr/media/File/pdf/WFSA%20tutorial%20333%20Breathing%20Systems%20in%20Anaesthesia.pdf.

Jaul, T.K., Mittall, G., 2013. Mapleson's breathing systems. Indian J. Anaesth. 57 (5), 507–515.

Kharasch, E.D., Powers, K.M., Artru, A.A., 2002. Comparison of Amsorb®, Sodalime, and Baralyme®Degradation of Volatile Anesthetics and Formation of Carbon Monoxide and Compound A in Swine *In Vivo*. Anesthesiology 96, 173–182.

MHRA, 2014. All anaesthetic breathing systems, anaesthetic machines and anaesthetic ventilators - inadequate ventilation (MDA/2010/036). Available from: https://www.gov.uk/drug-device-alerts/medical-device-alert-all-anaesthetic-breathing-systems-anaesthetic-machines-and-anaesthetic-ventilators-inadequate-ventilation.

SELF-ASSESSMENT QUESTIONS

Please check your eBook for additional self-assessment

MCQs

In the following lists, which of the statements (a) to (e) are true?

1. Adjustable pressure limiting (APL) valve in a breathing system

a. In the open position, a pressure of less than 1 cm H_2O (0.1 kPa) is needed to actuate the valve.

b. A pressure relief mechanism is activated at a pressure of 60 cm H_2O.

c. Is incorporated in the T-piece breathing system.

d. The dead space of the breathing system is reduced during spontaneous ventilation when excessive negative pressure from the scavenging system is applied through the APL valve.

e. Should be closed during controlled ventilation using a Bain breathing system and an intermittent blower ventilator.

2. Breathing systems

a. The fresh gas flow (FGF) rate required to prevent rebreathing of alveolar gas in the breathing system is a measure of the efficiency of a breathing system.

b. The reservoir bag limits the pressure build-up in a breathing system to about 40 cm H_2O.

c. An FGF of 150 mL/kg/min is needed in the Mapleson A system during spontaneous ventilation.

d. The inner tube in the Bain system delivers the FGF.

e. The Humphrey ADE system can be used for spontaneous ventilation only.

3. Dead space

a. The face mask in the Mapleson A breathing system has no effect on the dead space.

b. Disconnection of the inner tube at the patient's end in the Bain system results in an increase in dead space.

c. Failure of the unidirectional valves to close in the circle system has no effect on the system's dead space.

d. The anatomical dead space is about 150 mL.

e. Bohr's equation is used to measure the physiological dead space.

4. Concerning soda lime

a. 20% volume for volume of soda lime is sodium hydroxide (NaOH).

b. 90% is calcium carbonate ($CaCO_3$).

c. 1 kg of soda lime can absorb about 120 mL of carbon dioxide (CO_2).

d. The reaction with CO_2 is exothermic.

e. Soda lime fills half of the canister.

5. The Bain breathing system

a. Is an example of a Mapleson A system.

b. Requires an FGF of 70 mL/kg during spontaneous ventilation.

c. Is made of standard corrugated tubing.

d. Can be used in a T-piece system.

e. Can be used for both spontaneous and controlled ventilation.

6. T-piece breathing system

a. Can be used in paediatric practice only.

b. Mapleson F system is the E system plus an open-ended reservoir bag.

c. Is an efficient system.

d. With a constant FGF, a too small reservoir has no effect on the performance of the system.

e. The reservoir bag in Mapleson F provides a degree of continuous positive airway pressure (CPAP) during spontaneous ventilation.

7. **Which of the following are true and which are false?**

   a. The Magill classification is used to describe anaesthetic breathing systems.
   b. Modern anaesthetic breathing systems are constructed using antistatic materials.
   c. Efficiency of a breathing system is determined by the mode of ventilation of the patient.
   d. As long as the valve is present in a breathing system, its position is not important.
   e. Circle systems must only be used with very low FGFs.

8. **The circle breathing system**

   a. With low flow rates, substance A can be produced when sevoflurane is used.
   b. The Goldman vaporizer is an example of a VOC.

   c. Failure of the unidirectional valves to close leads to an enormous increase in the dead space.
   d. Patients should not be allowed to breathe spontaneously, because of the high resistance caused by the soda lime.
   e. Exhaustion of the soda lime can be detected by an end-tidal CO_2 rebreathing waveform.

9. **Regarding the circle system**

   a. A high oxygen/air FGF is needed in the first 15 minutes to wash out any CO_2 remaining in the breathing system.
   b. The pH of soda lime is highly acidic.
   c. The lower the FGF, the slower the exhaustion of soda lime granules.
   d. The Waters to-and-fro system is very efficient.
   e. Partially harmful substances can be produced when using soda lime.

Single best answer

10. **The APL valve**

    a. Is present in all breathing systems.
    b. Is actuated at only very high pressures when in the open position.
    c. Can act as a scavenging system.
    d. Scavenging systems can usually be attached to it.
    e. Is coloured bright yellow for safety reasons.

11. **Which breathing system would be most suitable for performing a gas induction of a spontaneously breathing adult patient?**

    a. Circle.
    b. Mapleson A.
    c. Mapleson C.
    d. Mapleson D.
    e. Mapleson F.

12. **If the inner tube of a Bain's (coaxial Mapleson D) breathing system became disconnected or perforated at the machine end, what classification of breathing system would it become?**

    a. Mapleson A.
    b. Mapleson B.
    c. Mapleson C.
    d. Mapleson D.
    e. Mapleson E.

13. **Approximately how much FGF is required to prevent rebreathing when using a Magill (Mapleson A) system for a 70-kg, spontaneously breathing patient?**

    a. 0.5 L/min.
    b. 4 L/min.
    c. 5 L/min.
    d. 10 L/min.
    e. 15 L/min.

14. **Which of the following statements regarding compound A is correct?**

    a. Studies show that compound A causes adverse effects in humans.
    b. Compound A formation increases if soda lime is allowed to become damp.
    c. Compound A causes a dose-dependent liver toxicity.
    d. Baralyme causes less formation of compound A.
    e. Compound A is only formed if sevoflurane is used.

Answers

1. APL valve in a breathing system
   a. *True.*
   b. *True. This is a safety feature in the design of the APL valve. If the APL valve is closed, a build-up of pressure within the breathing system puts the patient at the risk of barotrauma. A pressure relief mechanism is activated at a pressure of 60 cm H_2O, allowing the reduction of pressure within the system.*
   c. *False. There are no valves in the standard T-piece system. This is to keep resistance to a minimum. A recent modification exists where an APL valve is included before a closed-ended 500-mL reservoir bag. A pressure relief safety mechanism in the APL valve is actuated at a pressure of 30 cm H_2O. This design allows for effective scavenging.*
   d. *False. There is a huge increase in the dead space, resulting in rebreathing. This is because excessive negative pressure can lead the APL valve to remain open throughout breathing.*
   e. *True. When ventilation is controlled using a Bain breathing system and an intermittent blower ventilator, the APL valve must be closed completely. This is to prevent the escape of inhaled gases through the APL valve, leading to inadequate ventilation.*

2. Breathing systems
   a. *True. The FGF rate required to prevent rebreathing is a measure of the efficiency of a breathing system, e.g. in spontaneous breathing, the circle system is the most efficient system, whereas the Bain system is the least efficient.*
   b. *True. This is a safety feature to protect the patient from overpressure. Because of its high compliance, the reservoir bag can accommodate rises in pressure within the system better than other parts. Due to Laplace's law (pressure = 2 (tension)/radius), when the reservoir is overinflated, it can limit the pressure in the breathing system to about 40 cm H_2O.*
   c. *False. Mapleson A system is an efficient system during spontaneous breathing needing an FGF of about 70 mL/kg/min. Mapleson D needs an FGF of 150–200 mL/kg/min.*
   d. *True. The inner tube delivers the FGF as close as possible to the patient. The outer tube, which is connected to the reservoir bag, takes the exhaled gases.*
   e. *False. The Humphrey ADE system is a very versatile system and can be used for both spontaneous and controlled ventilation both for adults and in paediatrics.*

3. Dead space
   a. *False. The face mask increases the dead space in the Mapleson A breathing system. The dead space can increase up to 200 mL in adults.*
   b. *True. Disconnection of the inner tube, which delivers the FGF at the patient's end in the Bain system, leads to an increase in dead space and rebreathing.*
   c. *False. The unidirectional valves are essential for the performance of the circle system. Failure of the valves to close would lead to a significant increase in the dead space (expiratory valve) and in resistance (inspiratory valve).*
   d. *True. The anatomical dead space is that part of the respiratory system which takes no part in the gas exchange.*
   e. *True. $V_D/V_T = P_ACO_2 - P_ECO_2/P_ACO_2$ where V_D is dead space; V_T is tidal volume; P_ACO_2 is alveolar CO_2 tension; P_ECO_2 is mixed expired CO_2 tension. Normally $V_D/V_T = 0.25–0.35$.*

4. Concerning soda lime
   a. *False. NaOH constitutes about 5% of the soda lime.*
   b. *False. $CaCO_3$ is a product of the reaction between soda lime and CO_2.*

   $$CO_2 + 2NaOH \rightarrow Na_2CO_3 + H_2O + heat$$

   $$Na_2CO_3 + Ca(OH)_2 \rightarrow 2NaOH + CaCO_3$$

   c. *False. 1 kg of soda lime can absorb 120 L of CO_2.*
   d. *True. Heat is produced as a by-product of the reaction between CO_2 and NaOH.*
   e. *False. In order to achieve adequate CO_2 absorption, the canister should be well packed to avoid channelling and incomplete CO_2 absorption.*

5. The Bain breathing system
   a. *False. The Bain breathing system is an example of a Mapleson D system.*
   b. *False. An FGF of about 150–200 mL/kg/min is required to prevent rebreathing in the Bain system*

during spontaneous ventilation. This makes it an inefficient breathing system.

c. **False.** The Bain system is usually made of a coaxial tubing. A more recent design, a pair of parallel corrugated tubings, is also available.

d. **False.** The Bain breathing system is a Mapleson D system, whereas the T-piece system is a Mapleson E system. The Bain system has an APL valve, whereas the T-piece is a valveless system.

e. **True.** The Bain system can be used for spontaneous ventilation requiring an FGF of 150–200 mL/kg. It can also be used for controlled ventilation requiring an FGF of 70–100 mL/kg. During controlled ventilation, the APL valve is fully closed, the reservoir bag is removed and a ventilator like the Penlon Nuffield 200 with a 1-m length of tubing is connected instead.

6. T-piece breathing system

a. **False.** Although the T-piece breathing system is mainly used in paediatrics, it can be used in adults with a suitable FGF and reservoir volume. An FGF of 2.5–3 times the minute volume and a reservoir approximating the tidal volume are needed. Such a system is usually used in post-anaesthesia recovery units and for intensive care patients.

b. **True.** Jackson-Rees added a double-ended bag to the reservoir tubing of the Mapleson E, thus converting it to a Mapleson F. The bag acts as a visual monitor during spontaneous ventilation and can be used for assisted or controlled ventilation.

c. **False.** The T-piece system is not an efficient system as it requires an FGF of 2.5–3 times the minute volume to prevent rebreathing.

d. **False.** If the reservoir is too small, entrainment of ambient air will occur, resulting in dilution of the FGF.

e. **True.** Patients under the age of 6 years have a small functional residual capacity (FRC). General anaesthesia causes a further decrease in the FRC. The reservoir bag in the Mapleson F provides a degree of CPAP during spontaneous ventilation, helping to improve the FRC.

7. Which of the following are true or false?

a. **False.** Mapleson classification is used. The Mapleson A breathing system was described by Magill.

b. **False.** As modern anaesthetic agents are not flammable, modern breathing systems are not constructed using antistatic materials. They are normally made of plastic.

c. **True.** Efficiency of a breathing system differs during spontaneous and controlled ventilation; e.g. the Mapleson A system is more efficient during

spontaneous than during controlled ventilation, whereas the opposite is true of the D system.

d. **False.** The position of the valve in the breathing system is crucial in the function and efficiency of a breathing system.

e. **False.** The circle system can be used with low flows (e.g. 2–3 L/min) as well as very low flows (e.g. 0.5–1.5 L/min). This can be achieved safely with adequate monitoring of the inspired and exhaled concentration of the gases and vapours used.

8. The circle breathing system

a. **True.** Substance A can be produced when sevoflurane is used with soda lime under low flow rates. Newer designs of soda lime claim lesser or no production of substance A.

b. **False.** The Goldman vaporizer is a VIC vaporizer. It is positioned on the expiratory limb with minimal resistance to flow and no wicks.

c. **True.** The function of the unidirectional valves in the circle system is crucial for its function. Failure of the valve to close causes rebreathing resulting from the huge increase in the dead space of the system. This usually happens because of water vapour condensing on the valve.

d. **False.** The circle system can be used for both spontaneous and controlled ventilation. Soda lime increases the resistance to flow but is clinically insignificant.

e. **True.** As the soda lime gets exhausted, a rebreathing end-tidal CO_2 waveform can be detected. A dye is added that changes the granules' colour as they become exhausted.

9. Regarding circle system

a. **False.** High FGF (several L/min) is needed initially to denitrogenate the system and the FRC to avoid the build-up of unacceptable levels of nitrogen in the system. In closed-circle anaesthesia, a high FGF for up to 15 minutes, and in low-flow anaesthesia, a high FGF of up to 6 minutes are required, and these can later be reduced to 0.5–1 L/min. If no N_2O is used during anaesthesia, it is not necessary to eliminate nitrogen. A short period of high flow is needed to prime the system and the patient with the inhalational agent.

b. **False.** The pH of soda lime is highly alkaline, 13.5, because of the presence of calcium hydroxide ($Ca(OH)_2$), NaOH and small amounts, if any, of potassium hydroxide (KOH). This makes the soda lime a corrosive substance. Colour changes occur when the pH is less than 10.

c. **False.** The lower the FGF, the more rapidly soda lime granules are exhausted because most of the exhaled gases pass through the absorber with very little being discarded through the APL valve. For a 70- to 80-kg patient with a tidal volume of 500 mL, respiratory rate of 12 breaths/min and CO_2 production of 250 mL/min, using an FGF of 1 L/min, the soda lime will be exhausted in 5–7 hours of use. For the same patient but using an FGF of 3 L/min, the soda lime will be exhausted in 6–8 hours of use.

d. **False.** It is not an efficient system as the granules nearest to the patient are exhausted first, so increasing the dead space.

e. **True.** Substance A, nephrotoxic in rats, can be produced when sevoflurane is used with soda lime, although newer designs claim less or no substance A production. Carbon monoxide (CO) can occur when dry soda lime is used. Newer designs claim less or no CO production.

10. d.

11. b. This system would rapidly provide a high concentration of anaesthetic vapour to the patient with the minimum FGF required to prevent rebreathing.

12. c. Mapleson C breathing system would be created but with a very large increase in dead space.

13. c. Spontaneous ventilation using Mapleson A breathing system requires an FGF of 70–100 mL/kg/min to prevent rebreathing. For a 70-kg patient, this equates to between 4.9 and 7 L/min.

14. e.

Chapter 5

Tracheal tubes, tracheostomy tubes and airways

Tracheal tubes

Tracheal tubes provide a means of securing the patient's airway, allowing spontaneous and controlled ventilation. These disposable plastic tubes are made of polyvinyl chloride (PVC), which could be clear, ivory or siliconized. As plastic is not radio-opaque, tracheal tubes have a radio-opaque line running along their length, which enables their position to be determined on chest X-rays. The siliconized PVC aids the passage of suction catheters through the tube. In the past, tracheal tubes used to be made of rubber, allowing them to be reused after cleaning and autoclaving.

FEATURES OF TRACHEAL TUBES (Fig. 5.1)

Size

The 'size' of a tracheal tube refers to its **internal diameter** (ID), which is marked on the outside of the tube in millimetres. Narrower tubes increase the resistance to gas flow, therefore the largest possible ID should be used. This is especially important during spontaneous ventilation in which the patient's own respiratory effort must overcome the tube's resistance. A size 4-mm tracheal tube has 16 times more resistance to gas flow than a size 8-mm tube. Usually, a size 8.5–9-mm ID tube is selected for an average size adult male and a size 7.5–8-mm ID tube for an average size adult female. Paediatric sizes are determined on the basis of age and weight (Table 5.1). Tracheal tubes have both ID and outside diameter (OD) markings. There are various methods or formulae used to determine the size of paediatric tracheal tubes. A commonly used formula is:

$$\text{Internal diameter in mm} = \frac{\text{age in years}}{4} + 4$$

The **length** (taken from the tip of the tube) is marked in centimetres on the outside of the tube. The tube can be cut down to size to suit the individual patient. If the tube is cut too long, there is a significant risk of it advancing into one of the main bronchi (usually the right one [Fig. 5.2]). Black intubation depth markers located 3 cm proximal to the cuff can be seen in some designs (see Fig. 5.1). These assist in the accurate placement of the tracheal tube tip within the trachea. The vocal cords should be at the black mark in tubes with one mark or should be between marks if there are two such marks. However, these are only rough estimates, and correct tracheal tube position depth should always be confirmed by auscultation.

More recent designs have a small integrated high-resolution camera (Fig. 5.3) positioned at the tip of the

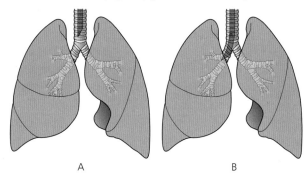

Fig. 5.2 (A) Correctly positioned tracheal tube. (B) The tracheal tube has been advanced too far, into the right main bronchus.

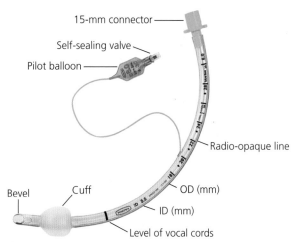

Fig. 5.1 Features of a cuffed tracheal tube. Some designs have the markings of implantation tested (IT) and Z-79 stands (the Z-79 Committee of the American National Standards Institute). *ID,* Internal diameter; *OD,* outside diameter. (Courtesy Smiths Medical, Ashford, Kent, UK.)

Labels in Fig. 5.1: 15-mm connector; Self-sealing valve; Pilot balloon; Radio-opaque line; Bevel; Cuff; OD (mm); ID (mm); Level of vocal cords

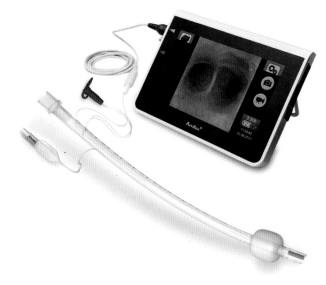

Fig. 5.3 The Ambu VivaSight-SL with an integrated high-resolution camera. An extra port is used to 'jet clean' by flushing saline to keep the camera lens clean. (Courtesy Ambu, Alconbury, Weald, Cambridgeshire, UK.)

Table 5.1 A guide to the size and length of oral tracheal tubes used in paediatric practice

Age	Weight (kg)	Size, ID (mm)	Length (cm)
Neonate	2–4	2.5–3.5	10–12
1–6 months	4–6	4.0–4.5	12–14
6–12 months	6–10	4.5–5.0	14–16
1–3 years	10–15	5.0–5.5	16–18
4–6 years	15–20	5.5–6.5	18–20
7–10 years	25–35	6.5–7.0	20–22
10–14 years	40–50	7.0–7.5	22–24

ID, Internal diameter.

tube, allowing continuous visual monitoring during intubation and positioning of the tube throughout the whole procedure.

The bevel

1. The bevel is left-facing and oval in most tube designs. A left-facing bevel improves the view of the vocal cords during laryngoscopy and intubation as the tube is inserted from the right-hand side.
2. Some designs incorporate a side hole just above and opposite the bevel, called a Murphy's eye. This enables ventilation to occur should the bevel become occluded by secretions, blood or the wall of the trachea (Fig. 5.4).

The cuff

1. Tracheal (oral or nasal) tubes can be either cuffed or uncuffed. The cuff, when inflated, provides an air-tight seal between the tube and the tracheal wall (Fig. 5.5). This air-tight seal protects the patient's airway from aspiration and allows efficient ventilation during intermittent positive pressure ventilation (IPPV). The cuff is connected to its pilot balloon, which has a self-sealing valve for injecting air. The pilot balloon also indicates whether the cuff is inflated or not. After intubation, the cuff is inflated until no gas leak can be heard during IPPV.
2. The narrowest point in the adult's airway is the glottis (which is hexagonal). In order to achieve an air-tight seal, cuffed tubes are used in adults.
3. The narrowest point in a child's airway is the cricoid cartilage. Since this is essentially circular, a correctly sized uncuffed tube will fit well. Because of the narrow upper airway in children, post-extubation subglottic oedema can be a problem. In order to minimize the risk, the presence of a small leak around the tube at an airway pressure of 15 cm H_2O is desirable.

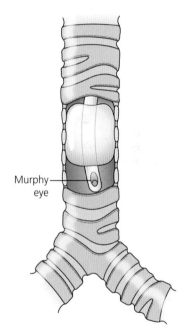

Murphy eye

Fig. 5.4 Diagram showing a tracheal tube with an obstructed bevel against the trachea wall but a patent Murphy's eye, thereby allowing ventilation.

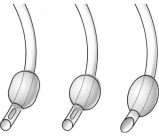

Fig. 5.5 Different types of tracheal tube cuffs. High volume *(left)*, intermediate volume *(centre)*, low volume *(right)*.

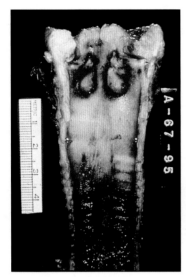

Fig. 5.6 A postmortem tracheal specimen. Note the black necrotic area, which was caused by long-term intubation with a high-pressure cuffed tube.

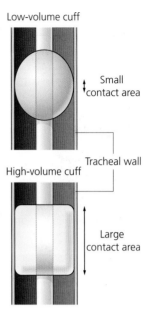

Fig. 5.7 Diagram illustrating how a low-volume cuff *(top)* maintains a seal against a relatively small area of tracheal wall compared to a high-volume cuff *(bottom)*.

4. Cuffs can be either:
   a. high pressure/low volume
   b. low pressure/high volume.

High-pressure/low-volume cuffs

1. These can prevent the passing of vomitus, secretions or blood into the lungs.
2. At the same time, they exert a high pressure on the tracheal wall. If left in position for long periods, they may cause necrosis of the tracheal mucosa (Fig. 5.6).

Low-pressure/high-volume cuffs

1. These exert minimal pressure on the tracheal wall as the pressure equilibrates over a wider area (Fig. 5.7). This allows the cuff to remain inflated for longer periods.
2. They are less capable of preventing the aspiration of vomitus or secretions. This is due to the possibility of wrinkles forming in the cuff.
   The pressure in the cuff should be checked at frequent and regular intervals (Figs. 5.8 and 5.9), maintaining a pressure of 15–20 mmHg (20–30 cm H$_2$O). The pressure may increase mainly because of diffusion of nitrous oxide into the cuff. Expansion of the air inside the cuff due to the increase in its temperature from room to body temperature and the diffusion of oxygen from the anaesthetic mixture (about 33%) into the air (21%) in the cuff can also lead to increase in the intracuff pressure. An increase in pressure of about 10–12 mmHg is expected

after 30 minutes of anaesthesia with 66% nitrous oxide. Some designs use cuff material (Soft Seal, Portex) that allows minimum diffusion of nitrous oxide into the cuff with a pressure increase of 1–2 mmHg only. The pressure may decrease because of a leak in the cuff or the pilot balloon's valve.
   Recent designs allow suction above the cuff (Fig. 5.10). A designated suction port runs along the wall of the tube to remove secretions above the cuff. This can reduce the incidence of ventilator-associated pneumonia.

Route of insertion

1. Tubes can be inserted orally or nasally (Fig. 5.11).
2. The indications for nasal intubation include:
   a. surgery where access via the mouth is necessary, e.g. maxilla-facial procedures.
   b. long-term ventilated patients in intensive care units. Patients tolerate a nasal tube better and cannot bite on the tube. However, long-term nasal intubation may cause sinus infection.
3. Nasal intubation is usually avoided, if possible, in children up to the age of 8–11 years. Hypertrophy of the adenoids in this age group increases the risk of profuse bleeding if nasal intubation is performed.
4. Ivory PVC nasotracheal tubes cause less trauma to the nasal mucosa.

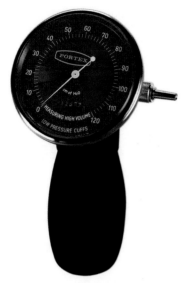

Fig. 5.8 Cuff pressure gauge. (Courtesy Smiths Medical, Ashford, Kent, UK.)

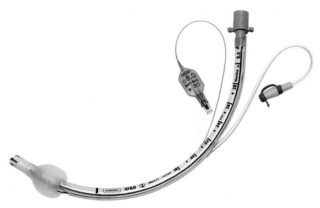

Fig. 5.10 Tracheal tube with suction above the cuff; Portex SACETT. Note the design of the top surface of the cuff, allowing the collection of secretion just distal to the suction port. (Courtesy Smiths Medical, Ashford, Kent, UK.)

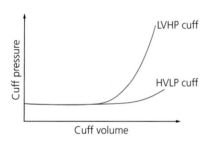

Fig. 5.9 Graph showing pressure changes in low-volume/high-pressure *(LVHP)* cuff and high-volume/low-pressure *(HVLP)* cuff. Note the steep rise in cuff pressure in the LVHP cuff when the cuff volume reaches a critical volume. A more gradual increase in pressure is seen in the HVLP cuff.

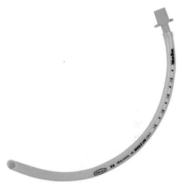

Fig. 5.11 A noncuffed oral/nasal tracheal tube. (Courtesy Smiths Medical, Ashford, Kent, UK.)

Connectors

These connect the tracheal tubes to the breathing system (or catheter mount). Various designs and modifications (Fig. 5.12) are available. They are made of plastic or metal and should have an adequate ID to reduce the resistance to gas flow.

On the breathing system end, the British Standard connector has a 15-mm diameter at the proximal end. An 8.5-mm diameter version exists for neonatal use. On the tracheal tube end, the connector has a diameter that depends on the size of the tracheal tube. Connectors designed for use with nasal tracheal tubes have a more acute angle than the oral ones (e.g. Magill's connector). Some designs have an extra port for suction.

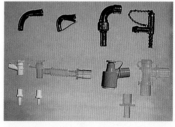

Fig. 5.12 A range of tracheal tube connectors. *Top row* from *left* to *right:* Magill oral, Magill nasal, Nosworthy, Cobb suction. (Note the Magill nasal connector has been supplied with a piece of wire threaded through it to demonstrate its patency.) *Bottom row:* Paediatric 8.5-mm connectors *(left)* and standard 15-mm connectors *(right).*

Problems in practice and safety features

1. Obstruction of the tracheal tube by kinking, herniation of the cuff, occlusion by secretions, foreign body or the bevel lying against the wall of the trachea.

2. Oesophageal or bronchial intubation.
3. Trauma and injury to the various tissues and structures during and after intubation.

Tracheal tubes
- Usually made of plastic.
- Oral or nasal (avoid nasal intubation in children).
- Cuffed or uncuffed.
- The cuff can be low pressure/high volume or high pressure/low volume.
- Recent designs incorporate high-definition camera and facility for suction above the cuff.

 Exam tip: It is important to understand the difference between low-pressure/high-volume and high-pressure/low-volume cuffs and their potential risks/benefits in clinical practice.

Specially designed tracheal tubes

ARMOURED/REINFORCED TRACHEAL TUBE

Armoured tracheal tubes are made of plastic or silicone rubber (Fig. 5.13). The walls of the armoured tube are thicker than ordinary tracheal tubes because they contain an embedded spiral of metal wire or tough nylon. They are used in anaesthesia for head and neck surgery. The spiral helps to prevent the kinking and occlusion of the tracheal tube when the head and/or neck is rotated or flexed, so giving it strength and flexibility at the same time. An introducer stylet is used to aid intubation.

Because of the spiral, it is not possible to cut the tube to the desired length. This increases the risk of bronchial intubation. Two markers, situated just above the cuff, are present on some designs. These indicate the correct position for the vocal cords.

POLAR AND RING, ADAIR AND ELWYN TRACHEAL TUBES

The **north-facing polar or the Ring, Adair and Elwyn (RAE) tube** is a preformed nasal cuffed or uncuffed tracheal tube (Fig. 5.14). It is used mainly during

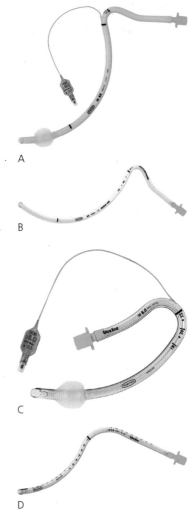

Fig. 5.14 Polar and Ring, Adair and Elwyn tracheal tubes: (A) cuffed nasal north facing, (B) non-cuffed nasal north facing, (C) cuffed oral south facing and (D) non-cuffed oral north facing. (Courtesy Smiths Medical, Ashford, Kent, UK.)

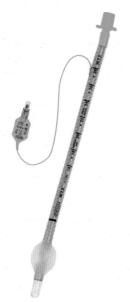

Fig. 5.13 Armoured cuffed tracheal tube. (Courtesy Smiths Medical, Ashford, Kent, UK.)

anaesthesia for maxillofacial procedures as it does not impede surgical access. Because of its design and shape, it lies over the nose and the forehead. It can be converted to an ordinary nasal tracheal tube by cutting it at the scissors mark just proximal to the pilot tube and reconnecting the 15-mm connector. An oral version of the polar tube exists. They can be made of ivory PVC or clear polyurethane.

The **south-facing polar or RAE tube** has a preformed shape to fit the mouth without kinking. It has a bend located just as the tube emerges, so the connections to the breathing system are at the level of the chin and not interfering with the surgical access. Such tubes can be either cuffed or uncuffed.

Because of its preformed shape, there is a higher risk of bronchial intubation than with ordinary tracheal tubes. The cuffed tracheal tube has one Murphy eye, whereas the uncuffed version has two eyes. Since the uncuffed version is mainly used in paediatric practice, two Murphy eyes ensure adequate ventilation should the tube prove too long.

The tube can be temporarily straightened to insert a suction catheter.

LASER-RESISTANT TRACHEAL TUBES

These tubes are used in anaesthesia for laser surgery on the larynx or trachea (Fig. 5.15). They are designed to withstand the effect of carbon dioxide and potassium-titanyl-phosphate (KTP) laser beams, avoiding the risk of fire or damage to the tracheal tube. One design has a flexible stainless steel body. Reflected beams from the tube are defocused to reduce the accidental laser strikes to healthy tissues. Other designs have a laser-resistant metal foil wrapped around the tube for protection (Fig. 5.16). The cuff is filled with methylene blue–coloured saline. If the laser manages to damage the cuff, the colouring will

help identify rupture and the saline will help prevent an airway fire.

Some designs have two cuffs. This ensures a tracheal seal should the upper cuff be damaged by laser. An air-filled cuff, hit by the laser beam, may ignite and so it is recommended that the cuffs are filled with saline instead of air.

Laser is an acronym for "*l*ight *a*mplification by the *s*timulated *e*mission of *r*adiation."

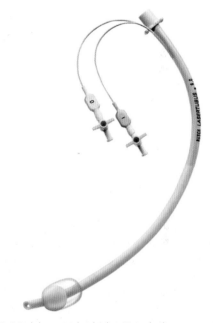

Fig. 5.16 Rüsch laser tracheal tube. Note the laser-protective wrapping and the two cuffs. (Image courtesy Teleflex Incorporated. © 2021. Teleflex Incorporated, Athlone, Ireland. All rights reserved.)

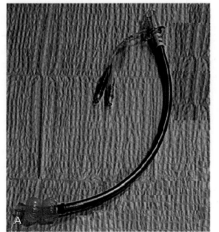

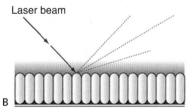

Laser beam

Fig. 5.15 (A) Stainless steel laser-resistant tracheal tube with two cuffs; (B) the reflected laser beam is defocused.

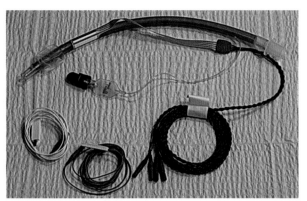

Fig. 5.17 Evoked potential tracheal tube. Note the electrodes (just above the cuff) with their cables. The other cable is earth.

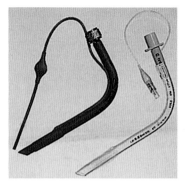

Fig. 5.19 The Oxford tracheal tube: red rubber *(left)* and plastic *(right)*.

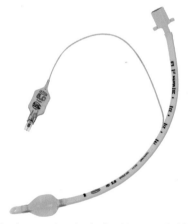

Fig. 5.18 Microlaryngeal tracheal tube. (Courtesy Smiths Medical, Ashford, Kent, UK.)

EVOKED POTENTIALS TRACHEAL TUBES (Fig. 5.17)

These tubes are used in a number of surgical procedures that have the risks of damage to nerves, e.g. thyroid surgery. Bipolar stainless steel contact electrical electrodes are embedded in the tracheal tubes above the cuff where they are in contact with the vocal cords. These electrodes are connected to a nerve stimulator. An additional earth electrode is attached to the skin of the patient.

The use of such tubes allows continuous nerve monitoring throughout surgery providing visual and audible warnings.

MICROLARYNGEAL TUBE

This tube allows better exposure and surgical access to the larynx. It has a small diameter (usually a 5-mm ID) with an adult-sized cuff (Fig. 5.18). Its length is sufficient

to allow nasal intubation if required. The tube is made of ivory PVC to reduce trauma to the nasal mucosa.

OXFORD TRACHEAL TUBE

This anatomically L-shaped tracheal tube is used in anaesthesia for head and neck surgery because it is non-kinking (Fig. 5.19). The tube can be made of rubber or plastic and can be cuffed or uncuffed. The bevel is oval and faces posteriorly, and an introducing stylet is supplied to aid the insertion of the tube. Its thick wall adds to the tube's external diameter, making it wider for a given ID. This is undesirable especially in paediatric anaesthesia.

The distance from the bevel to the curve of the tube is fixed. If the tube is too long, the problem cannot be corrected by withdrawing the tube and shortening it because this means losing its anatomical fit.

This tube is not widely used in the current anaesthetic practice.

Tracheostomy tracheal tubes

These are curved plastic tubes usually inserted through the second, third and fourth tracheal cartilage rings (Fig. 5.20).

Components
1. An introducer is used for insertion.
2. Wings are attached to the proximal part of the tube to fix it in place with a ribbon or suture. Some designs have an adjustable flange to fit the variable thickness of the subcutaneous tissues (Fig. 5.21).
3. They can be cuffed or uncuffed. The former has a pilot balloon.
4. The proximal end can have a standard 15-mm connector.

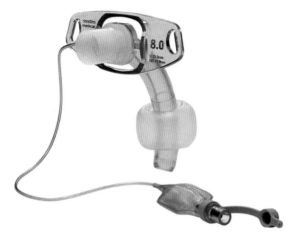

Fig. 5.20 BLUselect cuffed tracheostomy tube. (Courtesy Smiths Medical, Ashford, Kent, UK.)

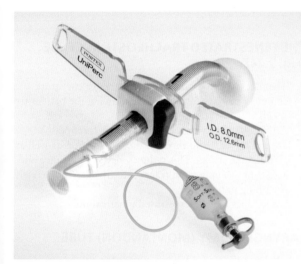

Fig. 5.21 Adjustable flange tracheostomy tube. (Courtesy Smiths Medical, Ashford, Kent, UK.)

5. The tip is usually cut square rather than bevelled. This decreases the risk of obstruction by lying against the tracheal wall.
6. Some designs have an additional suctioning lumen, which opens just above the cuff. The cuff shape is designed to allow the secretions above it to be suctioned effectively through the suctioning lumen (Fig. 5.22).
7. In patients with a difficult anatomy, some designs use a reinforced tube to prevent kinking (Fig. 5.23).
8. Some tubes have an inner cannula. Secretions can collect and dry out on the inner lumen of the tube, leading to obstruction. The internal cannula can be replaced instead of changing the complete tube in

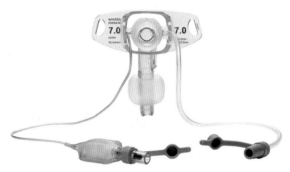

Fig. 5.22 Smith's Portex tracheostomy tube with an above-cuff suction facility.

such cases. The cannula leads to a slight reduction of the ID of the tube.
9. Different sizes of tracheostomy tubes are available to fit neonates to adults.
10. Older uncuffed metal tracheostomy tubes made of a non-irritant and bactericidal silver are rarely used in current practice. Some designs have a one-way flap valve and a window at the angle of the tube to allow the patient to speak.

Indications for tracheostomy
- Long-term ventilation.
- Upper airway obstruction that cannot be bypassed with an oral/nasal tracheal tube.
- Maintenance of an airway and to protect the lungs in patients with impaired pharyngeal or laryngeal reflexes and after major head and neck surgery (e.g. laryngectomy).
- Long-term control of excessive bronchial secretions especially in patients with a reduced level of consciousness.
- To facilitate weaning from a ventilator. This is due to a reduction in the sedation required, as the patients tolerate tracheostomy tubes better than tracheal tubes. Also there is a reduction in the anatomical dead space.

Benefits of tracheostomy
- Increased patient comfort.
- Less need for sedation.
- Improved access for oral hygiene.
- Possibility of oral nutrition.
- Bronchial suctioning aided.
- Reduced dead space.
- Reduced airway resistance.
- Reduced risk of glottic trauma.

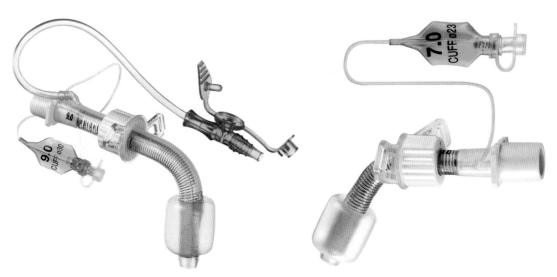

Fig. 5.23 The cuffed and reinforced Rüsch TracFlex Plus tube *(left)* and TracFlex Plus Subglottic tube *(right)* with above-cuff suction facility. (Image courtesy Teleflex Incorporated. © 2021.Teleflex Incorporated, Athlone, Ireland. All rights reserved.)

Problems in practice and safety features

Surgical tracheostomy has a mortality rate of <1% but has a total complications rate as high as 40%. The complications rate is higher in the intensive care unit and emergency patients.

The complications can be divided into:

1. Immediate:
   a. haemorrhage
   b. tube misplacement (e.g. into a main bronchus)
   c. occlusion of tube by cuff herniation
   d. occlusion of the tube tip against carina or tracheal wall
   e. pneumothorax.
2. Delayed:
   a. blockage of the tube by secretions, which can be sudden or gradual; this is rare with adequate humidification and suction
   b. infection of the stoma
   c. overinflation of the cuff leads to ulceration and distension of the trachea
   d. mucosal ulceration because of excessive cuff pressures, asymmetrical inflation of the cuff or tube migration
   e. surgical emphysema, pneumothorax and pnuemomediastinum.
3. Late:
   a. tracheal stenosis
   b. granulomata of the trachea may cause respiratory difficulty after extubation
   c. persistent sinus at the tracheostomy site
   d. tracheal dilatation
   e. tracheal stenosis at the cuff site
   f. scar formation.

THE FENESTRATED TRACHEOSTOMY TUBE (Fig. 5.24)

1. The fenestration (window) in the greater curvature channels air to the vocal cords, allowing the patient to speak.
2. After deflation of the cuff, the patient can breathe around the cuff and through the fenestration as well as through the stoma. This reduces airway resistance and assists in weaning from tracheostomy in spontaneously breathing patients.
3. Some tubes have a fenestrated inner cannula.

LARYNGECTOMY (MONTANDON) TUBE

This J-shaped cuffed tube is inserted through a tracheostomy stoma to facilitate IPPV during neck surgery (Fig. 5.25). It has the advantage of offering better surgical access by allowing the breathing system to be connected well away from the surgical field. Usually, it is replaced with a tracheostomy tube at the end of operation.

Tracheostomy tubes
- Can be plastic or metal, cuffed or uncuffed.
- The tip is cut horizontally.
- Used for long-term intubation.
- Some designs use an adjustable flange, reinforced tube and suction above the cuff.
- Speaking versions exist.

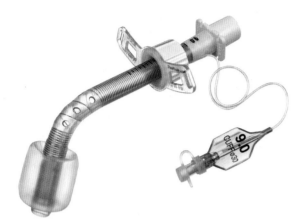

Fig. 5.24 The Rüsch TracFlex Plus Phonation to allow speech. (Image courtesy Teleflex Incorporated. © 2021. Teleflex Incorporated, Athlone, Ireland. All rights reserved.)

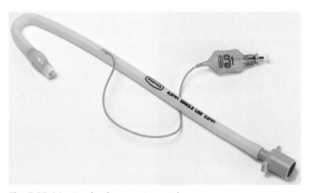

Fig. 5.25 Montandon laryngectomy tube.

TRACHEOSTOMY SPEAKING VALVE (Fig. 5.26)

This is a one-way speaking valve. It is fitted to the uncuffed tracheostomy tube or to the cuffed tracheostomy tube with its cuff deflated.

Tracheostomy button (Fig. 5.27)

Once a tracheostomy is removed after long-term use, this device is inserted into the stoma to maintain patency of the tract and to act as a route for tracheal suction.

PERCUTANEOUS TRACHEOSTOMY TUBES

These tubes are inserted between the first and second or second and third tracheal rings, usually at the bedside in the intensive care unit. Percutaneous tracheostomy tubes are becoming more popular and have fewer complications than the surgical technique.

1. If the patient is intubated, the tracheal tube is withdrawn until the tip is just below the vocal cords.

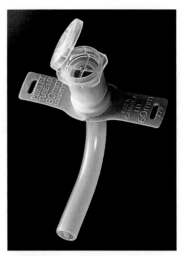

Fig. 5.26 A tracheostomy speaking valve mounted on an uncuffed tracheostomy tube.

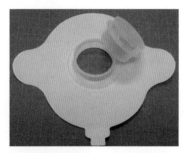

Fig. 5.27 Tracheostomy button and its skin dressing.

Then the cuff is inflated and rested on the vocal cords. A laryngeal mask can be used instead.
2. Through an introducing needle, a Seldinger guidewire is inserted into the trachea. A fibreoptic bronchoscope should be used throughout the procedure. It helps to ensure the initial puncture of the trachea is in the midline and free of the tracheal tube. It can also ensure that the posterior tracheal wall is not damaged during the procedure. Finally, it can assess the position of the tracheostomy tube relative to the carina.
3. A series of curved dilators can be used. The diameter of the stoma is serially increased until the desired diameter is achieved. A single curved dilator of a graduated diameter can be used instead (Fig. 5.28). A tracheostomy tube can then be inserted.
4. A pair of specially designed Griggs forceps are inserted over the guidewire instead of the dilator(s). These forceps are used to dilate the trachea. A tracheostomy tube is threaded over the guidewire and advanced into the trachea. The guidewire is then removed (Fig. 5.29).

5. An adjustable flange percutaneous tracheostomy is available. The flange can be adjusted to suit the patient's anatomy, e.g. in the obese patient. The flange can be moved away from the stoma site to aid in cleaning around the stoma.

6. The procedure can be performed in the intensive care unit with a lower incidence of complications than the conventional open surgical method (infection rate, subglottic stenosis and bleeding problems). The operative time is about half that of a formal surgical procedure.

7. Percutaneous tracheostomy can be performed faster using the dilating forceps technique compared to the dilator technique.

8. There is an increased risk of surgical emphysema due to air leaks from the trachea to the surrounding tissues. Loss of the airway, bleeding and incorrect placement of the needle are potential difficulties during the procedure. The risk of aspiration is increased when the tracheal tube has to be withdrawn at the start of the procedure.

9. Relative contraindications include enlarged thyroid gland, non-palpable cricoid cartilage, paediatric application, previous neck surgery and positive end expiratory pressure (PEEP) of more than 15 cm H_2O. The latter is because of the difficulty in applying a high PEEP during the process of insertion.

10. Reinsertion of a percutaneously fashioned tube can be more difficult than the surgical one as the stoma

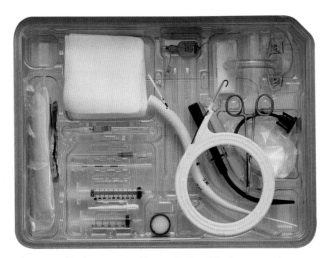

Fig. 5.28 BLUperc single dilator tracheostomy kit. (Courtesy Smiths Medical, Ashford, Kent, UK.)

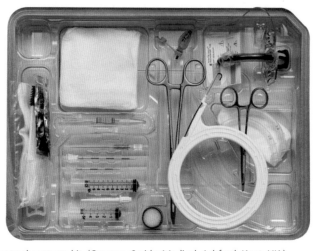

Fig. 5.29 BLUgriggs percutaneous tracheostomy kit. (Courtesy Smiths Medical, Ashford, Kent, UK.)

may close immediately. A track is formed after long-term intubation, and the tracheostomy tube can be removed. In order to protect the patency of the tract, a tracheostomy button (see Fig. 5.27) is inserted into the stoma. It also acts as a route for tracheal suction. Tracheostomy buttons are made of straight rigid plastic.

Minitracheostomy tube

This tube is inserted percutaneously into the trachea through the avascular cricothyroid membrane (Fig. 5.30).

Components

1. A siliconized PVC tube 10 cm in length with an ID of 4 mm. Some designs have lengths ranging from 3.5 to 7.5 cm with IDs from 2 to 6 mm.
2. The proximal end of the tube has a standard 15-mm connector that allows attachment to breathing systems. The proximal end also has wings used to secure the tube with the ribbon supplied.
3. A 2-cm, 16-G needle is used to puncture the cricothyroid cartilage. A 50-cm guidewire is used to help in the tracheal cannulation. A 10-mL syringe is used to aspirate air to confirm the correct placement of the needle.

4. A 7-cm curved dilator and a curved introducer are used to facilitate the insertion of the cricothyrotomy tube in some designs.

Mechanism of action

1. The Seldinger technique is used to insert the tube.
2. It is an effective method to clear tracheobronchial secretions in patients with an inefficient cough.
3. In an emergency, it can be used to administer oxygen in patients with upper airway obstruction that cannot be bypassed with a tracheal tube.

Problems in practice and safety features

Percutaneous insertion of minitracheostomy has the risk of:

1. pneumothorax,
2. perforation of the oesophagus,
3. severe haemorrhage,
4. ossification of the cricothyroid membrane, and
5. incorrect placement.

> **Minitracheostomy**
> - Tube inserted into the trachea through the cricothyroid membrane using the Seldinger technique.
> - Used for clearing secretions and maintaining an airway in an emergency.

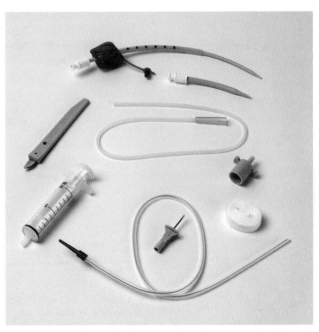

Fig. 5.30 The Portex minitracheostomy set inserted using Sledinger technique. (Courtesy Smiths Medical, Ashford, Kent, UK.)

Cricothyrotomy tube (Fig. 5.31)

This tube is used to maintain the airway in challenging situations such as on the battlefield or in a 'can't intubate, can't oxygenate' (CICO) emergency. It is inserted into the trachea through the cricothyroid cartilage.

Components

1. A scalpel and syringe.
2. A needle with a Veress design and a dilator. The needle has a 'red flag' indicator. This helps in locating the tissues.
3. A 6-mm cuffed tube.

Mechanism of action

1. After a 2-cm horizontal skin incision has been made, the needle is inserted perpendicular to the skin.
2. As the needle enters the trachea, the red indicator disappears. The needle is advanced carefully until the red reappears, indicating contact with the posterior wall of the trachea.
3. As the cricothyrotomy tube is advanced into the trachea, the needle and the dilator are removed.

Problems in practice and safety features

The cricothyrotomy tube has complications similar to the minitracheostomy tube.

> **Cricothyrotomy**
> - A cuffed 6-mm tube is inserted into the trachea through the cricothyroid cartilage.
> - A Veress needle is designed to locate the trachea.
> - Used in emergencies to establish an airway via 'Front of Neck access' (FONA).

Double lumen endobronchial tubes

During thoracic surgery, one lung needs to be deflated. This offers the surgeon easier and better access within the designated hemithorax. In order to achieve this, double lumen tubes are used, which allows the anaesthetist to selectively deflate one lung while maintaining standard ventilation of the other.

Components

1. The double lumen tube has two separate colour-coded lumens, each with its own bevel (Fig. 5.32). One lumen ends in the trachea and the other lumen ends in either the left or right main bronchus. Blue colour is usually used for the bronchial lumen.
2. Each lumen has its own cuff (tracheal and bronchial cuffs) and colour-coded pilot balloons; blue for the bronchial components. Both lumens and pilot balloons are labelled.
3. There are two curves to the tube: the standard anterior curve to fit into the oropharyngeal laryngeal tracheal airway and the second curve, either to the right or left, to fit into the right or left bronchus, respectively.
4. The proximal end of these tubes is connected to a Y-shaped catheter mount attached to the breathing system.
5. More recent designs have a high-definition camera positioned at the tip of the tracheal lumen. This allows visual confirmation of correct positioning during insertion of the tube. Since per-op tube displacement is a problem, the continuous real-time monitoring of the tube position is invaluable (Fig. 5.33). An extra port

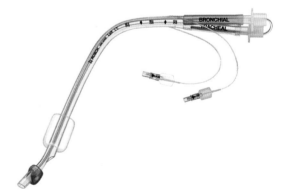

Fig. 5.32 Rüsch right-sided double lumen tube. Note the design of the bronchial cuff and its 'eye' to facilitate ventilation of right upper lobe. (Image courtesy Teleflex Incorporated. © 2021.Teleflex Incorporated, Athlone, Ireland. All rights reserved.)

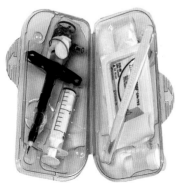

Fig. 5.31 Portex cricothyrotomy set. (Courtesy Smiths Medical, Ashford, Kent, UK.)

is used to 'jet clean' the camera lens by flushing saline, removing unwanted secretions.

Mechanism of action

1. Because of the differing anatomy of the main bronchi and their branches, both right and left versions of double lumen tubes must exist.
2. Once the tubes are correctly positioned, the anaesthetist can selectively ventilate one lung. So for procedures requiring that the right lung is deflated, a left-sided double lumen tube would be used that enabled selective ventilation of the left lung alone and vice versa.
3. It is desirable, when possible, to insert a left double lumen tube instead of a right one. This reduces the risk of upper lobe bronchus obstruction by the bronchial cuff in the right-sided version.
4. The right-sided version has an eye in the bronchial cuff to facilitate ventilation of the right upper lobe. The distance between the right upper lobe bronchus and the carina in an adult is only 2.5 cm, so there is a real risk of occluding it with the bronchial cuff. There is no eye in the left-sided version because the distance between the carina and the left upper lobe bronchus is about 5 cm, which is adequate to place the cuff.
5. The tubes come in different sizes to fit adult patients, but they do not come in paediatric sizes.

Tube positioning

1. The position of the tube should be checked by auscultation immediately after intubation and after positioning the patient for the operation. It is also recommended to use a bronchoscope to confirm correct positioning of the double lumen tube. Designs with a camera can visually confirm the position during insertion and throughout the procedure.
2. The tracheal cuff is inflated first until no leak is heard. At this point, both lungs can be ventilated. Next, the tracheal limb of the Y-catheter mount is clamped and disconnected from the tracheal lumen tube. Then the bronchial cuff is inflated with only a few millilitres of air until no leak is heard from the tracheal tube. At this stage, only the lung ventilated via the bronchial lumen should be ventilated. The ability to selectively ventilate the other lung should also be checked by clamping the bronchial limb of the Y-catheter mount and disconnecting it from the bronchial lumen having already reconnected the tracheal lumen. At this stage, only the lung ventilated via the tracheal lumen should be ventilated.

 Exam tip: A common question in the exams is how to check the position of a double lumen endobronchial tube.

The commonly used double lumen bronchial tubes are:

1. **Robertshaw** (rubber) tubes (Fig. 5.34).
2. **Single-use plastic** tubes. These tubes require an introducer for insertion. Some designs the facility of applying continuous positive airway pressure (CPAP) to the deflated lung to improve arterial oxygenation (Fig. 5.35).
3. **Carlens** (left-sided version) and **White** (right-sided version) tubes that use a carinal hook to aid final positioning of the tube (see Fig. 5.34). The hook can cause trauma to the larynx or carina. Because of the relatively small lumens (6 and 8 mm), the Carlens tube

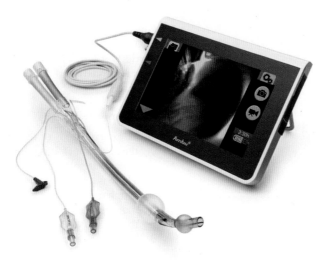

Fig. 5.33 The Ambu VivaSight-Dl double lumen tube with a high-definition camera at the tip of the tracheal lumen. This design is available as a left-sided double lumen tube only. (Courtesy Ambu, Alconbury, Weald, Cambridgeshire, UK.)

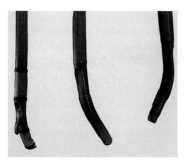

Fig. 5.34 White double lumen tube with carinal hook *(left)*. Left and right versions of the Robertshaw double lumen tube *(centre and right)*.

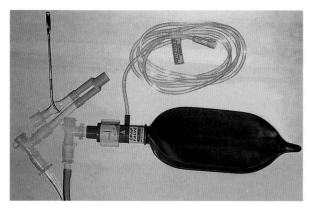

Fig. 5.35 Bronchocath double lumen tube with the bronchial lumen connected to a continuous positive airway pressure valve assembly. The disconnected limb of the Y-shaped catheter mount has been clamped.

causes an increase in airway resistance and difficulty in suctioning thick secretions.

> **Double lumen endobronchial tubes**
> - These tubes have two separate lumens, each with its own cuff and pilot tube.
> - There are two curves, anterior and lateral.
> - The right-sided version has an eye in the bronchial cuff to facilitate ventilation of the right upper lobe.
> - Commonly used tubes are the single-use tubes, Robertshaw tubes, and Carlens (and White) tubes. The latter has a carinal hook.

Endobronchial blocker

The endobronchial blocker is an alternative means to the double lumen tube for providing one-lung ventilation (Fig. 5.36).

Components

1. The endobronchial blocker catheter. This is a thin catheter that has a unique bifurcated distal end. The pair of colour-coded distal cuffs are inflated via their individual pilot balloon.
2. Multiport adaptor. This allows ergonomic alignment of the bronchoscope port and endobronchial blocker port to approach the single lumen tube. The fresh gas supply is also attached at an angle.

Mechanism of action

The patient is intubated with as large a single lumen standard tracheal tube as is possible. A specially designed multiport adapter is connected to the tube's standard 15-mm connector. The blocker is then advanced under direct vision of a narrow bronchoscope into the desired position, straddling the carina. The selected cuff is then inflated to block the corresponding main bronchus while maintaining ventilation to the contralateral side. Ventilation of the contralateral lung is maintained via the tracheal tube.

Oropharyngeal airways

This anatomically shaped airway is inserted through the mouth into the oropharynx above the tongue to maintain the patency of the upper airway (Fig. 5.37) in cases of upper airway obstruction caused by a decreased level of consciousness. Decreased consciousness can lead to loss of pharyngeal tone that can result in airway obstruction by the tongue, epiglottis, soft palate or pharyngeal tissues. There are various regularly used types of oropharyngeal airway. The most common type is the Guedel airway, named after its developer Arthur Guedel, an American anaesthetist who served in France during World War I. It is available in up to nine sizes, which have a standardized number coding (the smallest '000' to the largest '6').

Components

1. The curved body of the oropharyngeal airway contains the air channel. It is flattened anteroposteriorly and curved laterally.
2. There is a flange at the oral end to prevent the oropharyngeal airway from falling back into the mouth, so avoiding further posterior displacement into the pharynx.
3. The bite portion is straight and fits between the teeth. It is made of hard plastic to prevent occlusion of the air channel should the patient bite the oropharyngeal airway.

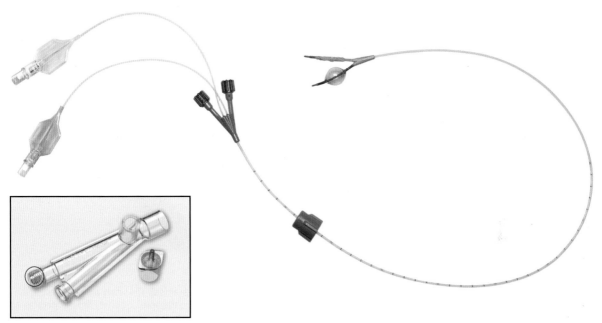

Fig. 5.36 The Rüsch EZ-Blocker endobronchial blocker (without adaptor). (Image courtesy Teleflex Incorporated. © 2021.Teleflex Incorporated, Athlone, Ireland. All rights reserved.)

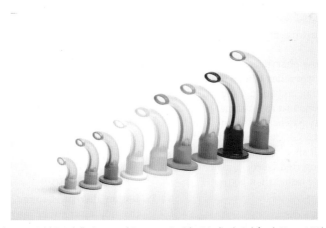

Fig. 5.37 Different sizes of oropharyngeal (Guedel) airways. (Courtesy Smiths Medical, Ashford, Kent, UK.)

Mechanism of action

1. The patient's airway is kept patent by preventing the tongue and epiglottis from falling backwards.
2. Oropharyngeal airways are designed in different sizes to fit the majority of patients from neonates to adults.
3. The air channel should be as large as possible in order to pass suction catheters.
4. As a good indication, a suitable Guedel airway size can be equivalent to either distance from the patient's incisors to the angle of the mandible (hard-to-hard method) or corner of the patient's mouth to the tragus of the ear (soft-to-soft method).
5. In adults, the Guedel airway is initially inserted upside down, with the curvature facing caudad. Once partially inserted, it is then rotated through 180 degrees and advanced until the bite block rests between the incisors. This method prevents the tongue being pushed back into the pharynx, causing further obstruction.
6. In children, it is often recommended that the Guedel airway is inserted the right way round, using a tongue depressor or laryngoscope to depress the tongue. This is done to minimize the risk of trauma to the oropharyngeal mucosa. The same technique can also be used in adults.

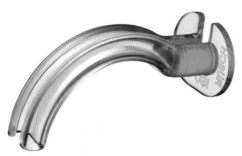

Fig. 5.38 Rüsch Berman oropharyngeal airway. (Image courtesy Teleflex Incorporated. © 2021.Teleflex Incorporated, Athlone, Ireland. All rights reserved.)

7. Berman airway is another type of oropharyngeal airway designed to assist with oral fibreoptic intubation (Fig. 5.38). It acts to guide the fibrescope around the back of the tongue to the larynx, with the purpose of both maintaining the patient's airway and acting as a bite block, thus preventing damage to the fibrescope. Unlike a Guedel airway, it has a side opening that allows it to be removed from the fibrescope prior to the railroading of the tracheal tube into the trachea.

Problems in practice and safety features

1. Trauma to the different tissues during insertion.
2. Trauma to the teeth and crowns/caps if the patient bites on it.
3. If inserted in a patient whose pharyngeal reflexes are not depressed enough, the gag reflex can be induced, which might lead to vomiting and laryngospasm.
4. They confer no protection against aspiration.
5. The degree to which airway patency has been increased after insertion of a Guedel airway should be assessed, not assumed. It should also always be remembered that a badly inserted Guedel airway can make airway patency worse rather than better.

> **Oropharyngeal airway**
> - Anatomically shaped.
> - Inserted through the mouth above the tongue into the oropharynx.
> - Maintains the patency of the upper airway.
> - Can cause trauma and injury to different structures.
> - Risk of gag reflex stimulation and vomiting.
> - Berman airway is designed to assist with oral fibreoptic intubation.

Nasopharyngeal airway

This airway is inserted through the nose into the nasopharynx, bypassing the mouth and the oropharynx. It can also be used to perform suctioning of the oropharynx.

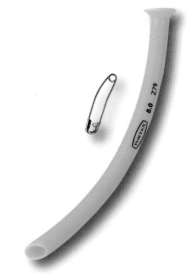

Fig. 5.39 Nasopharyngeal airway. The safety pin is to prevent the airway from migrating into the nose. (Courtesy Smiths Medical, Ashford, Kent, UK.)

The distal end is just above the epiglottis and below the base of the tongue (Fig. 5.39).

Components

1. The rounded curved body of the nasopharyngeal airway.
2. The bevel is left-facing.
3. The proximal end has a flange. In some designs, a 'safety pin' is provided to prevent the airway from migrating into the nose.

Mechanism of action

1. It is an alternative to the oropharyngeal airway when the mouth cannot be opened or an oral airway does not relieve the obstruction.
2. Nasotracheal suction can be performed using a catheter passed through the nasal airway.
3. It is better tolerated by semi-awake patients than the oral airway.
4. A lubricant is used to help in its insertion.
5. The size inserted can be estimated as size 6 for an average height female and size 7 for an average height male.
6. Once lubricated, it can be inserted through either nares, although the left-facing bevel is designed to ease insertion into the right nostril. On insertion, it should be passed backwards through the nasopharynx such that its distal end lies beyond the pharyngeal border of the soft palate but not beyond the epiglottis.

Problems in practice and safety features

1. Its use is not recommended when the patient has a bleeding disorder, is on anticoagulants, has nasal deformities or sepsis.
2. Excess force should not be used during insertion as a false passage may be created. There is a potential risk of intracranial placement in cases of basal skull fracture.
3. An airway that is too large can result in pressure necrosis of the nasal mucosa, whereas an airway that is too small may be ineffective at relieving airway obstruction.

> **Nasopharyngeal airway**
> - Inserted through the nose into the nasopharynx.
> - A useful alternative to the oropharyngeal airway.
> - Not recommended in coagulopathy, nasal sepsis and deformities.

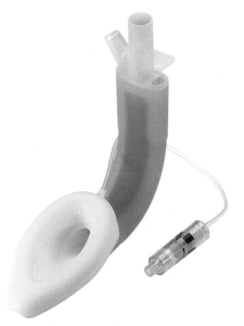

Fig. 5.40 The LMA Protector Airway with two gastric channels. (Image courtesy Teleflex Incorporated. © 2021.Teleflex Incorporated, Athlone, Ireland. All rights reserved.)

Supraglottic airway devices

The introduction of the LMA heralded an era of hands-free airway maintenance without the need for tracheal intubation. Many other airway devices (well over 100 designs) that lie outside the trachea and attempt to provide a leak-free seal for spontaneous ventilation, while some provide an adequate seal for positive pressure ventilation under normal conditions, have been used. These devices are collectively known as supraglottic airways devices (SADs). Worldwide, millions of such devices are used each year. SADs can be divided into:

- **First-generation SADs**
  These fit the description 'simple airway devices', including the original LMA Classic with only one ventilation channel. They may or may not protect against aspiration in the event of regurgitation but have no specific design features that lessen this risk.
- **Second-generation SADs**
  These have design features to reduce the risk of aspiration with a separation of ventilatory and gastric access channels; e.g. LMA ProSeal, LMA Supreme, AuraGain and i-gel. The LMA Protector Airway (Fig. 5.40) has dual gastric channels to aid in channelling gastric contents away from the airway. Such devices offer an oropharyngeal seal (first seal) and an oesophageal seal (second seal). Some designs have a 'bite block' to prevent the patient biting the tube and occluding it during emergence from anaesthesia.

SADs, in general, provide the following:

1. The ability to be placed without direct visualization of the larynx.
2. Increased speed and ease of placement when compared with tracheal intubation, both by experienced and less experienced operators.
3. Increased cardiovascular stability on insertion and emergence.
4. During emergence, improved oxygen saturation and lower frequency of coughing.
5. Minimal rise in intraocular pressure on insertion.
6. When the device is properly placed, it can act as a conduit for oral tracheal intubation due to the anatomical alignment of its aperture with the glottic opening.
7. In the 'can't intubate, can't ventilate' scenario, the decision to use such devices should be made early to gain time while attempts are made to secure a definite airway.
8. First-generation SADs normally provide little or no protection against aspiration of refluxed gastric contents and are therefore contraindicated in patients with full stomachs or prone to reflux. However, second-generation devices (e.g. LMA Protector, LMA ProSeal, LMA Supreme, AuraGain and i-gel) offer many improvements such as high

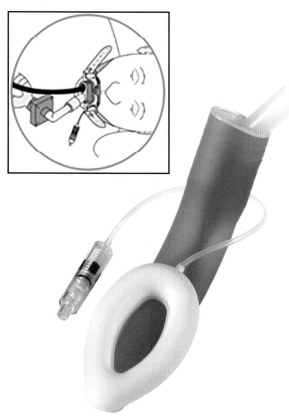

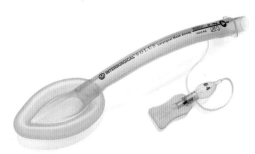

Fig. 5.42 Teleflex Classic Laryngeal Mask Airway size 4. (Courtesy Teleflex Incorporated. © 2013 Teleflex Incorporated, Dublin, Ireland. All rights reserved.)

Fig. 5.43 Single-use MRI compatible Solus laryngeal mask. (Image courtesy Intersurgical, Wokingham, UK.)

Laryngeal mask airway

This very useful device is frequently used as an alternative to either the face mask or tracheal tube during anaesthesia (Fig. 5.42).

Components

1. It has a transparent tube of wide ID. The proximal end is a standard 15-mm connection.
2. An elliptical cuff is found at the distal end. The cuff resembles a small face mask to form an air-tight seal around the posterior perimeter of the larynx and is inflated via a pilot balloon with a self-sealing valve. A nonmetallic self-sealing valve is available for use during magnetic resonance imaging (MRI) scans (Fig. 5.43).
3. The original design, LMA Classic, had two slits or bars at the junction between the tube and the cuff to prevent the epiglottis from obstructing the lumen of the laryngeal mask. Other designs, such as Intersurgical Solus, omit the bars with no adverse clinical effects.
4. A modified design, LMA ProSeal (second-generation SAD) has an additional lumen (drain tube) lateral to the airway tube and traverses the floor of the mask to open in the mask tip opposite the upper oesophageal sphincter, allowing blind passage of an orogastric tube and helping in the drainage of gastric air or secretions. Both tubes are contained within an integrated bite

Fig. 5.41 LMA Gastro Airway has a special channel allowing the insertion of an oesophago-gastro-duodenscopy scope along the airway channel. (Image courtesy Teleflex Incorporated. © 2021. Teleflex Incorporated, Athlone, Ireland. All rights reserved.)

cuff seal, second seal, gastric access and drain tube. These allow for rapid drainage of gastric fluids or secretions and reduce the risk of gastric gas insufflation during ventilation. Future indications might even be in emergency medicine, where gastric vacuity is unknown, and in cases of increased risk of regurgitation.

9. SADs would normally elicit airway reflexes such as the gag reflex and therefore require depression of pharyngeal reflexes by general or topical anaesthesia.
10. These devices are increasingly used in a variety of settings, including routine anaesthesia, emergency airway management, as an aid to intubation and during oesophago-gastro-duodenscopy (OGD) under general anaesthesia (Fig. 5.41).

 Exam tip: Classification of SADs is a common topic and how first-generation SADs differ from second-generation SADs.

which combines the best features of previous LMA versions and contains an elliptical and anatomically shaped curve, which facilitates insertion success and provides a double seal. A first seal is important for adequacy of gas exchange, better known as the oropharyngeal seal. It also incorporates a second seal, designed to reduce the risk of stomach insufflation during ventilation, to provide a passive conduit for (unexpected) regurgitation or active suctioning of gastric content and enhances the effectiveness of the first seal.

5. Low-cost disposable laryngeal masks have been introduced and are widely used.

Mechanism of action

1. A variety of techniques have been described for the insertion of the laryngeal mask. It should provide an adequate seal for spontaneous and mechanical ventilation with a minimal leak at a pressure of 20–25 cm H_2O. A seal pressure of up to 35 cm H_2O can be achieved with the LMA ProSeal.
2. The cuff is deflated and lubricated before use. It is inserted through the mouth. The cuff lies over the larynx.
3. Once the cuff is in position, it is inflated (Table 5.2). It is important to measure and monitor the cuff pressure throughout the procedure as the pressure can increase due to N_2O diffusion and warming of the inserted air. This can cause trauma to the surrounding tissues. *Cuff Pilot Technology* allows continuous cuff pressure monitoring (Fig. 5.45).
4. Partial inflation of the cuff before insertion is used by some anaesthetists.
5. The laryngeal masks have wide IDs in order to reduce the flow resistance to a minimum (e.g. the IDs of sizes 2, 3, 4 and 5 are 7, 10, 10 and 11.5 mm, respectively).

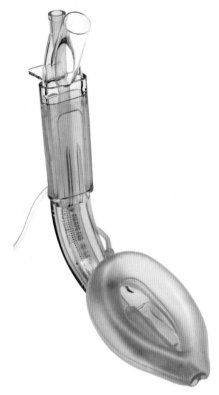

Fig. 5.44 Teleflex Single-use LMA-Unique. (© 2013 Teleflex Incorporated, Dublin, Ireland. All rights reserved.)

block. The cuff inflates in a three-dimensional manner with the elliptical cuff augmented by a second cuff behind the bowl, known as the rear boot or dorsal cuff. This design improves the seal pressure. A single-use version, LMA Supreme (Fig. 5.44), is available,

Table 5.2 The recommended sizes and cuff inflation volumes		
	Size of patient	**Cuff inflation volume**
Size 1	Neonates, infants up to 5 kg	Up to 4 mL
Size 1.5	Infants 5–10 kg	Up to 7 mL
Size 2	Infants/children 10–20 kg	Up to 10 mL
Size 2.5	Children 20–30 kg	Up to 14 mL
Size 3	Paediatric 30–50 kg	Up to 20 mL
Size 4	Adults 50–70 kg	Up to 30 mL
Size 5	Adults 70–100 kg	Up to 40 mL
Size 6	Large adults over 100 kg	Up to 60 mL

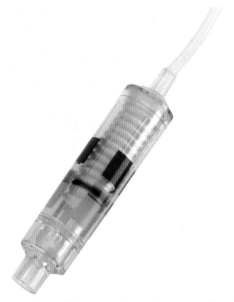

Fig. 5.45 Teleflex *Cuff Pilot Technology* used to monitor the cuff pressure; yellow zone indicates 0–40 cm H$_2$O, green zone indicates 40–60 cm H$_2$O, clear zone indicates 60–70 cm H$_2$O and red zone indicates 70+ cm H$_2$O pressures. (Image courtesy Teleflex Incorporated. © 2021. Teleflex Incorporated, Athlone, Ireland. All rights reserved.)

This makes them suitable for long procedures using a spontaneous ventilation technique.

6. It also has a role as an aid in difficult intubation. Once in position, it can be used to introduce a bougie or a narrow lumen tracheal tube into the trachea. Alternatively, the laryngeal mask may be used to guide passage of a fibreoptic bronchoscope into the trachea, thus allowing intubation of the trachea.

The **reinforced version** of the laryngeal mask is used for head and neck surgery (Fig. 5.46). The tubes, although flexible, are kink and crush resistant because of a stainless steel wire spiral in their wall. The tube can be moved during surgery without loss of the cuff's seal against the larynx. The breathing system can easily be connected at any angle from the mouth.

1. A throat pack can be used with the reinforced version.
2. The reinforced laryngeal masks have smaller IDs and longer lengths than the standard versions, causing an increase in flow resistance. This makes their use with spontaneous ventilation for prolonged periods less suitable.

Currently, there is a trend to use disposable single-use laryngeal masks (Fig. 5.47). Some have similar designs to the original LMA Classic such as Intavent Unique (Teleflex, Beaconsfield, Bucks, UK) and Intersurgical Solus laryngeal masks. Some have different designs such as the Ambu LMA device. Their clinical performance is similar to the original Classic LMA

with some achieving even better results and with fewer traumas.

The recommended safety checks before the use of laryngeal masks

- Inflate the cuff and look for signs of herniation.
- Check that the lumen of the tube is patent.
- The tube can be bent to 180 degrees without kinking or occlusion.
- Inspect the device for signs of dehiscence of the tube or mask aperture bars and cuff separations. In the reusable devices, look for signs of damage or weakness where the teeth were in contact with the tube.
- The device should also be inspected after removal from the patient for signs of bleeding.

The intubating laryngeal mask airway

The intubating laryngeal mask airway (ILMA) is a modification of the laryngeal mask designed to facilitate tracheal intubation with a tracheal tube either blindly or with a fibrescope while minimizing the requirements for head and neck manipulation. The specially designed laryngeal mask is inserted first (Fig. 5.48). A specially designed tracheal tube is then passed through the laryngeal mask through the vocal cords into the trachea. Single-use ILMA is available (Fig. 5.49).

Problems in practice and safety features

1. The laryngeal mask does not protect against the aspiration of gastric contents.
2. Despite the presence of the slits or bars, about 10% of patients develop airway obstruction because of down-folding of the epiglottis. Although clinically often insignificant, a higher proportion of obstructions by the epiglottis can be observed endoscopically. Down-folding of the epiglottis can occur in 20%–56% of patients with some having an airway obstruction.
3. The manufacturers recommend using the reusable laryngeal masks for a maximum of 40 times. The cuff is likely to perish after autoclaving. A record card that accompanies the laryngeal mask registers the number of autoclaving episodes.
4. Unlike the tracheal tube, rotation of the laryngeal mask may result in complete airway obstruction. In order to assess the orientation of the laryngeal

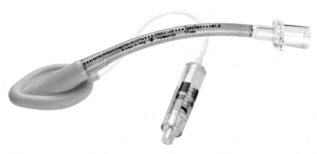

Fig. 5.46 Reinforced laryngeal mask. (Image courtesy Teleflex Incorporated. © 2021.Teleflex Incorporated, Athlone, Ireland. All rights reserved.)

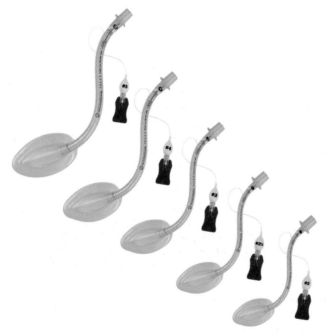

Fig. 5.47 Single-use reinforced laryngeal mask. (Courtesy Intersurgical, Wokingham, UK.)

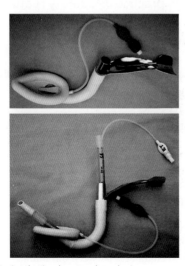

Fig. 5.48 The intubating laryngeal mask airway.

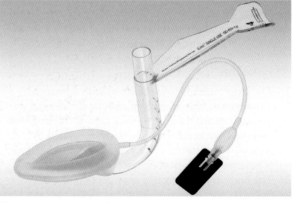

Fig. 5.49 Single-use intubating laryngeal mask airway. (Image courtesy Teleflex Incorporated. © 2021.Teleflex Incorporated, Athlone, Ireland. All rights reserved.)

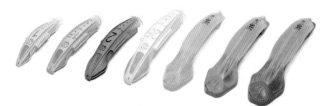

Fig. 5.50 The Intersurgical i-gel airway. (Courtesy Intersurgical, Wokingham, UK.)

mask when inserted, a black line is present on the tube. This should face the upper lip of the patient when the laryngeal mask is in position.

5. Cricoid pressure may prevent correct placement of the laryngeal mask.

> ### *Laryngeal masks*
> - Used instead of face masks or tracheal tubes during spontaneous and controlled ventilation, allowing hands-free anaesthesia.
> - Can be used as an aid in difficult intubation.
> - The reinforced version can be used for head and neck surgery.
> - Second-generation designs offer more protection against aspiration.
> - The ILMA allows blind tracheal intubation.
> - Single-use devices are commonly used.
> - It is important to measure and monitor cuff pressure.

---

i-Gel airway

The i-gel airway (Intersurgical, Wokingham, UK) is a single-use extraglottic airway that uses an anatomically designed mask to fit the perilaryngeal and hypopharyngeal structures without the use of an inflatable cuff (Fig. 5.50). As a second-generation SAD, it also incorporates a second drain tube.

Components

1. The large lumen is for ventilation with a proximal 15-mm connector. Distally, it ends in a non-inflatable gel-like cuff with a ridge at the superior anterior edge.
2. Two separate ventilation and gastric channels or lumens. The distal end of the integrated gastric lumen is positioned in the upper oesophagus.
3. The body is a wide oval in cross section.

Mechanism of action

1. The soft, gel-like plastic from which the i-gel is manufactured is intended to mould into place without the use of an inflatable cuff.

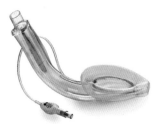

Fig. 5.51 The Ambu AuraGain airway. (Courtesy Ambu, Alconbury, Weald, Cambridgeshire, UK.)

2. The gastric channel allows direct suctioning or passage of a gastric tube.
3. The wide oval in cross section body is designed to prevent rotation and to act as an integral bite block.
4. The epiglottic blocking ridge is intended to reduce the possibility of epiglottic down-folding.
5. It is available in adult, paediatric and neonatal sizes 1–5.
6. It is intended for use with fasted patients, with both spontaneous and controlled ventilation, and can be used as a conduit for tracheal intubation.

Problems in practice and safety features

Despite its gastric channel, the i-gel does not offer absolute protection from aspiration of gastric contents.

AuraGain airway

The AuraGain (Ambu) is an anatomically curved, single-use, second-generation SAD (Fig. 5.51). It incorporates a gastric channel to allow drainage of gastric contents and the insertion of a wide-bore gastric tube, up to 16 FR. It is available in paediatric and adult sizes 1–6; the former for patients <5 kg and the latter for >100 kg body weight.

Its wide ventilation channel allows tracheal intubation, usually aided using a flexible fibreoptic scope. The ID of the ventilation channel is between 6.6 mm (size 1) and 12.9 mm (sizes 5 and 6). This allows the insertion of tracheal tube sizes of 3.5 mm (size 1) and 8 mm (sizes 5 and 6). The proximal end of the ventilation channel has a proximal 15-mm connector.

Using the AuraGain, high seal pressures up to 40 cm H$_2$O can be successfully achieved.

SUGGESTED FURTHER READING

Brimacombe, J., 2004. Laryngeal Mask Anesthesia: Principles and Practice, second ed. WB Saunders, Philadelphia.

Cook, T., Howes, B., 2011. Supraglottic airway devices: recent advances. Cont. Educ. Anaesth. Crit. Care 11 (2), 56–61.

Farrow, S., Farrow, C., Soni, N., 2012. Size matters: choosing the right tracheal tube. Anaesthesia 67, 815–822.

Frerk, C., Mitchell, V.S., McNarry, A.F., et al., 2015. Difficult Airway Society 2015 guidelines for management of unanticipated difficult intubation in adults. Br. J. Anaesthesia 115 (6), 827–848.

Haas, C.F., Eakin, R.M., Konkle, M.A., Blank, R., 2014. Endotracheal tubes: old and new. Respir. Care 59 (6), 933–955.

Van Zundert, T.C.R.V., Brimacombe, J.R., Ferson, D.Z., Bacon, D.R., Wilkinson, D.J., 2012. Archie Brain: celebrating 30 years of development in laryngeal mask airways. Anaesthesia 67 (12), 1375–1385.

SELF-ASSESSMENT QUESTIONS

Please check your eBook for additional self-assessment

MCQs

In the following lists, which of the statements (a) to (e) are true?

1. Concerning tracheal tubes
  a. The Ring, Adair and Elwyn (RAE) tracheal tube is ideal for microlaryngeal surgery.
  b. Preformed tracheal tubes have a higher risk of bronchial intubation.
  c. Laryngeal masks can be used in nasal surgery.
  d. RAE tubes stand for reinforced anaesthetic endotracheal tubes.
  e. The Oxford tracheal tube has a left-facing bevel.

2. Laryngeal masks
  a. They can prevent aspiration of gastric contents.
  b. The bars at the junction of the cuff and the tube prevent foreign bodies from entering the trachea.
  c. Because of its large internal diameter (ID), it can be used in spontaneously breathing patients for long periods of time.
  d. The reusable version can be autoclaved and used repeatedly for an unlimited number of times.
  e. The standard design can be used in magnetic resonance imaging (MRI).

3. Double lumen endobronchial tubes
  a. Robertshaw double lumen tubes have carinal hooks.
  b. The left-sided tubes have an eye in the bronchial cuff to facilitate ventilation of the left upper lobe.
  c. Carlens double lumen tubes have relatively small lumens.
  d. Continuous positive airway pressure (CPAP) can be applied to the deflated lung to improve oxygenation.
  e. Fibreoptic bronchoscopy can be used to ensure correct positioning of the tube.

4. Concerning the tracheal tube cuff during anaesthesia
  a. Low-pressure/high-volume cuffs prevent aspiration of gastric contents.
  b. The intracuff pressure can rise significantly because of the diffusion of the anaesthetic inhalational vapour.
  c. High-pressure/low-volume cuffs may cause necrosis of the tracheal mucosa if left in position for long periods.
  d. Low-volume cuffs have a smaller contact area with the tracheal wall than high-volume cuffs.
  e. The pressure in the cuff may decrease because of the diffusion of nitrous oxide.

5. Concerning tracheal tubes
  a. The ID is measured in centimetres.
  b. Red rubber tubes never have cuffs.
  c. Armoured tubes need to be cut to length.
  d. Tubes should have a Murphy eye to allow suction.
  e. The tip is cut square.

6. Concerning tracheal tubes
  a. Standard tracheal tubes have a right-facing bevel to improve view at laryngoscopy.
  b. Reinforced tubes have many rings of wire to prevent kinking.
  c. Microlaryngoscopy tubes differ from standard 5-mm tubes by having a larger cuff.
  d. Oxford tubes are kink-resistant.
  e. A standard paediatric tube is fitted with an 8.5-mm diameter connector.

7. Tracheostomy tubes
  a. Have a forward-facing bevel.
  b. Fenestrated tubes require an unfenestrated inner tube.
  c. Are available in uncuffed varieties.
  d. Insertion can cause surgical emphysema.
  e. Enlarged thyroid glands present an absolute contraindication to percutaneous tracheostomy insertion.

8. Concerning airway adjuncts
   a. Oropharyngeal airways are available in sizes 1–9.
   b. Berman airways have an opening on the side.
   c. Nasopharyngeal airways are placed so that the tip is superior to the border of the soft palate.
   d. Nasopharyngeal airways are easier to insert in the right nostril than the left.
   e. Nasopharyngeal airways should be taped in place.

Single best answer

9. Bronchial blockers
   a. Can be used only with a nasal tracheal tube.
   b. Should be used without a fibreoptic scope for guidance.
   c. Can be used for blocking only the right main bronchus.
   d. Can be used to easily suck out blood and secretions.
   e. Can have a 'hockey stick' design to aid directing placement.

10. A size 4 laryngeal mask airway Classic has an ID of
    a. 7 mm.
    b. 9 mm.
    c. 10 mm.
    d. 11.5 mm.
    e. 12 mm.

11. Which of the following statements regarding supraglottic airways is correct?
    a. Classic LMAs can be safely used in MRI scanners.
    b. i-Gels are available in seven sizes.
    c. LMAs cause airway obstruction by folding the epiglottis in 20% of insertions.
    d. For secondary intubation using an intubating LMA, a standard 6.0-mm tracheal tube is used.
    e. Cricoid pressure aids insertion of the intubating LMA.

Answers

1. *Concerning tracheal tubes*
   a. **False.** *An RAE tube is a normal size preformed tracheal tube. It does not allow good visibility of the larynx because of its large diameter. A microlaryngeal tracheal tube of 5–6 mm ID is more suitable for microlaryngeal surgery, allowing good visibility and access to the larynx.*
   b. **True.** *Because the shape of these tubes is fixed, they might not fit all patients of different sizes and shapes; e.g. a small, short-necked patient having an RAE tube inserted is at risk of an endobronchial tube position.*
   c. **True.** *Some anaesthetists use the laryngeal mask in nasal surgery with a throat pack. This technique has a higher risk of aspiration.*
   d. **False.** *RAE stands for the initials of the designers (Ring, Adair and Elwyn).*
   e. **False.** *The Oxford tube is one of the few tracheal tubes with a front-facing bevel. This might make intubation more difficult as it obscures the larynx.*

2. *Laryngeal masks*
   a. **False.** *Laryngeal masks do not completely protect the airway from the risks of aspiration.*
   b. **False.** *The bars in the cuff are designed to prevent the epiglottis from blocking the lumen of the tube.*
   c. **True.** *The laryngeal mask has a large ID in comparison with a tracheal tube. This reduces the resistance to breathing, which is of more importance during spontaneous breathing. This makes the laryngeal mask more suitable for use in spontaneously breathing patients for long periods of time.*
   d. **False.** *The reusable laryngeal mask can be autoclaved up to 40 times. The cuff is likely to perish after repeated autoclaving. A record should be kept of the number of autoclaves.*
   e. **False.** *The standard laryngeal mask has a metal component in the one-way inflating valve. This makes it unsuitable for use in MRI. A specially designed laryngeal mask with no metal parts is available for MRI use.*

3. *Double lumen endobronchial tubes*
   a. **False.** *The Robertshaw double lumen tube does not have a carinal hook. The Carlens double lumen tube has a carinal hook.*
   b. **False.** *Left-sided tubes do not have an eye in the bronchial cuff to facilitate ventilation of the left upper lobe. This is because the distance between the carina and the upper lobe bronchus is about 5 cm, which is enough for the bronchial cuff. Right-sided tubes have an eye to facilitate ventilation of the right upper lobe because the distance between the carina and the upper lobe bronchus is only 2.5 cm.*
   c. **True.** *Carlens double lumen tubes have relatively small lumens in comparison to the Robertshaw double lumen tube.*
   d. **True.** *CPAP can be applied to the deflated lung to improve oxygenation during one-lung anaesthesia.*
   e. **True.** *It is sometimes difficult to ensure correct positioning of the double lumen endobronchial tube. By using a fibreoptic bronchoscope, the position of the tube can be adjusted to ensure correct positioning.*

4. *Concerning the tracheal tube cuff during anaesthesia*
   a. **False.** *The design of the low-pressure/high-volume cuff allows wrinkles to be formed around the tracheal wall. The presence of the wrinkles allows aspiration of gastric contents to occur.*
   b. **False.** *The rise in the intracuff pressure is mainly due to the diffusion of N_2O. Minimal changes are due to diffusion of oxygen (from 21% to, say, 33%) and because of increase in the temperature of the air in the cuff (from 21°C to 37°C). The diffusion of inhalational agents causes minimal changes in pressure due to the low concentrations used (1%–2%). New design material cuffs prevent the diffusion of gases, thus preventing significant changes in pressure.*
   c. **True.** *The high pressures achieved by the high-pressure/low-volume cuffs, especially during nitrous oxide anaesthesia, can cause necrosis to the mucosa of the trachea if left in position for a long period.*
   d. **True.** *Because of the design of the low-volume cuffs, a seal can be maintained against a relatively small area of the tracheal wall. In the case of the high-volume/low-pressure cuffs, a large contact area on the tracheal wall is achieved.*
   e. **False.** *The pressure in the cuff may decrease because of a leak in the cuff or the pilot balloon's valve.*

5. *Concerning tracheal tubes*
   a. **False.** *The ID is measured in millimetres.*
   b. **False.**

c. **False.** An armoured tube should not be cut, as that will cut the spiral present in its wall. This increases the risk of tube kinking.

d. **False.** A Murphy eye allows pulmonary ventilation in the situation in which the bevel of the tube is occluded.

e. **False.** The bevel of the tube is usually left-facing to allow easier visualization of the vocal cords. The tracheostomy tube has a square-cut tip.

6. *Concerning tracheal tubes*

a. **False.** A left-facing bevel improves view at laryngoscopy.

b. **False.** Reinforced tubes have a spiral of wire running through the wall to resist crushing and kinking.

c. **True.**

d. **True.** They have a thicker than usual wall to prevent kinking, but this reduces ID.

e. **True.**

7. *Tracheostomy tubes*

a. **False.** Tracheostomy tubes are cut horizontally.

b. **False.** Fenestrated inner tubes can be used to allow phonation.

c. **True.**

d. **True.**

e. **False.** This is a relative contraindication; ultrasound or cross-sectional imaging should be considered to identify if percutaneous tracheostomy can be safely attempted.

8. *Concerning airway adjuncts*

a. **False.** Nine sizes are available, but they are numbered 000–6.

b. **True.**

c. **False.** The tip should be inferior to the soft palate.

d. **True.**

e. **False.** Nasopharyngeal airways do not require tape. A flanged end or safety pin prevents migration into the nose.

9. *e.*

10. *c.*

11. *b.*

Chapter 6

Face masks and oxygen delivery devices

Face masks and angle pieces

The face mask is designed to fit the face anatomically and comes in different sizes to fit patients of different age groups (from neonates to adults). It is connected to the breathing system via the angle piece.

Components

1. The body of the mask, which rests on an air-filled cuff (Fig. 6.1). Some paediatric designs do not have a cuff, e.g. Rendell–Baker (Fig. 6.2).
2. The proximal end of the mask has a 22-mm inlet connection to the angle piece.
3. Some designs have clamps for a harness to be attached.
4. The angle piece has a 90-degree bend with a 22-mm end to fit into a catheter mount or a breathing system.

Mechanism of action

1. They are made of transparent plastic. Previously, masks made of silicon rubber were used. The transparent plastic allows the detection of vomitus or secretions. It is also more acceptable to the patient during inhalational induction. Some masks are 'flavoured', e.g. strawberry flavour.
2. The cuff helps to ensure a snug fit over the face, covering the mouth and nose. It also helps to minimize the mask's pressure on the face. Cuffs can be either air-filled or made from a soft material.
3. The design of the interior of the mask determines the size of its contribution to apparatus dead space. The dead space may increase by up to 200 mL in adults. Paediatric masks are designed to reduce the dead space as much as possible.

Problems in practice and safety features

1. Excessive pressure by the mask may cause injury to the branches of the trigeminal or facial nerves.
2. Sometimes it is difficult to achieve an air-tight seal over the face. Edentulous patients and those with nasogastric tubes pose particular problems.
3. Imprecise application of the mask on the face can cause trauma to the eyes.

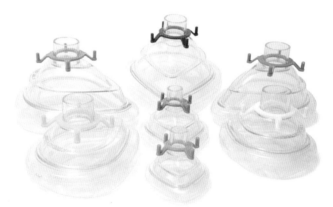

Fig. 6.1 A range of transparent face masks with air-filled cuffs. (Courtesy of Intersurgical, Wokingham, UK.)

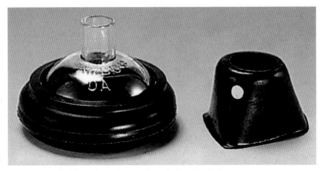

Fig. 6.2 Paediatric face masks. Ambu design *(left)* and Rendell–Baker design *(right)*.

Face masks
- Made of silicone rubber or plastic.
- Their design ensures a snug fit over the face of the patient.
- Cause an increase in dead space (up to 200 mL in adults).
- Can cause trauma to the eyes and facial nerves.

NASAL MASKS (INHALERS)

1. These masks are used during dental chair anaesthesia.
2. An example is the Goldman inhaler (Fig. 6.3), which has an inflatable cuff to fit the face and an adjustable pressure limiting (APL) valve at the proximal end. The mask is connected to tubing, which delivers the fresh gas flow (FGF).
3. Other designs have an inlet for delivering the inspired FGF and an outlet connected to tubing with a unidirectional valve for expired gases.

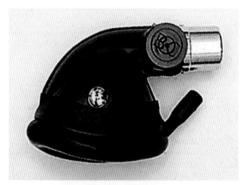

Fig. 6.3 The Goldman nasal inhaler.

Catheter mount

This is the flexible link between the breathing system tubing and the tracheal tube, face mask, supraglottic airway device or tracheostomy tube (Fig. 6.4). The length of the catheter mount varies from 45 to 170 mm.

Components

1. It has a corrugated disposable plastic tubing. Some catheter mounts have a concertina design, allowing their length to be adjusted.
2. The distal end is connected to either a 15-mm standard tracheal tube connector, usually in the shape of an angle piece, or a 22-mm mask fitting.
3. The proximal end has a 22-mm connector for attachment to the breathing system.
4. Some designs have a condenser humidifier built into them.
5. A gas sampling port is found in some designs.

Mechanism of action

1. The mount minimizes the transmission of accidental movements of the breathing system to the tracheal tube. Repeated movements of the tracheal tube can cause injury to the tracheal mucosa.
2. Some designs allow for suction or the introduction of a fibreoptic bronchoscope. This is done via a special port.

Problems in practice and safety features

1. The catheter mount contributes to the apparatus dead space. This is of particular importance in paediatric anaesthesia. The concertina design allows adjustment of the dead space from 25 to 60 mL.
2. Foreign bodies can lodge inside the catheter mount causing an unnoticed blockage of the breathing system. To minimize this risk, the catheter mount

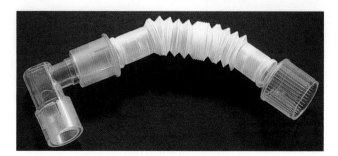

Fig. 6.4 Catheter mount.

should remain wrapped in its sterile packaging until needed.

Catheter mount
- Acts as an adapter between the tracheal tube and breathing system in addition to stabilizing the tracheal tube.
- It is made of plastic with different lengths available.
- Some have a condenser humidifier built in.
- Its length contributes to the apparatus dead space.
- Can be blocked by a foreign body.

Oxygen delivery devices

Currently, a variety of delivery devices are used. These devices differ in their ability to deliver a set fractional inspired oxygen concentration (FiO_2). The delivery devices can be divided into variable and fixed performance devices. The former devices deliver a fluctuating FiO_2 whereas the latter devices deliver a more constant and predictable FiO_2 (Table 6.1). The FiO_2 delivered to the patient is dependent on device- and patient-related factors. The FiO_2 delivered can be calculated by measuring the

end-tidal oxygen fraction in the nasopharynx using oxygraphy.

Variable performance masks (medium concentration [MC])

These masks are used to deliver oxygen-enriched air to the patient (Fig. 6.5). They are also called *low-flow delivery devices*. They are widely used in the hospital because of greater patient comfort, low cost, simplicity and the ability to manipulate the FiO_2 without changing the appliance. Their performance varies between patients and from

Table 6.1 Classification of the oxygen delivery systems

Variable performance devices	Fixed performance devices
Hudson face masks and partial rebreathing masks Nasal cannulae (prongs or spectacles) Nasal catheters	Venturi-operated devices Anaesthetic breathing systems with a suitably large reservoir

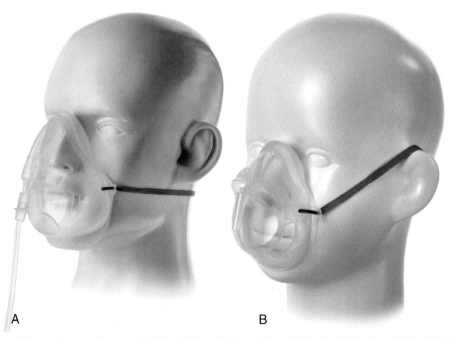

Fig. 6.5 (A) Adult variable performance face mask. (B) Paediatric variable performance face mask. (Courtesy Intersurgical, Wokingham, UK.)

Table 6.2 Factors that affect the delivered FiO_2 in the variable performance masks

High FiO_2 delivered	Low FiO_2 delivered
Low peak inspiratory flow rate	High peak inspiratory flow rate
Slow respiratory rate	Fast respiratory rate
High fresh oxygen flow rate	Low fresh oxygen flow rate
Tightly fitting face mask	Less tightly fitting face mask

breath to breath within the same patient. These systems have a limited reservoir capacity, so in order to function appropriately, the patient must inhale some ambient air to meet the inspiratory demands. The FiO_2 is determined by the oxygen flow rate, the size of the oxygen reservoir and the respiratory pattern (Table 6.2).

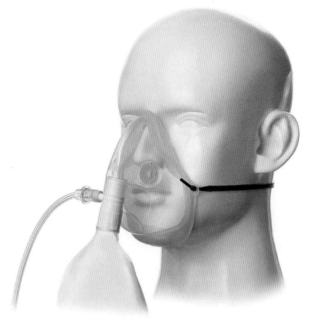

Fig. 6.6 A variable performance mask with a reservoir bag. (Courtesy Intersurgical, Wokingham, UK.)

Components

1. The plastic body of the mask has holes on both sides.
2. A port is connected to an oxygen supply.
3. Elastic band(s) fix(es) the mask to the patient's face.

Mechanism of action

1. Ambient air is entrained through the holes on both sides of the mask. The holes also allow exhaled gases to be vented out.
2. During the expiratory pause, the fresh oxygen supplied helps in venting out the exhaled gases through the side holes. The body of the mask (acting as a reservoir) is filled with a fresh oxygen supply and is available for the start of the next inspiration.
3. The final concentration of inspired oxygen depends on:
   a. the oxygen supply flow rate
   b. the pattern of ventilation: If there is a pause between expiration and inspiration, the mask fills with oxygen and a high concentration is available at the start of inspiration.
   c. the patient's inspiratory flow rate: During inspiration, oxygen is diluted by the air drawn in through the holes when the inspiratory flow rate exceeds the flow of oxygen supply. During normal tidal ventilation, the peak inspiratory flow rate is 20–30 L/min, which is higher than the oxygen supplied to the patient and the oxygen that is contained in the body of the mask, so some ambient air is inhaled to meet the demands, thus diluting the fresh oxygen supply. The peak inspiratory flow rate increases further during deep inspiration and during hyperventilation.
   d. how tight the mask fits on the face.
4. If there is no expiratory pause, alveolar gases may be rebreathed from the mask at the start of inspiration.
5. The rebreathing of CO_2 from the body of the mask (apparatus dead space of about 100 mL) is usually of little clinical significance in adults but may be a problem in some patients who are not able to compensate by increasing their alveolar ventilation. CO_2 elimination can be improved by increasing the fresh oxygen flow and is inversely related to the minute ventilation. The rebreathing is also increased when the mask body is large and when the resistance to flow from the side holes is high (when the mask is a good fit). The patients may experience a sense of warmth and humidity, indicating significant rebreathing.
6. A typical example of 4 L/min of oxygen flow delivers an FiO_2 of about 0.35–0.4, providing there is a normal respiratory pattern.
7. Adding a 600–800-mL bag to the mask will act as an extra reservoir (Fig. 6.6). Such masks are known as 'partial rebreathing masks' or 'nonrebreather masks'.

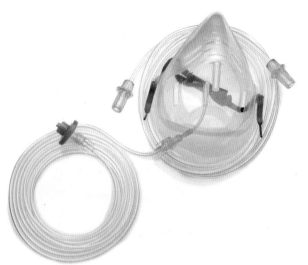

Fig. 6.7 A variable performance mask with an exhaled CO_2 monitoring port. (Courtesy Intersurgical, Wokingham, UK.)

A one-way valve is fitted between mask and reservoir to prevent rebreathing to ensure a 100% O_2 in the reservoir. The inspired oxygen is derived from the continuous fresh oxygen supply, oxygen present in the reservoir and the entrained ambient air. Higher variable FiO_2 (0.6–0.8) can be achieved with such masks.

8. Some designs have an extra port attached to the body of the mask, allowing it to be connected to a side-stream CO_2 monitor (Fig. 6.7). This allows it to sample the exhaled CO_2 so monitoring the patient's respiration, e.g. during sedation.

9. Similar masks can be used in patients with tracheostomy (Fig. 6.8). As with the face mask, similar factors will affect its performance. Care must be taken to humidify the inspired dry oxygen as the gases delivered bypass the nose and its humidification.

Problems in practice and safety features

These devices are used only when delivering a fixed oxygen concentration is not critical. Patients whose ventilation is dependent on a hypoxic drive must not receive oxygen from a variable performance mask.

> **Variable performance mask, MC mask**
> - Entrains ambient air.
> - The inspired oxygen concentration depends on the oxygen flow rate, pattern and rate of ventilation, maximum inspiratory flow rate and how well the mask fits the patient's face.
> - Adding a reservoir with a one-way valve can significantly increase FiO_2 delivered.

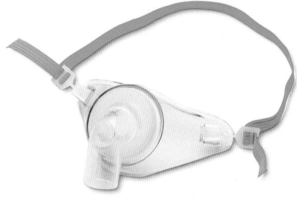

Fig. 6.8 Variable performance tracheostomy mask.

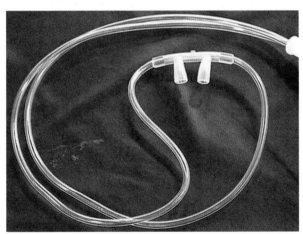

Fig. 6.9 Oxygen nasal cannula.

Nasal cannulae

Nasal cannulae are ideal for patients on long-term oxygen therapy (Fig. 6.9). A flow rate of 2–4 L/min delivers an FiO_2 of 0.28–0.36, respectively. Higher flow rates are uncomfortable. Humidifying oxygen allows higher flow rates to be used. They are available in various sizes suitable for adult and paediatric patients.

Components

1. It has two prongs that protrude about 1 cm into the nose. Different design prongs are available (straight, curved and flared).
2. These are held in place by an adjustable head strap.

Mechanism of action

1. There is entrainment of ambient air through the nostrils. The nasopharynx acts as a reservoir.

2. The FiO_2 achieved is proportional to:
   a. the flow rate of oxygen
   b. the patient's tidal volume, inspiratory flow and respiratory rate
   c. the volume of the nasopharynx.
3. Mouth breathing causes inspiratory air flow. This produces a Venturi effect in the posterior pharynx, entraining oxygen from the nose.
4. There is increased patient compliance with nasal cannulae compared with facial oxygen masks. The patient is able to speak, eat and drink.
5. Some designs have the facility to sample exhaled CO_2 in addition to delivering oxygen. One prong is used to deliver oxygen while the other prong samples the exhaled CO_2. When connected to a side-stream CO_2 monitor (Fig. 6.10), it is possible to monitor the patient's respiration, e.g. during sedation.

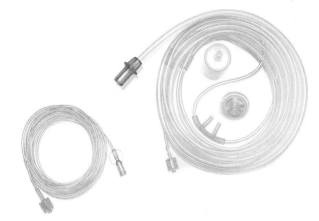

Fig. 6.10 Nasal cannula with exhaled CO_2 sampling. (Courtesy Intersurgical, Wokingham, UK.)

Problems in practice and safety features

The cannulae and the dry gas flow cause trauma and irritation to the nasal mucosa. They are not appropriate in patients with blocked nasal passages.

Nasal cannulae
- Entrainment of ambient air through the nostrils and during mouth breathing.
- The FiO_2 depends on the oxygen flow rate, tidal volume, inspiratory flow rate, respiratory rate and the volume of the nasopharynx.
- Better patient compliance compared with facial masks.

Nasal catheters

Nasal catheters comprise a single lumen catheter, which is lodged into the anterior naris (nostril) by a foam collar (Fig. 6.11). Oxygen flows of 2–3 L/min can be used. The catheter can be secured to the patient's face by using tape. It can be useful in patients undergoing certain surgical procedures, such as lacrimal surgery under regional anaesthesia. It should not be used when a nasal mucosal tear is suspected because of the risk of surgical emphysema.

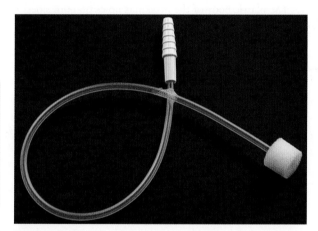

Fig. 6.11 Oxygen nasal catheter.

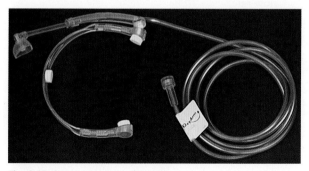

Fig. 6.12 Open oxygen supply system.

Open oxygen delivery systems

These are designed to offer the maximum comfort to patients while delivering variable FiO_2 concentrations. They fit around the patient's head like headphones, so making minimal physical contact (Fig. 6.12). Such systems are suitable for both nasal- and mouth-breathing patients. They may be more suitable for patients on long-term oxygen therapy.

A wide range of fresh oxygen flows can be used, so delivering a variable performance. As with the other devices of this kind, similar factors will affect its performance.

 Exam tip: It is important to understand how the variable performance devices function. Why are they termed 'variable'?

Fixed performance devices

VENTURI MASK

These masks are fixed performance devices (sometimes called *high-air-flow oxygen enrichment*, or HAFOE).

Components

1. The plastic body of the mask has holes on both sides.
2. The proximal end of the mask consists of a Venturi device. The Venturi devices are colour-coded (Table 6.3) and marked with the recommended oxygen flow rate to provide the desired oxygen concentration (Fig. 6.13).

Mechanism of action

1. The Venturi mask uses the Bernoulli principle, described in 1778 (*in order to maintain a constant flow, a fluid must increase its velocity as it flows through a constriction*), in delivering a predetermined and fixed concentration of oxygen to the patient. The size of the constriction determines the final concentration of oxygen for a given gas flow. This is achieved despite the patient's respiratory pattern by providing a higher gas flow than the peak inspiratory flow rate.
2. The Bernoulli effect can be written as:

$$P + \tfrac{1}{2}\rho v^2 = \kappa$$

where ϱ is the density, v is the velocity, P is the pressure and κ is a constant.
3. As the flow of oxygen passes through the constriction, a negative pressure is created. This causes the ambient air to be entrained and mixed with the oxygen flow (Fig. 6.14). The FiO_2 is dependent on the degree of air entrainment. Less entrainment ensures a higher FiO_2 is delivered. This can be achieved by using smaller entrainment apertures or bigger 'windows' to entrain ambient air. The smaller the orifice is, the greater the negative pressure generated, so the more ambient air entrained, the lower the FiO_2. The oxygen concentration can be 0.24, 0.28, 0.3, 0.35, 0.4, 0.5 or 0.6.

Table 6.3 Colour coding for Venturi devices in the United Kingdom

Colour	FiO$_2$	Recommended oxygen FGF L/min
Blue	0.24	2
White	0.28	4
Orange	0.31	6
Yellow	0.35	8
Red	0.40	10
Pink	0.50	15
Green	0.60	15

FGF, Fresh gas flow; *FiO$_2$*, Fractional inspired oxygen concentration.

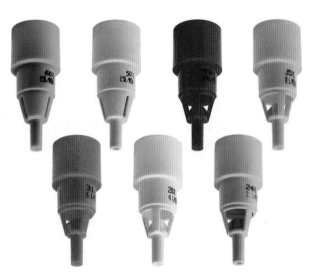

Fig. 6.13 Colour coding for Venturi devices in the United Kingdom, the set fractional inspired oxygen concentration and recommended fresh gas flow. (Courtesy Intersurgical, Wokingham, UK.)

4. The total energy during a fluid (gas or liquid) flow consists of the sum of kinetic and potential energy. The kinetic energy is related to the velocity of the flow, whereas the potential energy is related to the pressure. As the flow of fresh oxygen passes through the constricted orifice into the larger chamber, the velocity of the gas increases distal to the orifice, causing the kinetic energy to increase. As the total energy is constant, there is a decrease in the potential energy so a negative pressure is created. This causes the ambient air to be entrained and mixed with the oxygen flow. The FiO_2 is

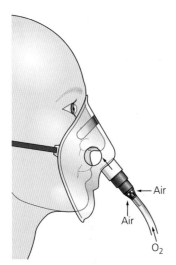

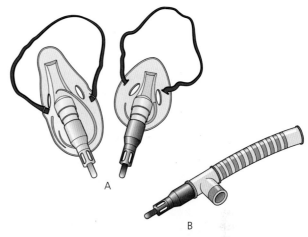

Fig. 6.16 (A) Adult and paediatric Venturi masks. (B) Venturi device as part of a breathing system.

Fig. 6.14 Mechanism of action of the fixed performance Venturi mask.

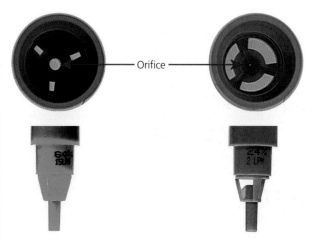

Orifice

Fig. 6.15 Detail of the Venturi device. Design for administering 60% oxygen *(left)* and 24% *(right)*. Note the difference in the recommended oxygen flow rates and the size of orifice and air entrainment apertures.

7. For example, a 24% oxygen Venturi mask has an air:oxygen entrainment ratio of 25:1. This means an oxygen flow of 2 L/min delivers a total flow of 50 L/min, well above the peak inspiratory flow rate.
8. The mask's side holes are used to vent the exhaled gases only (as above) in comparison to the side holes in the variable performance mask in which the side holes are used to entrain inspired air in addition to expel exhaled gases.
9. The Venturi face masks are designed for both adult and paediatric use (Fig. 6.16A).
10. The Venturi attachments, with a reservoir tubing, can be attached to a tracheal tube or a supraglottic airway device as part of a T-piece breathing system (Fig. 6.16B). This arrangement is usually used in postanaesthesia care units to deliver oxygen-enriched air to patients.
11. A more recent design is the *adjustable Venturi device*. The FiO_2 can be changed without changing the valve by changing the size of the entrainment window and adjusting the oxygen flow rate (Fig. 6.17).

Problems in practice and safety features

1. These masks are recommended when a fixed oxygen concentration is desired in patients whose ventilation is dependent on their hypoxic drive, such as those with chronic obstructive pulmonary disease. However, caution should be exercised as it has been shown that the average FiO_2 delivered in such masks is up to 5% above the expected value.
2. The Venturi mask with its Venturi device and the oxygen delivery tubing is often not well tolerated by patients because it is noisy and bulky.

Anaesthetic breathing systems are other examples of the fixed performance devices. The reservoir bag acts

dependent on the degree of air entrainment. Less entrainment ensures higher FiO_2 is delivered, and smaller entrainment apertures are one method of achieving this (see Fig. 6.15). The devices must be driven by the correct oxygen flow rate, calibrated for the aperture size if a predictable FiO_2 is to be achieved.
5. Because of the high FGF rate, the exhaled gases are rapidly flushed from the mask via its holes. Therefore there is no rebreathing and no increase in dead space.
6. These masks are recommended when a fixed oxygen concentration is desired in patients whose ventilation is dependent on the hypoxic drive.

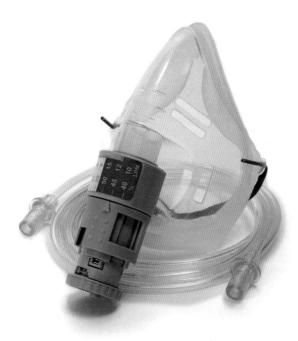

Fig. 6.17 Adjustable Venturi valve. (Courtesy Intersurgical, Wokingham, UK.)

to deliver a FGF that is greater than the patient's peak inspiratory flow rate.

Venturi mask
- Fixed performance device (HAFOE).
- Uses the Venturi principle to entrain ambient air.
- No rebreathing or increase in dead space.
- Changes in kinetic and potential energy during gas flow lead to negative pressure and air entrainment.

Humidified high-flow nasal oxygenation (Fig. 6.18)

This device delivers warm and humidified high inspiratory flow of accurate oxygen concentrations. It acts as a fixed performance device. Its use in intensive care, high dependency units, theatres and A&E has increased during the COVID pandemic in attempts to reduce the incidence of tracheal intubation and mechanical ventilation. It can also be used as part of a ventilation weaning strategy. It is also useful when preoxygenating a patient who may be difficult to intubate.

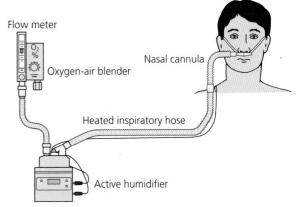

Fig. 6.18 Humidified high-flow nasal oxygenation.

Components
1. Air/oxygen blender to adjust FiO_2.
2. An active humidifier.
3. A single heated circuit of corrugated tubing.
4. A nasal cannula.

Mechanism of action
1. Flows of up to 70 L/min of warm (up to 37°C) and humidified gas (with an absolute humidity of 44 mg H_2O/L) of a more reliable FiO_2 are delivered to a patient via a nasal cannula.
2. It is thought that it produces a reduction of pharyngeal anatomical dead space with a moderate positive airway pressure (CPAP) effect of about 2.7–7.4 cm H_2O.
3. The above can lead to reduced work of breathing, improved oxygenation and ventilatory efficiency.
4. Such systems enhance patient comfort, mucociliary clearance and tolerance compared with other oxygen delivery systems.

Problems in practice and safety features
1. Contraindicated in recent nasal surgery and severe epistaxis.
2. Base of skull fracture and/or cerebrospinal fluid (CSF) leak.
3. High flows generate significant noise.
4. The heated, humidified gases can make the nose feel hot.

Humidified high-flow nasal oxygenation
- Humidified and warmed flows of up to 60 L/min.
- Accurate FiO_2 is delivered.
- Reduces work of breathing.
- Provides a moderate CPAP effect.

Exam tip: It is important to understand how the fixed devices function. A full knowledge of how the Venturi devices work is essential. Also a good understanding of high-flow humidified nasal oxygenation is needed.

SUGGESTED FURTHER READING

Estates and Facilities Alert NHSE/I – 2020/001, Issued 31 March 2020. Use of high flow Oxygen therapy devices (including wall CPAP and high flow face mask or nasal oxygen) during the Coronavirus epidemic – urgent patient safety notice; immediate attention required.

Medicines and Healthcare Products Regulatory Agency (MHRA), 2011. Medical Device alert: Oxygen Masks Manufactured by Lifecare Hospital Supplies Ltd.

MDA/2011/015) http://webarchive.nationalarchives.gov.uk/20141205150130/http://www.mhra.gov.uk/Publications/Safetywarnings/MedicalDeviceAlerts/CON108738.

Nishimura, M., 2015. High-flow nasal cannula oxygen therapy in adults. J. Intens. Care 3 (1), 15.

Renda, T., Corrado, A., Iskandar, G., Pelaia, G., Abdalla, K., Navalesi, P., 2018. High-flow nasal oxygen therapy in intensive care and anaesthesia. B. J. Anaesth. 120 (1), 18–27.

The Royal Children's Hospital Melbourne. Oxygen delivery. https://www.rch.org.au/rchcpg/hospital_clinical_guideline_index/Oxygen_delivery/

Waldau, T., Larsen, V.H., Bonde, J., 1998. Evaluation of five oxygen delivery devices in spontaneously breathing subjects by oxygraphy. Anaesthesia 53, 256–263.

SELF-ASSESSMENT QUESTIONS

Please check your eBook for additional self-assessment

MCQs

In the following lists, which of the statements (a) to (e) are true?

1. **Concerning the Venturi mask**
   a. Gas flow produced should be more than 20 L/min.
   b. Reducing the flow of oxygen from 12 to 8 L/min results in a reduction in oxygen concentration.
   c. With a constant oxygen supply flow, widening the orifice in the Venturi device increases the oxygen concentration delivered to the patient.
   d. There is rebreathing in the mask.
   e. The mask is a fixed performance device.

2. **High-air-flow oxygen enrichment face masks**
   a. Use the Venturi principle to deliver a fixed O_2 concentration to the patient.
   b. The size of the constriction of the Venturi has no effect on the final O_2 concentration delivered to the patient.
   c. The holes on the side of the mask are used to entrain ambient air.
   d. The gas flow delivered to the patient is more than the peak inspiratory flow rate.
   e. There is significant rebreathing.

3. **Face masks used during anaesthesia**
   a. The rubber mask is covered by carbon particles, which act as an antistatic measure.
   b. Masks have no effect on the apparatus dead space.
   c. The mask's cuff has to be checked and inflated before use.
   d. The dental nasal masks are also known as nasal inhalers.
   e. Masks have a 15-mm end to fit the catheter mount.

4. **Concerning the oxygen nasal cannula**
   a. Is a fixed performance device.
   b. Is a variable performance device.

   c. There is a Venturi effect in the posterior pharynx.
   d. An oxygen flow of 8 L/min is usually used in an adult.
   e. Has increased patient compliance.

5. **Variable performance masks**
   a. During slow and deep breathing, a higher FiO_2 can be achieved.
   b. Ambient air is not entrained into the mask.
   c. Alveolar gas rebreathing is not possible.
   d. Normal inspiratory peak flow rate is 20–30 L/min for an adult.
   e. Can be used safely on all patients.

6. **Regarding variable performance devices**
   a. They can offer greater patient compliance.
   b. They can deliver an FiO_2 that can vary from breath to breath in the same patient.
   c. The size of the medium concentration oxygen face mask has no effect on rebreathing and CO_2 elimination.
   d. Capnography can be used to measure the FiO_2 delivered to the patient.
   e. With a variable performance mask, the FiO_2 is higher when the face mask is a tight fit.

7. **Concerning fixed performance devices**
   a. Anaesthetic breathing systems with reservoirs are fixed performance devices.
   b. Distal to the constriction of a Venturi device, there is an increase in potential energy.
   c. In a Venturi mask, the higher the entrainment ratio, the higher the FiO_2.
   d. A nasal oxygen catheter is a fixed performance device.
   e. Venturi masks are very well tolerated by patients.

Single best answer

8. Catheter mounts
   a. Should have a 22-mm connector at the distal (patient) end.
   b. Should have a 15-mm connector at the proximal (machine) end.
   c. Gas sampling ports should always be built into the structure.
   d. Should never incorporate an angle piece.
   e. Should have a 15-mm connector at the distal (patient) end.

9. Average delivered oxygen percentage from a Venturi device can vary from the expected value by what percentage?
   a. 1%.
   b. 2%.
   c. 5%.
   d. 7.5%.
   e. 10%.

Answers

1. Concerning the Venturi mask
   a. **True.** *The Venturi mask is a fixed performance device. In order to achieve this, the flow delivered to the patient should be more than the peak inspiratory flow rate. A flow of more than 20 L/min is adequate.*
   b. **True.** *It is the flow rate of oxygen through the orifice that determines the final FiO_2 the patient receives. With a constant orifice, the amount of air entrained remains constant. So by reducing the oxygen flow rate from 12 to 8 L/min, less oxygen will be in the final mixture.*
   c. **True.** *The wider the orifice, the less the drop in pressure across the orifice and the less the entrainment of the ambient air, hence the less the dilution of the O_2, resulting in an increase in oxygen concentration delivered to the patient. The opposite is also correct.*
   d. **False.** *There is no rebreathing in the mask because of the high fresh gas flow (FGF) rates, causing the exhaled gases to be flushed from the mask through the side holes.*
   e. **True.** *The Venturi mask is a fixed performance device that delivers a constant concentration of oxygen in spite of the patient's respiratory pattern, by providing a higher gas flow than the peak inspiratory flow rate.*

2. High-air-flow oxygen enrichment face masks
   a. **True.** *Laminar flow through a constriction causes a decrease in pressure at the constriction. This leads to entrainment of ambient air leading to mixture of fixed oxygen concentration.*
   b. **False.** *It is the size of the orifice that determines the degree of decrease in pressure at the constriction. This determines the amount of ambient air being entrained, hence the final concentration of oxygen.*
   c. **False.** *In such a mask, the holes are used to expel the exhaled gases. Ambient air is not entrained in such a mask because of the high gas flows. The holes in a variable performance mask are used to entrain ambient air.*
   d. **True.** *The gas flow generated is higher than the peak inspiratory flow rate. This allows the delivery of a fixed oxygen concentration to the patient regardless of the inspiratory flow rate. It also prevents rebreathing.*

   e. **False.** *There is no rebreathing because of the high flows delivered to the patient. The exhaled gases are expelled through the holes in the mask.*

3. Face masks used during anaesthesia
   a. **True.** *Carbon particles prevent the build-up of static electricity. The rubber face masks and the rubber tubings used in anaesthesia are covered with carbon. With modern anaesthetic practice in which no flammable drugs are used, its significance has all but disappeared.*
   b. **False.** *Face masks can have a significant effect on the apparatus dead space if the wrong size is chosen. In an adult, the dead space can increase by about 200 mL. It is of more importance in paediatric practice.*
   c. **True.** *The cuff of the face mask is designed to ensure a snug fit over the patient's face and to minimize the mask's pressure on the face. Ensuring that the cuff is inflated before use is therefore important.*
   d. **True.** *Nasal inhalers are nasal masks used during dental anaesthesia, allowing good surgical access to the mouth. The Goldman nasal inhaler is an example.*
   e. **False.** *The face masks have a 22-mm end to fit the angle piece or catheter mount.*

4. Concerning the oxygen nasal cannula
   a. **False.** *It is not a fixed performance device. The final FiO_2 depends on the flow rate of oxygen, tidal volume, inspiratory flow, respiratory rate and the volume of the nasopharynx.*
   b. **True.** *See above.*
   c. **True.** *During mouth breathing, the inspiratory air flow produces a Venturi effect in the posterior pharynx, entraining oxygen from the nose.*
   d. **False.** *It is uncomfortable for the patient to have higher flows than 1–4 L/min.*
   e. **True.** *Patients tolerate the nasal cannula for much longer periods than a face mask. Patients are capable of eating, drinking and speaking despite the cannula.*

5. Variable performance masks
   a. **True.** *This allows FGF during the expiratory pause to fill the mask ready for the following inspiration. In tachypnoea (fast and shallow breathing), the opposite occurs when there is not enough time for the FGF to fill the mask.*

b. **False.** The maximum inspiratory flow rate is much higher than the FGF, so ambient air is entrained into the mask through the side holes.

c. **False.** During tachypnoea, there is not enough time for the FGF to fill the mask and expel the exhaled gases. This leads to rebreathing of the exhaled gases.

d. **True.**

e. **False.** As their performance is variable, the FiO_2 the patient is getting is uncertain. Patients who are dependent on their hypoxic drive require a fixed performance mask.

6. Regarding variable performance devices

a. **True.** These devices are better tolerated by patients because they are more comfortable. They also offer simplicity, low cost and the ability to manipulate the FiO_2 without changing the appliance.

b. **True.** The FiO_2 delivered can vary from one breath to another in the same patient. This is because of changes in the inspiratory flow rate and respiratory pattern. These lead to changes in the amount of air entrained, so altering the FiO_2.

c. **False.** Rebreathing is increased when the mask body is large. In addition, the high inspiratory resistance of the side holes increases the rebreathing. CO_2 elimination can be improved by increasing the fresh oxygen flow and is inversely related to the minute ventilation.

d. **False.** Oxygraphy can be used to measure the FiO_2 by measuring the end-tidal oxygen fraction in the nasopharynx.

e. **True.** The tighter the fit of the face mask, the higher the FiO_2. Low peak inspiratory flow rate, slow respiratory rate and a higher oxygen flow rate can also increase the FiO_2.

7. Concerning fixed performance devices

a. **True.** Anaesthetic breathing systems are fixed performance devices. The reservoir bag acts to deliver an FGF that is greater than the patient's peak inspiratory flow rate.

b. **False.** The potential energy is related to the pressure, whereas the kinetic energy is related to the velocity of the flow. As the flow of fresh oxygen supply passes through the constricted orifice into the larger chamber, the velocity of the gas increases distal to the orifice, causing the kinetic energy to increase. As the total energy is constant, there is a decrease in the potential energy, so a negative pressure is created. This causes the ambient air to be entrained and mixed with the oxygen flow.

c. **False.** The higher the entrainment ratio, the lower the FiO_2 delivered. This is because of the 'dilution' of the 100% oxygen fresh flow by ambient air.

d. **False.** Nasal catheters are variable performance devices.

e. **False.** Venturi masks are not very well tolerated by patients because of the noise and bulkiness of the masks and the attachments.

8. e.

9. c.

Chapter 7

Laryngoscopes and tracheal intubation equipment

Laryngoscopes

These devices are used to perform direct laryngoscopy and to aid in tracheal intubation (Fig. 7.1). They can also be used to visualize the larynx or pharynx for suctioning, removal of foreign body, placing of nasogastric tube and throat packs.

Components

1. The handle houses the power source (batteries) and is designed in different sizes.
2. The blade is fitted to the handle and can be either curved or straight. There is a wide range of designs for both curved and straight blades (Fig. 7.2).

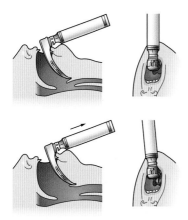

Fig. 7.1 Performing direct laryngoscopy. The vocal cords are visualized by lifting the laryngoscope in an upward and forward direction *(see arrow)*.

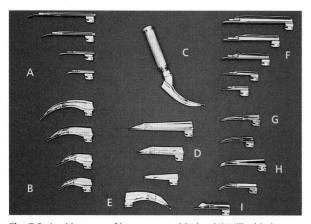

Fig. 7.2 A wide range of laryngoscope blades. (A) Miller blades (large, adult, infant, premature); (B) Macintosh blades (large, adult, child, baby); (C) Macintosh polio blade; (D) Soper blades (adult, child, baby); (E) left-handed Macintosh blade; (F) Wisconsin blades (large, adult, child, baby, neonate); (G) Robertshaw blades (infant, neonate); (H) Seward blades (child, baby); (I) Oxford infant blade.

Mechanism of action

1. Usually the straight blade is used for intubating neonates and infants. The blade is advanced over the posterior border of the relatively large, floppy, V-shaped epiglottis, which is then lifted directly in order to view the larynx (Fig. 7.3B). Larger-size straight blades can be used in adults.
2. The curved blade (**Macintosh blade**) is designed to fit into the oral and oropharyngeal cavity. It is inserted through the right angle of the mouth and advanced gradually, pushing the tongue to the left and away from the view until the tip of the blade reaches the vallecula. The blade has a small bulbous tip to help lift the larynx (Fig. 7.3A). The laryngoscope is lifted upwards, elevating the larynx and allowing the vocal cords to be seen. The Macintosh blade is made in five sizes: neonate (0), infant (1), child (2), adult (3) and large adult (4).
3. In the standard designs (colour-coded black) (Fig. 7.4), the light source is a bulb screwed/positioned onto the blade and an electrical connection is made when the blade is opened and ready for use. In more recent designs, the bulb is placed in the handle and the light is transmitted to the tip of the blade by means of fibreoptics (colour-coded green). Opening the blade turns the light on by forcing the bulb down to contact the battery terminal. Acrylic fibre is used in the disposable blades. The two systems are not cross-compatible.
4. A left-sided Macintosh blade is available. It is used in patients with right-sided facial deformities, making the use of the right-sided blade difficult (Fig. 7.5).
5. The **McCoy laryngoscope** (Penlon Ltd, Abingdon, UK) is based on the standard Macintosh blade. It has a hinged tip that is operated by the lever mechanism present on the back of the handle. It is suited for both routine use and in cases of difficult intubation (Fig. 7.6). Another McCoy design based on the Seward blade (Fig. 7.7) is also available.

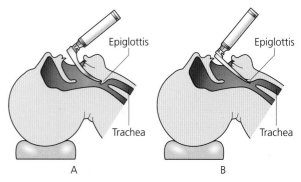

Fig. 7.3 Use of the laryngoscope with (A) curved and (B) straight blade.

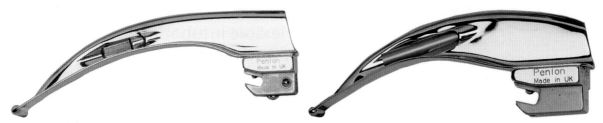

Fig. 7.4 Conventional standard laryngoscope blade with the light bulb mounted on the blade *(left)*; fibreoptics laryngoscope blade with the bulb mounted on the handle *(right)*. (Courtesy Penlon, Abingdon, UK.)

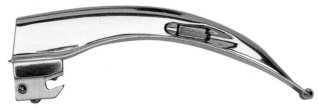

Fig. 7.5 Penlon left-sided Macintosh blade. (Courtesy Penlon, Abingdon, UK.)

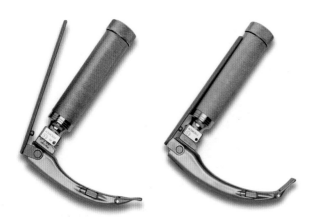

Fig. 7.6 Penlon Macintosh McCoy blade. (Courtesy Penlon, Abingdon, UK.)

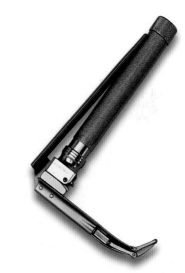

Fig. 7.7 Penlon Seward McCoy blade. (Courtesy Penlon, Abingdon, UK.)

6. A modified design called the Flexiblade exists in which the whole distal half of the blade can be manoeuvred rather than just the tip, as in the McCoy. This can be achieved using a lever on the front of the handle.
7. The blades are designed to be interchangeable among different manufacturers and laryngoscope handles. Two international standards are used: ISO 7376/2009 (green system) and ISO 7376/1 (black system) with a coloured marking placed on the blade and handle. The two systems have different dimension hinges and with different light source positions. The 'green system' is the most commonly used fitting standard.
8. Magnetic resonance imaging (MRI) compatible laryngoscope handles and blades are available.

Problems in practice and safety features

1. The risk of trauma and bruising to the different structures (e.g. epiglottis) is higher with the straight blade.
2. It is of vital importance to check the function of the laryngoscope before anaesthesia has commenced. Reduction in power or total failure due to the corrosion at the electrical contact point is possible.
3. Patients with large amounts of breast tissue present difficulty during intubation. Insertion of the blade into the mouth is restricted by the breast tissue, impinging on the handle. To overcome this problem, specially designed blades are used such as the polio blade (Fig. 7.2). The polio blade is at about 120 degrees to the handle, allowing laryngoscopy without restriction. The polio

blade was first designed to intubate patients ventilated in the iron lung during the poliomyelitis epidemic in the 1950s. A Macintosh laryngoscope blade attached to a short handle can also be useful in this situation.

4. To prevent cross-infection among patients, a disposable blade (Fig. 7.8) is used.
5. Laryngoscope handles must be appropriately decontaminated between patients to prevent cross-infection.

> **Laryngoscopes**
> - Consist of a handle and a blade. The latter can be straight or curved.
> - The bulb is either in the blade or in the handle.
> - Different designs and shapes exist.

Exam tip: It is important to have knowledge about the different design laryngoscope blades and their advantages and disadvantages. An understanding of the difference between a fibreoptic laryngoscope blade and a standard blade with a mounted light bulb is important.

Flexible intubation videoscope/bronchoscopes

These devices have made a huge impact on airway management in anaesthesia and intensive care. Single-use portable devices with their high-resolution monitor screens are becoming more popular (Fig. 7.9) over the traditional fibreoptic scopes. As single-use devices, the need for cleaning/sterilization and continuous maintenance has been eliminated. They are used to perform oral or nasal tracheal intubation (Figs. 7.10 and 7.11); to evaluate the airway in trauma, tumour, infection and inhalational injury; to confirm tube placement (tracheal, endobronchial, double lumen or tracheostomy tubes) and to perform tracheobronchial toilet.

The Ambu aScope 4 Broncho Regular consists of an insertion cord of 600 mm length and 5 mm diameter with a digital camera and 2 light-emitting diode (LED) light sources at its distal tip, offering an 85-degree viewing field. Other sizes are available: *slim* 3.8-mm diameter and *large* 5.8-mm diameter.

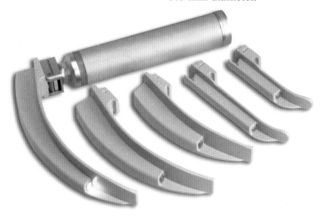

Fig. 7.8 Intersurgical fibreoptic single-use plastic laryngoscope blade with the handle. From *left* to *right*: Macintosh blade sizes 4, 3 and 2; Miller blade sizes 1 and 0. (Courtesy Intersurgical, Wokingham, UK.)

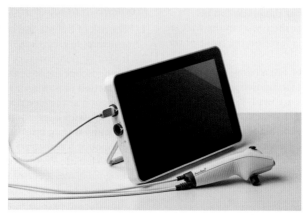

Fig. 7.9 Ambu aScope 4 Broncho Regular endoscope. (Courtesy Ambu, Alconbury, Weald, Cambridgeshire, UK.)

The lightweight handheld control unit consists of the following:

a. tip deflection control lever. This allows the distal part of the cord to bend with an angle range up to180 degrees upwards and 180 degrees downwards.

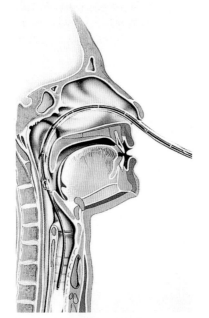

Fig. 7.10 Performing fibreoptic nasal intubation.

b. button that activates the suction with a suction port that can be connected to an external suction device. A purpose-built, closed-loop container can be attached to collect any aspirated samples.

c. a working channel (2.2-mm diameter) port with Luer-Lok allows the installation of fluids or local anaesthetic. Its distal end is positioned at the distal tip of the cord.

A tracheal tube can be attached to the proximal end of the cord using the 'retention rings/discs'. It can be railroaded into the trachea to facilitate intubation. A size 6.0-mm ID tracheal tube or larger can be used. A double lumen tracheal tube of 41 Fr size or larger can also be used.

The unit is attached to a high-definition monitor screen via a separate cable.

Other equipment may be needed, e.g. endoscopic face mask, oral airway, bite block, defogging agent.

Videolaryngoscopes (rigid indirect laryngoscopes)

These devices have revolutionized airway management in the elective and emergency settings. Advances in miniaturized, high-resolution, digital cameras with LED illumination have superseded the original fibreoptic technology. This has led to a new generation of 'crossover' devices. Some videolaryngoscopes offer both direct and indirect

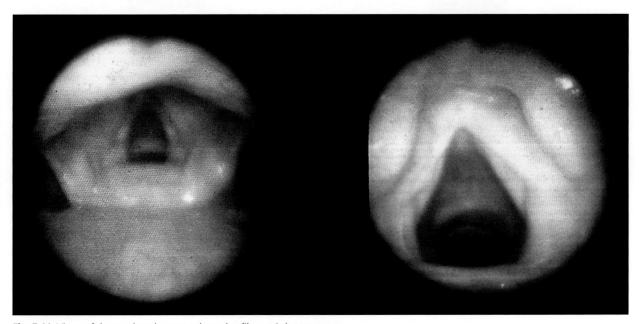

Fig. 7.11 Views of the vocal cords as seen through a fibreoptic laryngoscope.

laryngoscopy while some offer only indirect laryngoscopy. They have the combined features of both the flexible 'fibreoptic' scopes and the standard rigid laryngoscopes. The digital cameras used offer wide views, allowing the user to see around corners during difficult intubations.

Currently, there are many different designs ranging in their sizes, being single-use or reusable, utilizing a conventional Macintosh blade type so allowing direct laryngoscopy (Fig. 7.12, i-View, Intersurgical) to nonconventional acutely angled or J-shaped blades. They also differ in their portability, recording ability, power source (mains or battery) and display/viewing choice (either as part of the device with direct viewing through an eyepiece or separate attached or remote screen monitor).

However, depending on how the tracheal tube is steered, they can be divided into two groups:

1. *Guided* or *channelled* videolaryngoscopes with a channel that guides the tracheal tube into the trachea (Figs. 7.13 and 7.14).
2. Nonguided or nonchannelled videolaryngoscopes allow visualization of the larynx with the anaesthetist steering the tube into the trachea using a stylet (Fig. 7.15).

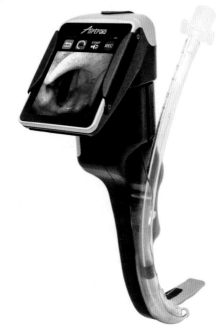

Fig. 7.13 Teleflex Airtraq is a guided or channelled videolaryngoscope. (Image courtesy Teleflex Incorporated. © 2021. Teleflex Incorporated, Athlone, Ireland. All rights reserved.)

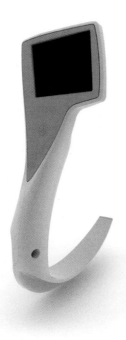

Fig. 7.12 Intersurgical i-View with the Macintosh blade design. (Courtesy Intersurgical, Wokingham, UK.)

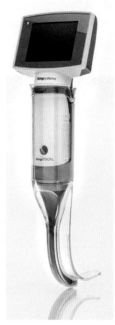

Fig. 7.14 Ambu King Vision is a guided or channeled videolaryngoscope. (Courtesy Ambu, Alconbury, Weald, Cambridgeshire, UK.)

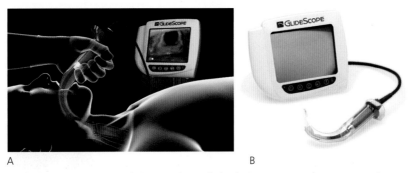

A   B

Fig. 7.15 Verathon Medical Glidescope is a nonguided or nonchannelled videolaryngoscope. (Courtesy Verathon Medical UK Ltd.)

Videolaryngoscopes improve the view of the glottis, as the camera eye is only centimetres away from the glottis. Their use requires minimal neck movement and can make laryngoscopy and successful tracheal intubation easier. These devices can be used both in difficult tracheal intubation (e.g. anterior larynx and limited neck extension) and routine tracheal intubation. Following local anaesthesia to the airway, they can also be used in awake intubation. Such devices may well supersede the classic laryngoscopes. However, a learning curve is needed before their routine use.

Magill forceps

These forceps are designed for ease of use within the mouth and oropharynx. Their curved design allows manipulation in the oropharynx without the operator's hand being in line of sight. Magill forceps come in small or large sizes (Fig. 7.16). During tracheal intubation, they can be used to direct the tracheal tube towards the larynx and vocal cords.

Care should be taken to protect the tracheal tube cuff from being damaged by the forceps.

Other uses include the insertion and removal of throat packs, manipulating nasogastric tubes, and removal of foreign bodies in the oropharynx and larynx.

Introducer, bougie, bite guard, local anaesthetic spray, Endotrol tube and Nosworthy airway

1. A local anaesthetic spray is used to coat the laryngeal and tracheal mucosa, usually with lidocaine. This decreases the stimulus of intubation.

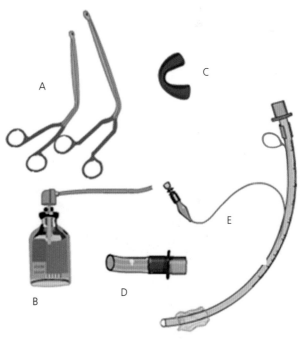

Fig. 7.16 Intubation aids. (A) Magill forceps, (B) local anaesthetic spray, (C) bite guard, (D) Nosworthy airway and (E) Endotrol tube.

2. A bite guard protects the front upper teeth during direct laryngoscopy.
3. The Endotrol tube (Shiley, Minneapolis, MN, USA) has a ring-pull on its inner curvature connected to the distal end of the tube. During intubation, the ring-pull can be used to adjust the curvature of the tube.
4. The Nosworthy airway (Smiths Medical, Ashford, Kent, UK) is an example of the many modifications that exist in oropharyngeal airway design. This airway allows the connection of a catheter mount and a breathing system.

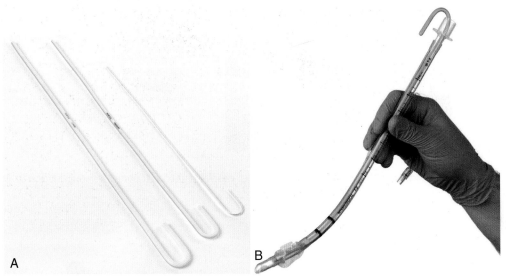

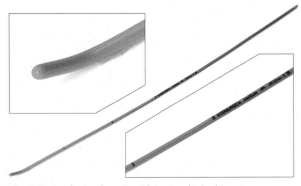

Fig. 7.17 (A) Examples of introducers or stylets and (B) introducer in tracheal tube.

Fig. 7.18 Intubating bougie with its Coudé tip. (Courtesy Intersurgical. Wokingham, UK.)

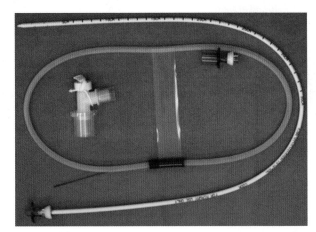

Fig. 7.19 The airway exchange catheter.

5. An introducer or stylet (Fig. 7.17) is used to adjust the curvature of a tracheal tube to help direct it through the vocal cords.
6. A gum elastic bougie is used when it is difficult to visualize the vocal cords. First the bougie is inserted through the vocal cords, then the tracheal tube is railroaded over it. As the bougie is inserted into the trachea, the tracheal rings can be felt as ridges in contrast to the smooth oesophagus. Currently, single-use intubating bougies are widely used (Fig. 7.18).
7. The airway exchange catheter (AEC) (Cook Medical, Limerick, Ireland) (Fig. 7.19) allows the exchange of tracheal tubes. It is a long hollow tube that can be inserted through a tracheal tube. This can then be withdrawn, and another tracheal tube is inserted over it. Specially designed, detachable, 15-mm male taper fit and Luer-Lok connectors can be used to provide temporary oxygenation.

8. The Aintree intubation catheter (Cook Medical, Limerick, Ireland) (Fig. 7.20). This catheter is designed to be used with a fibrescope being passed through a laryngeal mask or other supraglottic airway device. It allows any appropriate size of tracheal tube to be inserted into the trachea which would otherwise be limited by the size of tube that could be passed through the supraglottic airway.

Retrograde intubation set (Fig. 7.21)

This set is used to assist in placement of a tracheal tube when a difficult intubation is encountered.

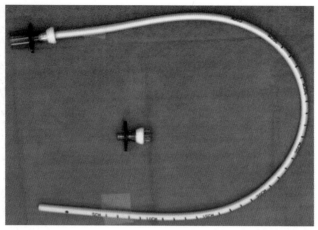

Fig. 7.20 The Aintree intubation catheter.

Components

1. It has an introducer needle (18 G and 5 cm in length).
2. A guidewire that has a J-shaped end.
3. It has a 14-G 70-cm hollow guiding catheter with distal sideports. The proximal end has a 15-mm connector.

Mechanism of action

1. The introducer needle is inserted through the cricothyroid membrane.
2. The guidewire is advanced in a retrograde (cephalic) direction to exit orally or nasally.
3. The hollow guiding catheter is then introduced in an antegrade direction into the trachea. The proximal end of the catheter can be connected to an oxygen supply.
4. A tracheal tube (5 mm or larger) can be introduced over the guiding catheter into the trachea.

Problems in practice and safety features

1. Pneumothorax.
2. Haemorrhage.
3. Failure.

> **Retrograde intubation kit**
> - The introducer needle is inserted through the cricothyroid.
> - The guidewire is advanced in a cephalic direction.
> - Pneumothorax and haemorrhage are potential complications.

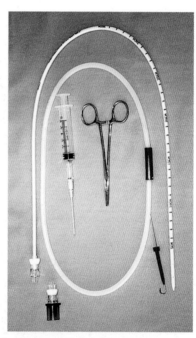

Fig. 7.21 The Cook retrograde intubation set.

SUGGESTED FURTHER READING

Cook, T.M., Boniface, N.J., Seller, C., et al., 2018. Universal videolaryngoscopy: a structured approach to conversion to videolaryngoscopy for all intubations in an anaesthetic and intensive care department. Br. J. Anaesth. 120 (1), 173–180.

Medical Device Alert MDA/2019/044. Issued: 12 December 2019 at 12:00. BritePro Solo and BriteBlade Pro single-use fibre optic laryngoscope blades and handles – risk of choking. Available from: https://www.gov.uk/drug-device-alerts/britepro-solo-and-briteblade-pro-single-use-fibre-optic-laryngoscope-blades-and-handles-risk-of-choking-mda-2019-044.

NICE. Video laryngoscopes to help intubation in people with difficult airways Medtech innovation briefing. Published: 19 December 2018. Available from: www.nice.org.uk/guidance/mib167. https://www.nice.org.uk/advice/mib167/resources/video-laryngoscopes-to-help-intubation-in-people-with-difficult-airways-pdf-2285963582135749.

Norris, A., Heidegger, T., 2016. Limitations of videolaryngoscopy. Br. J. Anaesth. 117 (2), 148–150.

Welsh Health Circular, 2020. Policy on single-use and reusable laryngoscopes. Available from: https://gov.wales/sites/default/files/publications/2020-09/policy-on-single-use-and-reusable-laryngoscopes.pdf.

Zaouter, C., Calderon, J., Hemmerling, T.M., 2015. Videolaryngoscopy as a new standard of care. Br. J. Anaesth. 114 (2), 181–183.

SELF-ASSESSMENT QUESTIONS

Please check your eBook for additional self-assessment

MCQs

In the following lists, which of the statements (a) to (e) are true?

1. Laryngoscopes
a. Straight blade laryngoscopes are only used in neonates and infants.
b. The left-sided Macintosh blade is designed for a left-handed anaesthetist.
c. The Macintosh blade is designed to elevate the larynx.
d. The Macintosh polio blade can be used in patients with large breasts.
e. The McCoy laryngoscope can improve the view of the larynx.

2. Light failure during laryngoscopy can be caused by
a. Battery failure.
b. A loose bulb.
c. The wrong-sized blade having been used.
d. A blown bulb.
e. Inadequate connection due to corrosion.

3. Concerning retrograde intubation
a. The introducer needle is inserted at the level of the second and third tracheal cartilages.
b. It is a very safe procedure with no complications.
c. A guidewire is inserted in a cephalic direction.
d. Supplemental oxygen can be administered.
e. A tracheal tube (5 mm or larger) can be introduced over the guiding catheter into the trachea.

Single best answer

4. Videolaryngoscopes
a. Are designed for retrograde intubation.
b. Utilize a screen to display the larynx.
c. Ensure safe intubation.
d. Cannot be used in paediatric patients.
e. Need no power supply.

Answers

1. Laryngoscopes
   a. *False. Straight blade laryngoscopes can be used for adults, neonates and infants. Because of the shape and size of the larynx in small children, it is usually easier to intubate with a straight-blade laryngoscope. The latter can be used in adults, but the curved blade laryngoscope is usually used.*
   b. *False. The left-sided Macintosh blade is designed to be used in cases of difficult access to the right side of the mouth or tongue, e.g. trauma or tumour.*
   c. *True. The Macintosh curved blade is designed to elevate the larynx, thus allowing better visualization of the vocal cords.*
   d. *True. The polio blade was designed during the polio epidemic in the 1950s to overcome the problem of intubating patients who were in an 'iron lung'. In current practice, it can be used in patients with large breasts where the breasts do not get in the way of the handle.*
   e. *True. By using the hinged blade tip, the larynx is further elevated. This improves the view of the larynx.*

2. Light failure during laryngoscopy
   a. *True.*
   b. *True.*
   c. *False. This should not cause light failure. It may, however, cause a worse view of the larynx.*
   d. *True.*
   e. *True. This usually happens in the traditional laryngoscope design where the handle needs good contact with the blade for the current to flow from the batteries to the bulb in the blade. Corrosion at that junction can cause light failure. Laryngoscopes using fibreoptics do not suffer from this problem as the bulb is situated in the handle.*

3. Concerning retrograde intubation
   a. *False. The needle is inserted through the cricothyroid membrane.*
   b. *False. Retrograde intubation can cause haemorrhage or pneumothorax.*
   c. *True. The guidewire is inserted in a retrograde cephalic direction to exit through the mouth or nose.*
   d. *True. Oxygen can be given through the proximal end of the guiding catheter.*
   e. *True.*

4. *b.*

Chapter 8

Ventilators

Ventilators are used to provide controlled ventilation to maintain oxygenation and removal of carbon dioxide. Many of them have the facilities to provide multiple ventilatory modes that can lead to some confusion. They can be used in the operating theatre, intensive care unit (ICU), during transport of critically ill patients and at home (e.g. for patients requiring nocturnal respiratory assistance).

Positive pressure ventilators are overwhelmingly used in current clinical practice where a positive pressure within the breathing system is created, driving the gas into the patient's lungs. Negative pressure ventilators mimic the normal physiology by generating a negative intrathoracic pressure, allowing gas flow into the lungs, but their use in current practice is limited.

In this chapter, we will describe the basic functions of the ventilators, attempt to classify them and define the characteristics of the ideal ventilator. A selection of the commonly used ventilators in current practice is described in more detail. Only positive pressure ventilators are described.

The basic variables in any ventilator are:

- **Tidal volume** (mL/breath), which can be delivered either as a *fixed volume* (e.g. 500 mL) with variable peak airway pressures or a *fixed pressure* (e.g. 12–15 cm H_2O) with variable volumes.
- **Respiratory rate** (breaths/min) can be set either by the *ventilator* (mandatory breaths) or by the *patient* (triggered breaths). These options allow different ventilatory modes:
    o *Control mode* when the ventilator does all the work of breathing, delivering the set and mandatory breaths only.
    o *Spontaneous breathing mode* when the patient does all the work of breathing, triggering all the breaths. The ventilator may provide supplementary oxygen or continuous positive airway pressure (CPAP) (see Chapter 13).
    o *Support mode* when the patient triggers the ventilator to deliver a breath. Here the patient does some of the work of breathing, but the ventilator offers support and does most of it.
- **Minute volume** is the volume of gas inhaled or exhaled from patient's lungs per **minute**. It is the product of tidal volume and respiratory rate. In some of the advanced modes of ventilation on modern intensive care ventilators, it is possible to set the minute volume directly and the ventilator will deliver variable tidal volumes and breathing rate depending on the lung mechanics.
- **I:E ratio** is the ratio of inspiratory time to expiratory time. The operator in mandatory ventilation can set this either directly or indirectly through adjusting

inspiratory time or respiratory rate. In spontaneous mode, the patient determines the I:E ratio. This can be very important to set appropriately in patients with acute respiratory distress syndrome (ARDS) or acute severe asthma.

The common ventilatory modes used are described in the following box.

Using the variables, tidal volume (fixed volume or fixed pressure) and respiratory rate (patient or ventilator), these ventilator modes can be derived:
- *Volume Control (VC):* the desired tidal volume is delivered regardless of the measured peak airway pressure. The latter is dependent on the lung compliance.
- *Pressure Control (PC):* the desired positive pressure is reached, delivering a compliance-dependent variable volume.
- *Pressure Support (PS):* the ventilator augments the patient's spontaneous breaths. The ventilator functions as a demand flow system that support the patient's spontaneous breathing efforts with a set PS. The PS setting defines the applied pressure. The patient determines the breath timing.
- *All of the above can be incorporated into one mode in modern ventilators.*

Classification of ventilators

There are many ways of classifying ventilators (Table 8.1).
1. *Power source:* ventilators can be:
    a. *Electrically powered:* use standard mains electrical output.
    b. *Pneumatically powered:* use high-pressure gas input to power the gas.
    c. *Pneumatically powered microprocessor-controlled:* both above power sources are required; electrical power is required to power a microprocessor within the ventilator that adds further control options to the gas flow such as pressure waveform.
2. *Pressure generation:* as previously described, a ventilator can either be:
    a. *Positive pressure:* gas is pushed into the lungs, generating positive pressure within the lungs to cause chest expansion. Airway pressure is higher than atmospheric pressure, so exhalation occurs due to this pressure gradient as well as the elastic recoil of the lungs and chest wall.
    b. *Negative pressure:*

Table 8.1 Summary of the methods used in classifying ventilators	
Power source	Electrically powered Pneumatically powered Pneumatically powered microprocessor-controlled
Pressure generation	Positive pressure Negative pressure

Control system	Open and closed loops systems
	Pneumatic circuit:
	  Internal: single or double
	  External

Suitability for use	Operating theatre Intensive care unit Both
Paediatric practice	Yes/no
Drive mechanisms	Flow devices Volume displacement devices
Output control mechanism	Proportional solenoid valve Digital on/off valves

i. *Tank ventilator or 'iron lung':* gas is pumped out of the airtight tank to generate a vacuum around the body, decreasing intrapulmonary pressure and leading to chest expansion. As the vacuum is released, elastic recoil of the chest leads to expiration.

ii. *Cuirass ventilator:* an upper body shell or cuirass generates negative pressure only around the chest. This technique has been improved by the ability to generate two pressures, biphasic cuirass ventilation. This allows control of expiration as well as inspiration, and therefore the I:E ratio and respiratory rate.

3. *Control system:*
   a. *Closed- and open-loop systems:* in closed-loop systems, microprocessors allow feedback loops between the control variable (such as tidal volume) as set by the operator and the measured control variable (exhaled tidal volume). If the two differ, for example, due to a leak, the ventilator can adjust to achieve the desired expired tidal volume by increasing the volume delivered. Open-loop systems deliver ventilation as set by the operator but do not measure or adjust.
   b. *Pneumatic circuit:* the means of delivering gas flow from a high-pressure gas source to the patient can be either:
      i. *Internal*

- Single: the gas from the high-pressure source flows directly to the patient (e.g. modern ICU ventilators)
- Double: the power source causes gas flow to compress a chamber such as bellows or 'bag-in-a-chamber'. The gas in the chamber is then delivered to the patient.
   ii. *External:* tubing goes from the ventilator to the patient.
4. *Suitability for use* in a theatre and/or an intensive care unit.
5. *Suitability for paediatric practice.*
6. *Drive mechanism:* the internal hardware that converts electrical power or gas pressure into a breath to the patient.
   a. *Flow devices:* compressors driven by pistons, rotating blades, diaphragms or bellows move atmospheric pressure gas into a higher pressure storage chamber, which is then delivered as a breath. Blowers generate high flows of gas as the direct ventilator output.
   b. *Volume displacement devices:* the volume of gas to be delivered to the patient is displaced by a moving part such as a piston or spring-loaded bellows.
7. *Output control mechanism:* valves regulate gas flow to and from the patient.
   a. *Proportional solenoid valve:* opens in very small increments dependent upon flow required.
   b. *Digital on/off valves:* a collection of valves whereby each one is either fully open or closed. Each valve produces a certain flow by controlling the opening/closing of a specifically sized orifice.

 Exam tip: A basic understanding of the classification of ventilators is important.

Characteristics of the ideal ventilator

1. The ventilator should be simple, portable, robust and economical to purchase and use. If compressed gas is used to drive the ventilator, a significant wastage of the compressed gas is expected. Some ventilators use a Venturi to drive the bellows to reduce the use of compressed oxygen.
2. It should be versatile and supply tidal volumes up to 1500 mL with a respiratory rate of up to 60 breaths/min and variable I:E ratio. It can be used with different breathing systems. It can deliver any gas or vapour mixture. The addition of positive end expiratory pressure (PEEP) should be possible.

3. It should monitor the airway pressure, inspired and exhaled minute and tidal volume, respiratory rate and inspired oxygen concentration.
4. There should be facilities to provide humidification. Drugs can be nebulized through it.
5. Disconnection, high airway pressure and power failure alarms should be present.
6. There should be the facility to provide other ventilatory modes, e.g. SIMV, CPAP and PS.
7. It should be easy to clean and sterilize.
   Some of the commonly used ventilators are described as follows.

Bag in bottle ventilator

Modern anaesthetic machines often incorporate a bag in bottle ventilator. Stand-alone designs are available for use in other settings, e.g. postanaesthesia care units.

Components

1. A driving unit consisting of:
   a. a chamber (Fig. 8.1) with a tidal volume range of 0–1500 mL (a paediatric version with a range of 0–400 mL exists)
   b. an ascending bellows accommodating the fresh gas flow (FGF).
2. A control unit with a variety of controls, displays and alarms: the tidal volume, respiratory rate (6–40 breaths/min), I:E ratio, airway pressure and power supply (Fig. 8.2).

Mechanism of action

1. It is a time-cycled ventilator that is pneumatically powered and electronically controlled.
2. The fresh gas is accommodated in the bellows.

3. Compressed air is used as the driving gas (Fig. 8.3). On entering the chamber, the compressed air forces the bellows down, delivering the fresh gas to the patient.
4. The driving gas and the fresh gas remain separate.
5. The volume of the driving gas reaching the chamber is equal to the tidal volume.
6. Although it is not desirable, some designs feature a descending bellows instead.

Problems in practice and safety features

1. Positive pressure in the standing bellows causes a PEEP of 2–4 cm H_2O.

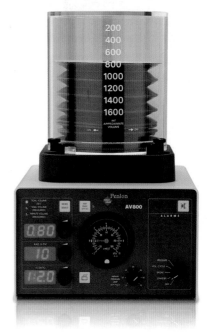

Fig. 8.1 Bag in bottle AV800 ventilator. (Courtesy Penlon Ltd, Abingdon, UK.)

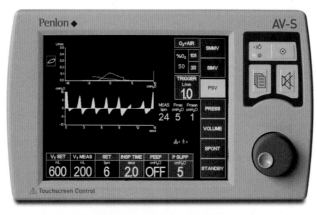

Fig. 8.2 Control panel of Penlon AV-S ventilator. (Courtesy Penlon, Abingdon, UK.)

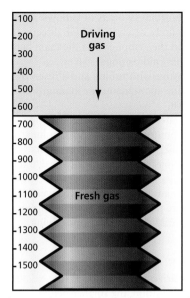

Fig. 8.3 Mechanism of action of the bag in bottle ventilator.

2. The ascending bellows collapses to an empty position and remains stationary in cases of disconnection or leak.
3. The descending bellows hangs down to a fully expanded position in a case of disconnection and may continue to move almost normally in a case of leakage.

Bag in bottle ventilator
- Uses ascending bellows and is a time-cycled ventilator.
- Consists of driving and control units.
- Fresh gas is within the bellows, whereas the driving gas is within the chamber.

Penlon Anaesthesia Nuffield Ventilator Series 200

This is an intermittent blower ventilator. It is small, compact, versatile and easy to use with patients of different sizes, ages and lung compliances. It can be used with different breathing systems (Fig. 8.4). It is a volume-preset, time-cycled, flow generator in adult use. In paediatric use, it is a pressure-preset, time-cycled flow generator.

Components

1. The control module consists of an airway pressure gauge (cm H_2O), inspiratory and expiratory time dials (seconds), inspiratory flow rate dial (L/s) and an on/off switch. Underneath the control module there are connections for the driving gas supply and the valve

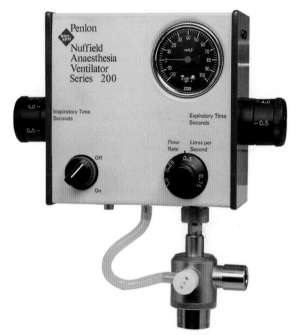

Fig. 8.4 The Penlon Nuffield 200 ventilator. (Courtesy Penlon Ltd, Abingdon, UK.)

block. Tubing connects the valve block to the airway pressure gauge.
2. The valve block has three ports:
   a. a port for tubing to connect to the breathing system reservoir bag mount
   b. an exhaust port that can be connected to the scavenging system
   c. a pressure relief valve that opens at 60 cm H_2O.
3. The valve block can be changed to a paediatric (Newton) valve.

Mechanism of action

1. The ventilator is powered by a driving gas independent from the FGF. The commonly used driving gas is oxygen (at about 400 kPa) supplied from the compressed oxygen outlets on the anaesthetic machine. The driving gas should not reach the patient as it dilutes the FGF, lightening the depth of anaesthesia.
2. It can be used with different breathing systems such as Bain, Humphrey ADE, T-piece and the circle. In the Bain and circle systems, the reservoir bag is replaced by the tubing delivering the driving gas from the ventilator. The adjustable pressure limiting (APL) valve of the breathing system must be fully closed during ventilation.
3. The inspiratory and expiratory times can be adjusted to the desired I:E ratio. The tidal volume is determined by adjusting the inspiratory time and inspiratory flow rate controls. The inflation pressure is adjusted by the inspiratory flow rate control.

4. With its standard valve, the ventilator acts as a time-cycled flow generator to deliver a minimal tidal volume of 50 mL. When the valve is changed to a paediatric (Newton) valve, the ventilator changes to a time-cycled pressure generator capable of delivering tidal volumes between 10 and 300 mL. This makes it capable of ventilating premature babies and neonates. It is recommended that the Newton valve is used for children of less than 20 kg body weight.
5. A PEEP valve may be fitted to the exhaust port.

Problems in practice and safety features

1. The ventilator continues to cycle despite breathing system disconnection without an alarm.
2. Requires high flows of driving gas.

Penlon Nuffield Anaesthesia Ventilator Series 200
- An intermittent blower with a pressure gauge and inspiratory and expiratory time and flow controls.
- Powered by a driving gas.
- Can be used for both adults and paediatric patients.
- Can be used with different breathing systems.

Manley MP3 ventilator

The Manley MP3 ventilator is a minute volume divider (time-cycled pressure generator). All the FGF (the minute volume) is delivered to the patient divided into readily set tidal volumes (Fig. 8.5). It is rarely used in current practice.

Components

1. Rubber tubing delivers the FGF from the anaesthetic machine to the ventilator.

2. The machine has two sets of bellows. A smaller time-cycling bellows receives the FGF directly from the gas source and then empties into the main bellows.
3. It has three unidirectional valves.
4. An APL valve with tubing and a reservoir bag is used during spontaneous or manually controlled ventilation.
5. The ventilator has a pressure gauge (up to 100 cm H_2O), inspiratory time dial, tidal volume adjuster (up to 1000 mL) and two knobs to change the mode of ventilation from and to controlled and spontaneous (or manually controlled) ventilation. The inflation pressure is adjusted by sliding the weight to an appropriate position along its rail. The expiratory block is easily removed for autoclaving.

Mechanism of action

1. The FGF drives the ventilator.
2. During inspiration, the smaller bellows receives the FGF, while the main bellows delivers its contents to the patient. The inspiratory time dial controls the extent of filling of the smaller bellows before it empties into the main bellows.
3. During expiration, the smaller bellows delivers its contents to the main bellows until the predetermined tidal volume is reached to start inspiration again.
4. Using the ventilator in the spontaneous (manual) ventilation mode changes it to a Mapleson D breathing system.

Problems in practice and safety features

1. The ventilator ceases to cycle and function when the FGF is disconnected. This allows rapid detection of gas supply failure.
2. Ventilating patients with poor pulmonary compliance is not easily achieved.
3. It generates back pressure in the back bar as it cycles.

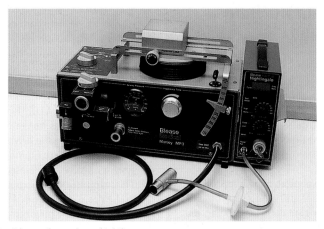

Fig. 8.5 The Blease Manley MP3 with ventilator alarm *(right)*.

4. The emergency oxygen flush in the anaesthetic machine should not be activated while ventilating a patient with the Manley.

Manley MP3 ventilator
- It is a minute volume divider.
- Consists of two sets of bellows, three unidirectional valves, an APL valve and a reservoir bag.
- Acts as a Mapleson D breathing system during spontaneous ventilation.

 Exam tip: The bag in bottle ventilator is the most commonly used type of ventilator in the operating theatre. It is important to have a good understanding of its components and functions.

SERVO-U ventilator

The SERVO-U is a versatile intensive care ventilator capable of being used for paediatric and adult patients. It is fully transportable, utilizing at least two 12-V batteries when mains electricity is not available. It is not intended for use with inhalational anaesthetics; however, it can be used with intravenous anaesthetics in the theatre setting if required. It can also be used to ventilate patients with a tight-fitting nasal mask or prong, face mask or hood instead of a standard endotracheal tube or tracheostomy. This is termed *non-invasive ventilation (NIV)*. Leaks are compensated for during NIV.

The most modern versions have advanced tools to safely perform lung recruitment, utilizing software that regulates PEEP and aims to maintain lung compliance.

Neurally adjusted ventilatory assist (NAVA) uses a specially adapted nasogastric tube that detects the phrenic nerve impulses to the diaphragm. This enhances the ability of the ventilator to match the respiratory efforts of the patient by timing its assisted breaths.

Components (Fig. 8.6)
1. It has a 'patient unit' where gases are mixed and administered.
2. The ventilator has a 'graphical user interface' where settings are made and ventilation is monitored.

Mechanism of action
1. Gas flow from the oxygen and air inlets is regulated by their respective gas modules.
2. Oxygen concentration is measured by an oxygen cell.
3. The pressure of the delivered gas mixture is measured by the inspiratory pressure transducer.
4. The patient's expiratory gas flow is measured by ultrasonic transducers and the pressure measured by the expiratory pressure transducer.
5. PEEP in the patient system is regulated by the expiratory valve.
   There are various modes of ventilation available:
1. *SIMV.* The ventilator provides mandatory breaths, which are synchronized with the patient's respiratory effort (if present). The type of mandatory breath supplied depends on the setting selected. Usually one of the following is selected:

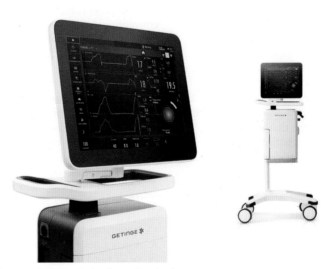

Fig. 8.6 SERVO-U ventilator. (Courtesy Getinge, Gothenburg, Sweden.)

a. *Pressure-regulated volume control* (PRVC): a preset tidal volume is delivered but limited to 5 cm H_2O below the set upper pressure limit. This automatically limits barotrauma if the upper pressure limit is appropriately set. The flow during inspiration is decelerating. The patient can trigger extra breaths.

b. *Volume control:* a preset tidal volume and respiratory rate are selected. The breath is delivered with constant flow during a preset inspiratory time. The set tidal volume will always be delivered despite high airway pressures if the patient's lungs are not compliant. To prevent excessive pressures being generated in this situation, the upper pressure limit must be set to a suitable level to prevent barotrauma.

c. *Pressure control:* a PC level above PEEP is selected. The delivered tidal volume is dependent upon the patient's lung compliance and airway resistance together with the tubing and endotracheal tube's resistance. PC ventilation is preferred when there is a leak in the breathing system (e.g. uncuffed endotracheal tube) or where barotrauma is to be avoided (e.g. acute lung injury). If the resistance or compliance improves quickly, there is a risk of excessive tidal volumes being delivered (volutrauma) unless the PC setting is reduced.

2. *Supported ventilation modes:* once the patient has enough respiratory drive to trigger the ventilator, usually one of the following modes is selected in addition to the PEEP setting:

a. *Volume support:* assures a set tidal volume by supplying the required PS needed to achieve that tidal volume. It allows patients to wean from ventilatory support themselves as their lungs' compliance and inspiratory muscle strength improves. This is shown by a gradual reduction in the peak airway pressure measured by the ventilator. Once the support is minimal, extubation can be considered.

b. *Pressure support (PS):* the patient's breath is supported with a set constant pressure above PEEP. This will give a tidal volume that is dependent on the lung compliance and patient's inspiratory muscle strength. The pressure support setting needs reviewing regularly to allow the patient to wean from respiratory support.

c. *CPAP:* a continuous positive pressure is maintained in the airways similar to that developed with a conventional CPAP flow generator (see Chapter 13). This differs from the conventional CPAP flow generator by allowing measurement of tidal volume, minute volume and respiratory rate, and trends can be observed also.

Problems in practice and safety features

1. A comprehensive alarm system is featured.
2. A mainstream carbon dioxide analyser is available that allows continuous inspiratory and expiratory monitoring of CO_2 to be displayed if required.
3. Multiple battery modules (from two to six) can be loaded on the ventilator if a long transport journey is anticipated, allowing extended use. It is recommended at least two battery modules are loaded for even the shortest transport.
4. The ventilator is heavier (23 kg) than a dedicated transport ventilator.

SERVO-U ventilator
- Versatile ICU ventilator suitable for both paediatric and adult use, including NIV.
- Wide range of controls, displays and alarms.
- Portable with battery power.

High-frequency jet ventilator

This ventilator reduces the extent of the side effects of conventional intermittent positive pressure ventilation (IPPV). It generates low tidal volumes at a high frequency, leading to lower peak airway pressures with better maintenance of the cardiac output and less antidiuretic hormone production and fluid retention. High-frequency jet ventilation is better tolerated by alert patients than conventional IPPV (Fig. 8.7). It is frequently used in anaesthesia for ear, nose and throat (ENT) surgery.

Components

1. A Venturi injector is used: for example, attached directly to a surgical suspension laryngoscope, or a cannula positioned in a tracheal tube (Fig. 8.8B), or a cannula positioned in the trachea via the cricothyroid membrane or a modified tracheal tube with two additional small lumens opening distally (Figs. 8.8A and 8.9).
2. Solenoid valves are used to deliver the jet gas.
3. Dials and display are used for driving pressure, frequency and inspiratory time. These determine the volume of gas delivered to the patient.
4. It has a built-in peristaltic pump for nebulizing drugs or distilled water for humidifying the jet gas.

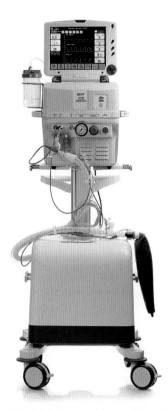

Fig. 8.7 The JV100 B high-frequency jet ventilator. (Courtesy Treaton, Ekaterinburg, Russia.)

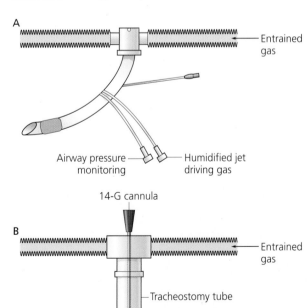

Fig. 8.8 (A) A jet tracheal tube with two additional lumens for the jet driving gas and airway pressure monitoring. (B) A 14-G cannula positioned within a tracheostomy tube through which the jet driving gas can be administered.

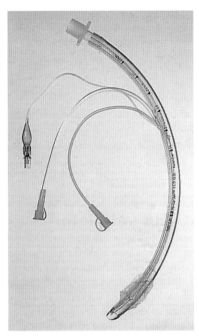

Fig. 8.9 The Mallinckrodt Hi-Lo Jet cuffed tracheal tube. An uncuffed version also exists.

5. High-flow air/oxygen or nitrous oxide/oxygen blender determines the mix of the jet gas.

Mechanism of action

1. Frequencies of 20–500 cycles/min can be selected, with minute volumes ranging from 5 to 60 L/min. A typical starting frequency is 100 cycles/min.
2. It is a time-cycled ventilator delivering gas in small jet pulsations. The inspiratory time is adjustable from 20% to 50% of the cycle.
3. The fresh gas leaving the narrow injector at a very high velocity causes entrainment of gas. The amount of entrained gas is uncertain making measurement of tidal volume and FiO_2 difficult.
4. The jet and entrained gases impact into the much larger volume of relatively immobile gases in the airway, causing them to move forward.
5. Expiration is passive. PEEP occurs automatically at a respiratory rate of over 100 breaths/min. Additional PEEP can be added by means of a PEEP valve.

Problems in practice and safety features

1. Barotrauma can still occur as expiration is dependent on passive lung and chest wall recoil driving the gas out through the tracheal tube.

2. High-pressure (35–40 cm H_2O) and system malfunction alarms are featured.

High-frequency jet ventilator

- Time-cycled ventilator.
- A Venturi injector is used.
- Built-in peristaltic pump for humidification.
- Frequencies of 20–500 cycles/min. Minute volumes of 5–60 L/min.

ParaPAC Plus ventilator

This is a portable ventilator used during the transport of critically ill patients and emergencies (Fig. 8.10). It allows controlled ventilation (with synchronized mandatory minute ventilation [SMMV], CMMV), CPAP (see Chapter 13) and spontaneous ventilation.

It is a gas-powered, time-cycled ventilator. ParaPAC plus ventilator allows synchronization of ventilation with external cardiac massage during cardiopulmonary resuscitation. It can be used both in adult and paediatric (above 10 kg body weight) practice.

Components

1. It has a variety of controls including:
   a. function switch: ventilator, demand and CPAP
   b. tidal volume with a range of 70–1000 mL
   c. frequency with a range of 8–40/min
   d. CPAP flow with a range of 0.5–35 L/min O_2 and up to a pressure of 16 cm H_2O
   e. adjustable inspiratory relief pressure with an audible alarm (20–60 cm H_2O)
   f. air mix dial to control FiO_2 at either 0.5 or 1.0
   g. PEEP control dial with a range of up to 20 cm H_2O
2. Inflation pressure manometer display measures the airway pressure, being luminous in the dark.
3. 120-cm polyester or silicone 15-mm corrugated tubing with a one-way valve delivers gases to the patient.
4. A separate port for the connection of a CPAP/oxygen delivery system to the patient.
5. Tubing delivers the oxygen to the ventilator.

Mechanism of action

1. The source of power is dry, filtered, oil-free pressurized gas (280–600 kPa) at 65 L/min. Using an FiO_2 of 0.5 reduces gas consumption by the ventilator by almost 70%.
2. In the FiO_2 0.5 (air mix) mode, the ventilator uses a high-efficiency entrainment device to mix ambient air with the supply gas in the ratio of approximately 2:1.
3. In addition to the various modes controlled by the function switch, if pressed, it can also deliver a single breath.
4. A visual indicator flashes when a spontaneous breath is detected.
5. During controlled ventilation, if the patient makes a spontaneous breath, this causes the ventilator to operate in an SMMV mode. Any superimposed mandatory ventilatory attempts are synchronized with the breathing pattern.
6. A built-in PEEP valve facility.

Problems in practice and safety features

1. Colour coding the tidal volume and frequency controls allow quick set-up for various patient groups.
2. An adjustable inspiratory pressure relief mechanism with a range of 20–60 cm H_2O reduces the risk of overpressure and barotrauma.
3. There are audible and visual low-pressure (disconnection) and high-pressure (obstruction) alarms.
4. It has a colour-coded supply gas failure alarm.

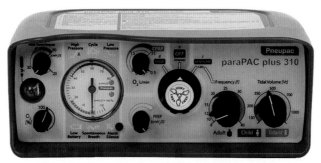

Fig. 8.10 ParaPAC plus 310 portable ventilator. (Courtesy Smiths Medical, Ashford, Kent, UK.)

5. The ventilator is magnetic resonance imaging (MRI) compatible.

VentiPAC Plus
- Portable ventilator powered by pressurized gas.
- Controls include tidal volume, frequency and PEEP.
- An FiO$_2$ of 0.5 or 1.0 can be delivered.
- It has a demand valve, allowing spontaneous breathes during controlled ventilation.
- MRI compatible.

Pneupac VR1 Emergency ventilator (Fig. 8.11)

This is a lightweight, handheld, time-cycled, gas-powered, flow generator ventilator. It is designed for use in emergency and during transport. It is MRI compatible up to 3 Tesla.

Components
1. It has a tidal volume/frequency control.
2. Auto/manual control has a manual trigger and push button.
3. Air mix switch allows the delivery of oxygen at 100% or 50% concentrations.
4. Patient valve connects to catheter mount/filter or face mask.
5. It has a gas supply input.

Mechanism of action
1. The source of power is pressurized oxygen (280–1034 kPa). Using air mix prolongs the duration of use from an oxygen cylinder.
2. A constant I:E ratio of 1:2 with flow rates of 11–32 L/min.
3. An optional patient demand facility is incorporated, allowing synchronization between patient and ventilator.
4. The linked manual controls allow the manual triggering of a single-controlled ventilation. This allows the ventilator to be used in a variety of chest compression/ventilation options in cardiac life support.
5. Suitable for children (above 10 kg body weight) and adults.

Problems in practice and safety features
1. Pressure relief valve designed to operate at 40 cm H$_2$O.
2. The manual control triggers a single ventilation equivalent to the volume of ventilation delivered in automatic ventilation. It is not a purge action so it cannot stack breaths and is therefore inherently much safer for the patient.

Pneupac VR1 Emergency ventilator
- Handheld, time-cycled, gas-powered flow generator ventilator.
- Used in emergency and transport.
- MRI compatible up to 3 Tesla.
- Various controls.
- Can be used in children and adults.

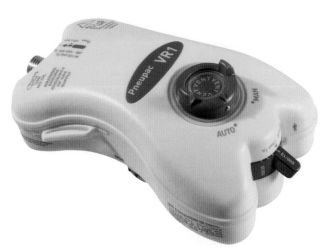

Fig. 8.11 Pneupac VR1 Emergency Ventilator. (Courtesy Smiths Medical, Ashford, Kent, UK.)

Venturi injector device

A manually controlled Venturi ventilation device that is used during rigid bronchoscopy (Fig. 8.12). The anaesthetist and the surgeon share the airway. General anaesthesia is maintained intravenously. It is also used for emergency ventilation using narrow bore airway devices as a rescue method in the 'can't intubate, can't oxygenate' (CICO) scenario.

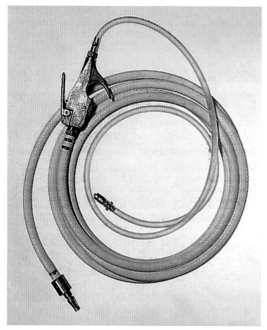

Fig. 8.12 The manually controlled injector. In practice this is connected to a rigid bronchoscope.

Components

1. A high-pressure oxygen source functions at about 400 kPa (from the anaesthetic machine or direct from a pipeline).
2. It has an on/off trigger.
3. Connection tubing can withstand high pressures.
4. A needle is of suitable gauge, which allows good air entrainment without creating excessive airway pressures.

Mechanism of action

1. The high-pressure oxygen is injected intermittently through the needle placed at the proximal end of the bronchoscope or a cricothyroid needle.
2. This creates a Venturi effect, entraining atmospheric air and inflating the lungs with oxygen-enriched air.
3. Oxygenation and carbon dioxide elimination are achieved with airway pressures of 25–30 cm H_2O.

Problems in practice and safety features

1. Barotrauma is possible. Airway pressure monitoring is not available. As exhalation is passive, it is essential to allow full exhalation before delivering the next breath to avoid air stacking and barotrauma.
2. Gastric distension can occur should ventilation commence before the distal end of the bronchoscope is beyond the larynx.

Venturi injector device
- Manually controlled Venturi used during rigid bronchoscopy and rescue ventilation.
- High-pressure oxygen injected through a needle entraining air.

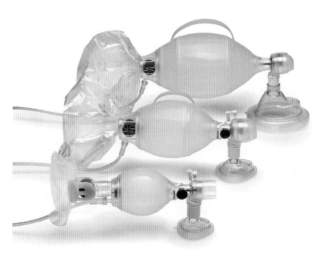

Fig. 8.13 A range of self-inflating resuscitation bags with oxygen reservoirs and face masks. (Courtesy Ambu, Alconbury, Weald, Cambridgeshire, UK.)

Self-inflating bag and mask

This disposable device offers a means of providing manual IPPV. It is portable and is used during resuscitation, transport and short-term ventilation (Fig. 8.13). It can be used with or without a pressurized gas supply.

Components

1. Self-inflating bag with a connection for added oxygen. The bag is usually made of clear silicone.
2. A one-way valve with three ports:
   a. inspiratory inlet allowing the entry of fresh gas during inspiration
   b. expiratory outlet allowing the exit of exhaled gas
   c. connection to the face mask or tracheal tube and marked 'patient'.
3. A reservoir for oxygen to increase the FiO_2 delivered to the patient.

Mechanism of action

1. The non-rebreathing valve (Ambu valve; artificial manual breathing unit) incorporates a silicone rubber membrane (Fig. 8.14). It has a small dead space and low resistance to flow. At a flow of 25 L/min, an inspiratory resistance of 0.4 cm H_2O and an expiratory resistance of 0.6 cm H_2O are achieved. The valve can easily be dismantled for cleaning and sterilization.
2. The valve acts as a spillover valve, allowing excess inspiratory gas to be channelled directly to the expiratory outlet, bypassing the patient port.
3. The valve is suitable for both IPPV and spontaneous ventilation.

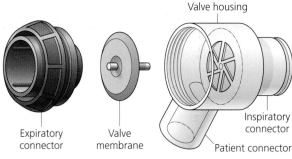

Valve housing

Expiratory connector

Valve membrane

Inspiratory connector

Patient connector

Fig. 8.14 An Ambu valve disassembled. (Courtesy Ambu, Alconbury, Weald, Cambridgeshire, UK.)

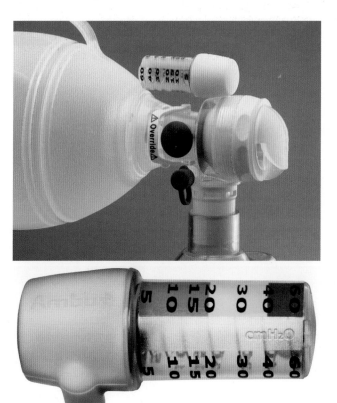

Fig. 8.15 Pressure manometer attached to a self-inflating bag. (Courtesy Ambu, Alconbury, Weald, Cambridgeshire, UK.)

4. The shape of the self-inflating bag is automatically restored after compression. This allows fresh gas to be drawn from the reservoir.
5. A paediatric version exists with a smaller inflating bag and a pressure relief valve.
6. A pressure manometer can be added to the bag to monitor airway pressure. This reduces lung barotrauma due to high inflation pressures (Fig. 8.15).

Self-inflating bag

- Compact, portable, self-inflating bag with a one-way valve.
- Oxygen reservoir can be added to increase FiO_2.
- Paediatric versions exist.

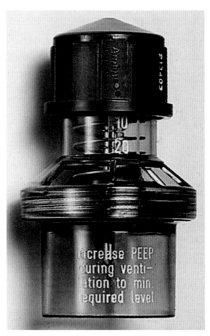

Fig. 8.16 The Ambu positive end expiratory pressure *(PEEP)* valve.

PEEP valve

This valve is used during IPPV to increase the functional residual capacity (FRC) to improve the patient's oxygenation.

It is a spring-loaded unidirectional valve positioned on the expiratory side of the a ventilator breathing system or a self-inflating bag with a standard 22-mm connector. By adjusting the valve knob, a PEEP of between 0 and 20 cm H_2O can be achieved (Figs. 8.16 and 8. 17).

The valve provides almost constant expiratory resistance over a very wide range of flow rates.

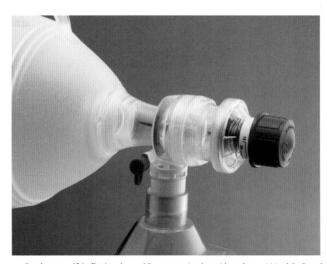

Fig. 8.17 The Ambu PEEP valve attached to a self-inflating bag. (Courtesy Ambu, Alconbury, Weald, Cambridgeshire, UK.)

SUGGESTED FURTHER READING

Chatburn, R.L., 2007. Classification of ventilator modes: update and proposal for implementation. Respir. Care 3, 301–323.

Chatburn, R.L., El-Khatib, M., Mireles-Cabodevila, E., 2014. A taxonomy for mechanical ventilation: 10 fundamental maxims. Respir. Care 59, 11.

Kacmarek, R.M., 2011. The mechanical ventilator: past, present, and future. Respir. Care 56 (8), 1170–1180.

Merck, 2007. Overview of Mechanical Ventilation. Available from: http://www.merckmanuals.com/professional/critical_care_medicine/respiratory_failure_and_mechanical_ventilation/overview_of_mechanical_ventilation.html.

Specifications for Rapidly Manufactured Ventilator System, 2020. MHRA. Available from: https://www.gov.uk/government/publications/specification-for-ventilators-to-be-used-in-uk-hospitals-during-the-coronavirus-covid-19-outbreak/rapidly-manufactured-ventilator-system-rmvs.

Van der Staay, M., Chatburn, R.L., 2018. Advanced modes of mechanical ventilation and optimal targeting schemes. Intensive Care Med. Exp. 6, 30.

SELF-ASSESSMENT QUESTIONS

Please check your eBook for additional self-assessment

MCQs

In the following lists, which of the following statements (a) to (e) are true?

1. Bag in bottle ventilator
a. The fresh gas flow (FGF) is the driving gas at the same time.
b. Is a minute volume divider.
c. The bellows can be either ascending or descending.
d. With a leak, the ascending bellows may continue to move almost normally.
e. Can be used only for adult patients.

2. Manley ventilator
a. Is a minute volume divider.
b. Has one set of bellows.
c. During controlled ventilation, it is safe to activate the emergency oxygen flush device of the anaesthetic machine.
d. A pressure-monitoring ventilator alarm is attached to the expiratory limb.
e. It acts as a Mapleson D system during spontaneous ventilation mode.

3. Bag in bottle ventilator
a. It is a time-cycled ventilator.
b. There is some mixing of the fresh gas and driving gas.

c. For safety reasons, the descending bellows design is preferred.
d. A small positive end expiratory pressure (PEEP) is expected.
e. The driving gas volume in the chamber equals the tidal volume.

4. Regarding classification of ventilators
a. A pressure generator ventilator can compensate for changes in lung compliance.
b. A flow generator ventilator cannot compensate for leaks in the system.
c. A time-cycling ventilator is affected by the lung compliance.
d. The duration of inspiration in a pressure-cycling ventilator is not affected by the compliance of the lungs.
e. A pressure generator ventilator can compensate, to a degree, for leaks in the system.

5. High-frequency jet ventilation
a. The fractional inspired oxygen concentration (FiO_2) can easily be measured.
b. Frequencies of up to 500 Hz can be achieved.
c. The cardiac output is better maintained than conventional intermittent positive pressure ventilation.
d. Can be used both in anaesthesia and intensive care.
e. Because of the lower peak airway pressures, there is no risk of barotrauma.

Single best answer

6. **Concerning pressure-control versus volume-control ventilation**
   a. Volume control will provide a set tidal volume.
   b. Pressure control will provide a set tidal volume.
   c. Lung compliance is irrelevant with pressure control.
   d. Paediatric ventilation never uses pressure control ventilation.
   e. Barotrauma is prevented by volume control ventilation.

Answers

1. Bag in bottle ventilator
   a. *False. The driving gas is separate from the FGF. The driving gas is usually either oxygen or, more economically, air. There is no mixing between the driving gas and the FGF. The volume of the driving gas reaching the chamber is equal to the tidal volume.*
   b. *False. The tidal volume and respiratory rate can be adjusted separately in a bag in bottle ventilator.*
   c. *True. Most of the bag in bottle ventilators use ascending bellows. This adds to the safety of the system as the bellows will collapse if there is a leak.*
   d. *False. See c.*
   e. *False. The ventilator can be used for both adults and children. A different size bellows can be used for different age groups.*

2. Manley ventilator
   a. *True. The tidal volume can be set in a Manley ventilator. The whole FGF (minute volume) is delivered to the patient according to the set tidal volume, thus dividing the minute volume.*
   b. *False. There are two sets of bellows in a Manley ventilator, the time-cycling bellows and the main bellows.*
   c. *False. As it is a minute volume divider and the FGF is the driving gas (see a above), activating the emergency oxygen flush will lead to considerable increase in the minute volume.*
   d. *False. The pressure-monitoring alarm should be attached to the inspiratory limb and not the expiratory limb. A Wright spirometer can be attached to the expiratory limb to measure the tidal volume.*

   e. *True. During the spontaneous (manual) breathing mode, the Manley ventilator acts as a Mapleson D system.*

3. Bag in bottle ventilator
   a. *True. The inspiratory and expiratory periods can be determined by adjusting the I:E ratio and the respiratory rate. So, for example, with a rate of 10 breaths/min and an I:E ratio of 1:2, each breath lasts for 6 seconds with an inspiration of 2 seconds and an expiration of 4 seconds.*
   b. *False. There is no mixing between the fresh gas and the driving gas as they are completely separate.*
   c. *False. In case of a leak in the system, the descending bellows will not collapse. The opposite occurs with the ascending bellows.*
   d. *True. A PEEP of 2–4 cm H_2O is expected due to the compliance of the bellows.*
   e. *True.*

4. Regarding classification of ventilators
   a. *False. A pressure generator ventilator cannot compensate for changes in lung compliance. It cycles when the set pressure has been reached. This can be a larger or smaller tidal volume depending on the lung compliance.*
   b. *True. It will deliver the set flow whether there is a leak or not.*
   c. *False. The ventilator will cycle with time regardless of the compliance.*
   d. *False. In a lung with low compliance, the inspiration will be shorter because the pressure will be reached more quickly, leading the ventilator to cycle and vice versa.*
   e. *True. The ventilator will continue to deliver gases, despite the leak, until a preset pressure has been reached.*

5. High-frequency jet ventilation
   a. **False.** *The ventilator uses the Venturi principle to entrain ambient air. The amount of entrainment is uncertain, making the measurement of the FiO_2 difficult.*
   b. **False.** *Frequencies of up to 500/min (not Hz, i.e. per second) can be achieved with a high-frequency jet ventilator.*
   c. **True.** *Because of the lower intrathoracic pressures generated during high-frequency jet ventilation, causing a lesser effect on the venous return, the cardiac output is better maintained.*

   d. **True.** *It can be used both in anaesthesia and intensive care, e.g. in the management of bronchopleural fistula.*
   e. **False.** *Although the risk is reduced, there is still a risk of barotrauma.*

6. *a.*

Chapter 9

Humidification and filtration

Inhaling dry gases can cause damage to the cells lining the respiratory tract, impairing ciliary function. Within a short period of just 10 minutes of ventilation with dry gases, cilia function will be disrupted. This increases the patient's susceptibility to respiratory tract infection. Inhaling dry gases has been shown to contribute to the cause of ventilator-associated pneumonia (VAP). A decrease in body temperature (due to the loss of the latent heat of vaporization) occurs as the respiratory tract humidifies the dry gases. It is thought that humidifying and warming inspired dry gas accounts for about 15% of the body's total basal heat expenditure.

Air, fully saturated with water vapour, has an absolute humidity of about 44 mg/L at 37°C. During nasal breathing at rest, inspired gases become heated to 36°C with a relative humidity of about 80%–90% by the time they reach the carina largely because of heat transfer in the nose. Mouth breathing reduces this to 60%–70% relative humidity. The humidifying property of soda lime can achieve an absolute humidity of 29 mg/L when used with the circle breathing system.

The *isothermic boundary point* is where 37°C and 100% humidity have been achieved. Normally it is a few centimetres distal to the carina. Insertion of a tracheal or tracheostomy tube bypasses the upper airway and moves the isothermic boundary distally. A similar effect happens when cold and dry gases are inhaled, as a greater proportion of the airways have to participate in heat and moisture exchange to achieve full saturation. Relative humidity in the operating theatre is usually measured with a hair hygrometer.

> ***Absolute humidity*** is the mass of water vapour per unit volume of gas measured in mg/L (at a specific temperature).
>
> ***Relative humidity*** is the ratio of the actual mass of water vapour in a volume of gas to the mass of water vapour required to saturate that volume of gas at a given temperature. It is expressed as a percentage.
>
> Relative humidity can also be calculated as the water vapour pressure over the saturated water vapour pressure.

> ***Characteristics of the ideal humidifier***
> - Capable of providing adequate levels of humidification.
> - Has low resistance to flow and low dead space.
> - Provides microbiological protection to the patient.
> - Maintenance of body temperature.
> - Safe and convenient to use.
> - Economical.

Heat and moisture exchanger humidifiers

Also known as 'artificial noses'! Heat and moist exchanger (HME) humidifiers are compact, inexpensive, passive and effective humidifiers for most clinical situations (Figs. 9.1 and 9.2). The British Standard describes them as 'devices intended to retain a portion of the patient's expired moisture and heat and return it to the respiratory tract during inspiration'.

The efficiency of an HME is gauged by the proportion of heat and moisture it returns to the patient. Adequate humidification is achieved with a relative humidity of 60%–70%. Inspired gases are warmed to temperatures of between 29°C and 34°C. HMEs should be able to deliver an absolute humidity of a minimum of 30 g/m³ water vapour at 30°C. HMEs are easy and convenient to use with no need for an external power source.

They are positioned between the breathing system and the catheter mount, which in turn is connected to the patient's mask, tracheal tube or supraglottic airway device (SGA).

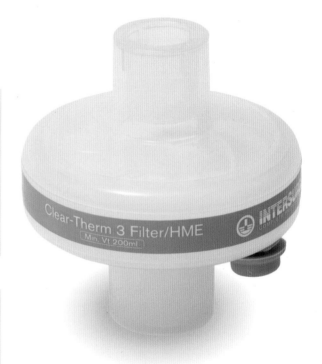

Fig. 9.1 The Clear-Therm HME (with filtration properties). (Courtesy Intersurgical, Wokingham, UK.)

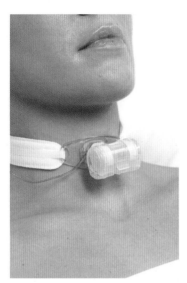

Fig. 9.2 The Thermovent T tracheostomy heat and moisture exchanger. (Courtesy Smiths Medical, Ashford, Kent, UK.)

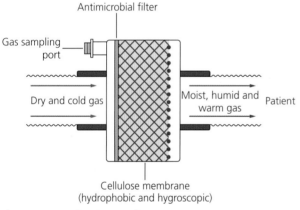

Fig. 9.3 Heat and moisture exchanger.

Components

1. Two ports that are designed to accept 15- and 22-mm size tubings and connections. Some designs have provision for connection of a sampling tube for gas and vapour concentration monitoring.
2. The head/housing contains a medium (Fig. 9.3), which can be:
   a. Hydrophobic (water repelling), such as aluminium or coated glass fibres to provide simple and cheap but less efficient HME. This medium has low thermal conductivity maintaining high temperature gradients.
   b. Hygroscopic (water retaining), such as paper or foam impregnated with calcium chloride or lithium chloride to provide better efficiency.
   c. Combined hygroscopic–hydrophobic to provide best efficiency.

Mechanism of action

1. In the hydrophobic HME, warm humidified exhaled gases pass through the humidifier, causing water vapour to condense on the cooler HME medium. The condensed water is evaporated and returned to the patient with the next inspiration of dry and cold gases, humidifying them. There is no addition of water over and above that previously exhaled.
2. In the hygroscopic version, the low thermal medium preserves the moisture by a chemical reaction with the salts, resulting in the chemical affinity to attract water particles, making it more efficient.
3. The greater the temperature difference between each side of the HME, the greater the potential for heat and moisture to be transferred during exhalation and inspiration.
4. The HME humidifier requires about 5–20 minutes before it reaches its optimal ability to humidify dry gases.
5. Some designs with a pore size of about 0.2 μm can filter out bacteria, viruses and particles from the gas flow in either direction, as discussed later. They are called heat and moisture exchanging filters (HMEFs).
6. Their volumes range from 7.8 mL (paediatric practice) to 100 mL. This increases the apparatus dead space.
7. The performance of the HME is affected by:
   a. water vapour content and temperature of the inspired and exhaled gases
   b. inspiratory and expiratory flow rates affecting the time the gas is in contact with the HME medium, hence the heat and moisture exchange
   c. the volume and efficiency of the HME medium: the larger the medium, the greater the performance. Low thermal conductivity, i.e. poor heat conduction, helps to maintain a greater temperature difference across the HME, increasing the potential performance.

Problems in practice and safety features

1. The estimated increase in resistance to flow due to these humidifiers ranges from 0.1 to 2.0 cm H₂O depending on the flow rate and the device used. Obstruction of the HME with mucus or because of the expansion of saturated heat exchanging material may occur and can result in dangerous increases in resistance.
2. It is recommended that they are used for a maximum of 24 hours and for single patient use only. There is a risk of increased airway resistance because of the accumulation of water in the filter housing if used for longer periods.
3. The humidifying efficiency decreases when large tidal and/or minute volumes are used.

4. For the HME to function adequately, a two-way gas flow is required.
5. For optimal function, HME must be placed in the breathing system close to the patient.
6. Generally, when aerosolized medications are administered, HMEs need to be removed from the breathing system to avoid aerosol deposition in the medium. However, some HMEs are designed to accept aerosolization.

> **Heat and moisture exchanger humidifiers**
> - Water vapour present in the exhaled gases is condensed or preserved on the medium. It is evaporated and returned to the patient with the following inspiration.
> - A relative humidity of 60%–70% can be achieved.
> - Some designs incorporate a filter.
> - Apparatus dead space and airway resistance is increased.
> - The water vapour content and temperature of gases, flow rate of gases and the volume of the medium affect performance of HMEs.

 Exam tip: The HME is a very popular topic in the exams. Know how they function and their advantages and limitations.

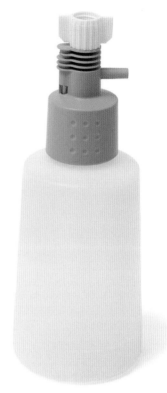

Fig. 9.4 Bubble humidifier. (Courtesy Intersurgical, Wokingham, UK.)

Bubble humidifier (Fig. 9.4)

This is an active humidifier in which the fresh gas flow (FGF) is simply bubbled through a sterile water container/bottle. The small bubbles gain humidity as they rise to the surface of the water. Such humidifiers are used with low-flow oxygen delivery devices, e.g. nasal cannulae. They are not very efficient due to the water losing latent heat of vaporization, so cooling it and making it less volatile, so reducing the amount of vapour produced.

Hot water bath humidifier

This provides active humidification by adding water vapour to a flow of gas in addition to the humidification efforts of the patient. It is used to deliver relative humidities higher than the heat moisture exchange humidifier. It is usually used in intensive care units (Fig. 9.5).

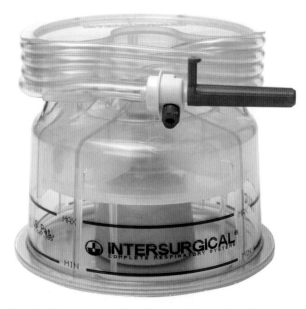

Fig. 9.5 Hot water humidifier. (Courtesy Intersurgical, Wokingham, UK.)

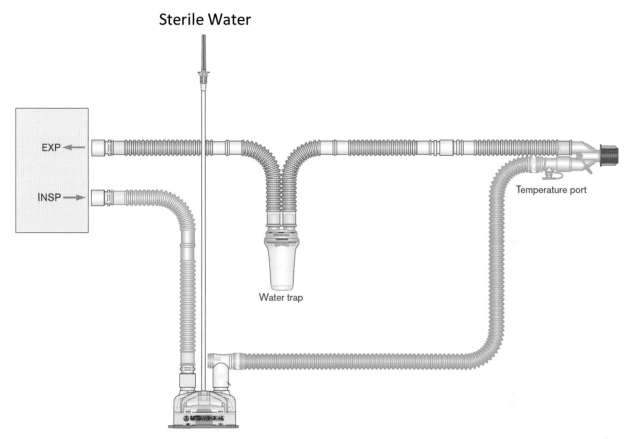

Fig. 9.6 Hot water humidifier breathing system. (Courtesy Intersurgical, Wokingham, UK.)

Components (Fig. 9.6)

1. It contains a disposable reservoir of sterile water with an inlet and outlet for inspired gases. Heated sterile water partly fills the container.
2. A thermostatically controlled heating element with temperature sensors, both in the reservoir and in the breathing system. The feedback temperature sensor is located close to the patient.
3. Tubing is used to deliver the humidified and warm gases to the patient. It should be as short as possible. A water trap is positioned between the patient and the humidifier along the tubing. The trap is positioned lower than the level of the patient.

Mechanism of action

1. Powered by electricity, the water is heated to between 45°C and 60°C (Fig. 9.7).
2. Dry cold FGF gas enters the container. This allows FGF to pass over the water surface, bubble through the water or come into contact with wicks dipped in the water, thereby dramatically increasing the surface area

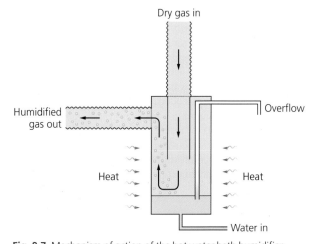

Fig. 9.7 Mechanism of action of the hot water bath humidifier.

available for evaporation. Some gas passes far from the water surface, gaining minimal saturation and heat.

3. The container has a large surface area for vaporization. This is to ensure that the gas is fully saturated at the temperature of the water bath. The amount of gas effectively bypassing the water surface should be minimal.

4. The tubing has poor thermal insulation properties, causing a decrease in the temperature of inspired gases. This is partly compensated for by the release of the heat of condensation.

5. By raising the temperature in the humidifier above body temperature, it is possible to deliver gases at 37°C and fully saturated. The temperature of gases at the patient's end is measured by a thermistor. Via a feedback mechanism, the thermistor controls the temperature of water in the container.

6. The temperature of gases at the patient's end depends on the surface area available for vaporization, the flow rate and the amount of cooling and condensation taking place in the inspiratory tubing.

7. Some designs have heated elements placed in the inspiratory and expiratory limb of the breathing system to maintain the temperature and prevent rainout (condensation) within the tube.

8. Some designs have an expiratory limb made from material that is permeable to water vapour.

Problems in practice and safety features

1. The humidifier, which is electrically powered, should be safe to use with no risk of scalding, overhydration and electric shock. A second backup thermostat cuts in should the first thermostat malfunction.

2. The humidifier and water trap(s) should be positioned below the level of the tracheal tube to prevent flooding of the airway by condensed water.

3. Colonization of the water by bacteria can be prevented by increasing the temperature to 60°C. This poses greater risk of scalding.

4. The humidifier is large, expensive and can be awkward to use.

5. There are more connections in a ventilator set-up, and so the risk of disconnections or leaks increases.

> **Hot water bath humidifier**
> - Consists of a container with a thermostatically controlled heating element and tubing with water traps.
> - The temperature of water in the container, via a feedback mechanism, is controlled by a thermistor at the patient's end.
> - Full saturation at 37°C can be achieved.
> - Colonization by bacteria is a problem.

Nebulizers (Fig. 9.8)

These produce a mist of microdroplets of water suspended in a gaseous medium. The quantity of water droplets delivered is not limited by gas temperature (as is the case with vapour). The smaller the droplets, the more stable they are. Droplets of 2–5 μm deposit in the tracheobronchial tree, whereas 0.5–1-μm droplets deposit in the alveoli. In addition to delivering water, nebulizers are used to deliver medications to peripheral airways and radioactive isotopes in diagnostic lung ventilation imaging.

There are three types of nebulizers: gas driven, spinning disc and ultrasonic.

GAS-DRIVEN (JET) NEBULIZER

Components

1. A capillary tube has the bottom end immersed in a water container.

2. The top end of the capillary tube is close to a Venturi constriction (Fig. 9.9).

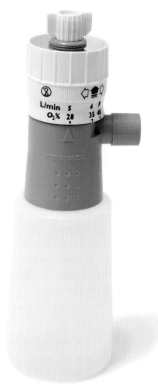

Fig. 9.8 Gas-driven nebulizer. (Courtesy Intersurgical, Wokingham, UK.)

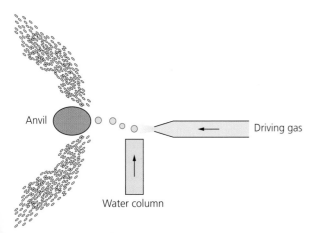

Anvil

Driving gas

Water column

Fig. 9.9 Mechanism of action of a gas-driven nebulizer.

Bacterial and viral filters (Fig. 9.10)

These minimize the risk of cross-transmission of bacteria and/or viruses among patients using the same anaesthetic breathing systems. The British Standard defines them as 'devices intended to reduce transmission of particulates, including microorganisms, in breathing systems'. It is thought that the incidence of bleeding after orotracheal intubation is 86%. The filter should be positioned as close to the patient as possible, e.g. on the disposable catheter mount, to protect the rest of the breathing system, ventilator and anaesthetic machine. It is recommended that a new filter should be used for each patient. A humidification element can be added, producing an HMEF (see Fig. 9.1).

Mechanism of action

1. A high-pressure gas flows through the Venturi, creating a negative pressure.
2. Water is drawn up through the capillary tube and broken into a fine spray. Even smaller droplets can be achieved as the spray hits an anvil or a baffle.
3. The majority of the droplets are in the range of 2–4 μm. These droplets tend to deposit on the pharynx and upper airway with a small amount reaching the bronchial level. This nebulizer is also capable of producing larger droplets of up to 20 μm. Droplets with diameters of 5 μm or more fall back into the container, leaving droplets of 4 μm or less to float out with the FGF.
4. The device is compact, making it easy to place close to the patient.

SPINNING DISC NEBULIZER

This is a motor-driven spinning disc throwing out microdroplets of water by centrifugal force. The water impinges onto the disc after being drawn from a reservoir via a tube over which the disc is mounted.

ULTRASONIC NEBULIZER

A transducer head vibrates at an ultrasonic frequency (e.g. 3 MHz). The transducer can be immersed into water or water can be dropped onto it, producing droplets less than 1–2 μm. Droplets of 1 μm or less are deposited in alveoli and lower airways. This is a highly efficient method of humidifying and delivering drugs to the airway. There is a risk of overhydration especially in children.

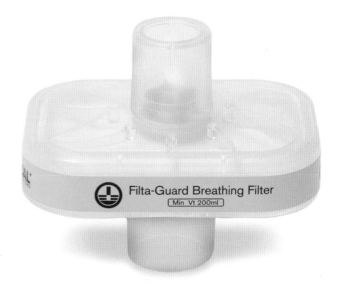

Filta-Guard Breathing Filter
Min Vt 200ml

Fig. 9.10 The Filta-Guard breathing filter. (Courtesy Intersurgical, Wokingham, UK.)

Characteristics of the ideal filter

- Efficient: the filter should be effective against both air- and liquid-borne microorganisms. A filtration action of 99.99%–99.999% should be achieved. This allows between 100 and 10 microorganisms to pass through the filter, respectively, after a 10^6 microorganism challenge. The filter should be effective bidirectionally.
- Minimal dead space, particularly for paediatric practice.
- Minimum resistance, especially when wet.
- Not affected by anaesthetic agents and does not affect the anaesthetic agents.
- Effective when either wet or dry. It should completely prevent the passage of contaminated body liquids (blood, saliva and other liquids) that may be present or generated in the breathing system.
- User friendly, lightweight, not bulky and nontraumatic to the patient.
- Disposable.
- Provides some humidification if no other methods are being used. Adequate humidification usually can be achieved by the addition of a hygroscopic element to the device.
- Transparent.
- Cost effective.

Size of microorganisms

Microorganism	Size (µm)
Hepatitis virus	0.02
Adenovirus	0.07
HIV	0.08
COVID-19 corona virus	0.05–0.1
Mycobacterium tuberculosis	0.3
Staphylococcus aureus	1.0
Cytomegalovirus	0.1

Components

1. Two ports are designed to accept 15- and 22-mm size tubings and connections.
2. A sampling port measures the gases'/agents' concentrations positioned on the anaesthetic breathing system side.
3. The filtration element can be either a felt-like electrostatic material or a pleated hydrophobic material.

Mechanism of action

There are five main mechanisms by which filtration can be achieved on a fibre:

1. *Direct interception:* large particles (=1 µm), such as dust and large bacteria, are physically prevented from passing through the pores of the filter because of their large size.
2. *Inertial impaction:* smaller particles (0.5–1 µm) collide with the filter medium because of their inertia. They tend to continue in straight lines, carried along by their own momentum rather than following the path of least resistance taken by the gas. The particles are held by Van der Waals electrostatic forces.
3. *Diffusional interception:* very small particles (<0.5 µm), such as viruses, are captured because they undergo considerable Brownian motion (i.e. random movement) because of their very small mass. This movement increases their apparent diameter so that they are more likely to be captured by the filter element.
4. *Electrostatic attraction:* this can be very important but it is difficult to measure as it requires knowing the charge on the particles and on the fibres. Increasing the charge on either the particles or the fibres increases the filtration efficiency. Charged particles are attracted to oppositely charged fibres by coulombic attraction.
5. *Gravitational settling:* this affects large particles (>5 µm). The rate of settling depends on the balance between the effect of gravity on the particle and the buoyancy of the particle. In filters used in anaesthesia, it has minimal effect as most of the settling occurs before the particles reach the filter.

ELECTROSTATIC FILTERS (Fig. 9.11)

1. The element used is subjected to an electric field producing a felt-like material with high polarity. One type of fibre becomes positively charged and the other type negatively charged. Usually two polymer fibres (modacrylic and polyprolyne) are used.
2. A flat layer of filter material can be used as the resistance to gas flow is lower per unit area.
3. These filters rely on the electrical charge to attract oppositely charged particles from the gas flow. They have a filtration efficiency of 99.99%.
4. The electrical charge increases the efficiency of the filter when the element is dry but can deteriorate rapidly when it is wet. The resistance to flow increases when the element is wet.
5. The electrical charge on the filter fibres decays with time so it has a limited life.
6. A hygroscopic layer can be added to the filter in order to provide humidification. In such an HMEF, the pressure drop across the element and thus the resistance to breathing will also increase with gradual absorption of water.

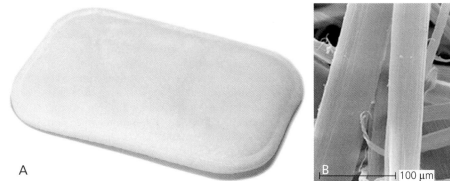
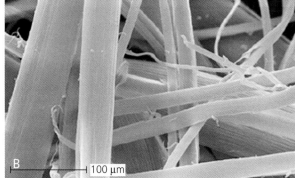

Fig. 9.11 (A) Electrostatic filter pad. (B) Microscopic view of an electrostatic filter. (A, Courtesy Intersurgical, Wokingham, UK.)

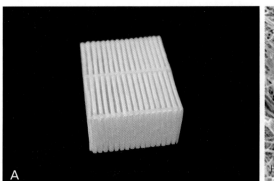
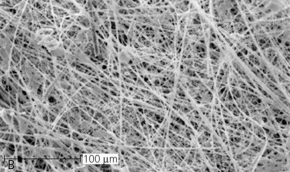

Fig. 9.12 (A) Pleated membrane. (B) Microscopic view of a hydrophobic filter. (A, Courtesy Intersurgical, Wokingham, UK.)

PLEATED HYDROPHOBIC FILTERS (Fig. 9.12)

1. The very small pore size filter membrane provides adequate filtration over longer periods of time. These filters rely on the naturally occurring electrostatic interactions to remove the particles. A filtration efficiency of 99.999% can be achieved.
2. To achieve minimal pressure drop across the device with such a small pore size, thereby allowing high gas flows while retaining low resistance, a large surface area is required. Pleated paper filters made of inorganic fibres are used to achieve this.
3. The forces between individual liquid water molecules are stronger than those between the water molecules and the hydrophobic membrane. This leads to the collection of water on the surface of the membrane with no absorption. Such a filter can successfully prevent the passage of water under pressures as high as 60 cm H_2O.

4. Although hydrophobic filters provide some humidification, a hygroscopic element can be added to improve humidification.
5. Currently, no evidence shows any type of filter is clinically superior to another.

> **Bacterial and viral filters**
> - Can achieve a filtration efficiency of 99.99%–99.999%.
> - Electrostatic filters rely on an electrical charge to attract oppositely charged particles. Their efficiency is reduced when wet, and they have a limited lifespan.
> - Hydrophobic pleated filters can repel water even under high pressures. They have a longer lifespan.

 Exam tip: As breathing filters (plus HME) are universally used in the operating theatre, a good understanding of the different types used and how they function is important.

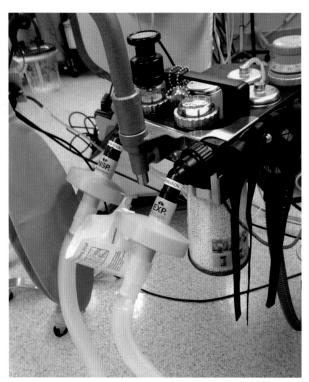

Fig. 9.13 Vapour-Clean activated charcoal filters in position in the circle breathing system. (Courtesy Dynasthetics.)

VAPOUR-CLEAN FILTERS

These filters are made of activated charcoal filters to remove traces of the volatile agents from an anaesthetic machine. They are used in the preparation of a 'vapour-free' anaesthetic machine when dealing with malignant hyperthermia susceptible patients. Using such filters, very low concentrations can be achieved within less than 2 minutes compared to up to 100 minutes when not used. The concentrations remained below the 5 ppm threshold for more than 60 minutes. It is recommended that filters are positioned on both the inspiratory and expiratory limbs of the circle breathing system (Fig. 9.13).

SUGGESTED FURTHER READING

Al Ashry, H.S., Modrykamien, A.M., 2014. Humidification during mechanical ventilation in the adult patient. BioMed Res. Int. 2014, 12.

Ball, D.R., 2015. Humidification devices. Anaesth. Intens. Care Med. 16 (8), 378–380.

McNulty, G., Eyre, L., 2015. Humidification in anaesthesia and critical care. Br. J. Anaesth. 15 (3), 131–135.

MHRA. Risk of using different airway humidification devices simultaneously. Available from: https://www.en gland.nhs.uk/patientsafety/wp-content/uploads/sites/32 /2015/12/psa-humidification-devices.pdf.

SELF-ASSESSMENT QUESTIONS

Please check your eBook for additional self-assessment

MCQs

In the following lists, which of the statements (a) to (e) are true?

1. Nebulizers

a. The gas-driven nebulizer can deliver much smaller droplets than the ultrasonic nebulizer.
b. There is a risk of drowning.
c. The temperature of the gas determines the amount of water delivered.
d. The smaller the droplets are, the more stable they are.
e. Droplets of 1 μm or less are deposited in the alveoli and lower airways.

2. Humidity

a. Humidity is measured using a hair hygrometer.
b. Air fully saturated with water vapour has a relative humidity of about 44 mg/L at 37°C.
c. Using the circle breathing system, some humidification can be achieved despite using dry fresh gas flow.
d. Relative humidity is the ratio of the mass of water vapour in a given volume of air to the mass of water vapour required to saturate the same volume at the same temperature.
e. The ideal relative humidity in the operating theatre is about 45%–55%.

3. Bacterial and viral filters

a. Particles of less than 0.5 μm can be captured by direct interception.
b. They can achieve a filtration action of 99.999%.
c. They should be effective when either wet or dry.
d. The filtration element used can be either an electrostatic or a pleated hydrophobic material.
e. The hydrophobic filter has a more limited lifespan than the electrostatic filter.

4. Hot water bath humidifiers

a. Heating the water improves the performance.
b. Because of its efficiency, the surface area for vaporization does not have to be large.
c. There is a risk of scalding to the patient.
d. Temperature in the humidifier is usually kept below body temperature.
e. The temperature of water in the container is controlled by a feedback mechanism using a thermistor, which measures the temperature of the gases at the patient's end.

5. Heat and moisture exchanger (HME) humidifiers

a. Inspired gases are warmed from 29°C to 34°C.
b. Performance is improved by increasing the volume of the medium.
c. An absolute humidity of 60%–70% can be achieved.
d. At high flows, the performance is reduced.
e. Performance is affected by the temperature of the inspired and exhaled gases.

6. Which of the following statements are true

a. Mucus can cause obstruction of the HME.
b. 2–5-μm-sized nebulized droplets are deposited in the alveoli.
c. HMEs should deliver a minimum of 300 g of water vapour at 30°C.
d. A relative humidity of 80% at the carina can be achieved during normal breathing.
e. HME requires some time before it reaches its optimal ability to humidify dry gases.

Answers

1. Nebulizers
   a. *False. The ultrasonic nebulizer can deliver very much smaller droplets. Droplets of 2–4 μm can be delivered by the gas-driven nebulizer. Droplets of less than 1–2 μm in size can be delivered by the ultrasonic nebulizer.*
   b. *True. This is especially so in children using the ultrasonic nebulizer.*
   c. *False. The temperature of the gas has no effect on the quantity of water droplets delivered. The temperature of the gas is of more importance in the humidifier.*
   d. *True. Very small droplets generated by the ultrasonic nebulizer are very stable and can be deposited in the alveoli and lower airways.*
   e. *True. See d.*

2. Humidity
   a. *True. The hair hygrometer is used to measure relative humidity between 15% and 85%. It is commonly used in the operating theatre. The length of the hair increases with the increase in ambient humidity. This causes a pointer to move over a chart, measuring the relative humidity.*
   b. *False. It should be absolute humidity and not relative humidity. Relative humidity is measured as a percentage.*
   c. *True. Water is produced as a product of the reaction between CO_2 and NaOH. An absolute humidity of 29 mg/L at 37°C can be achieved.*
   d. *True.*
   e. *True. A high relative humidity is uncomfortable for the staff in the operating theatre. Too low a relative humidity can lead to the build-up of static electricity, increasing the risk of ignition.*

3. Bacterial and viral filters
   a. *False. Such small particles are captured by diffusional interception. Direct interception can capture particles with sizes equal to or more than 1 μm.*
   b. *True. Hydrophobic filters can achieve a filtration action of 99.999%. Electrostatic filters can achieve 99.99%, which is thought to be adequate for routine use during anaesthesia.*
   c. *True. Hydrophobic filters are effective both when dry and wet. Electrostatic filters become less effective when wet.*
   d. *True.*
   e. *False. The electrostatic filter has a more limited lifespan than the hydrophobic filter. The efficacy of the electrostatic filter decreases as the electrical charge on the filter fibres decays.*

4. Hot water bath humidifiers
   a. *True. This is due to the loss of latent heat of vaporization as more water changes into vapour. The lower the water temperature, the less vapour is produced.*
   b. *False. A large surface area is needed to improve efficiency.*
   c. *True. A faulty thermostat can cause overheating of the water. There is usually a second thermostat to prevent this.*
   d. *False. The temperature of the humidifier is usually kept above body temperature. A large amount of heat is lost as the vapour and gases pass through the plastic tubings.*
   e. *True.*

5. HME humidifiers
   a. *True.*
   b. *True. The larger the volume of the medium, the better the performance of the HME. This is because of the larger surface area of contact between the gas and the medium.*
   c. *False. A relative, not absolute, humidity of 60%–70% can be achieved.*
   d. *True. At high flows, the time the gas is in contact with the medium is reduced, so decreasing the performance of the HME. The opposite is also correct.*
   e. *True. The higher the temperature of the gases, the better the performance of the HME.*

6. Which of the following statements are true
   a. *True. Mucus can cause obstruction of the HME, resulting in dangerous increases in resistance.*
   b. *False. 2–5-μm nebulized droplets are deposited in the tracheobronchial tree. Smaller droplets of 0.5–1 μm are deposited in the alveoli.*
   c. *False. HME should deliver a minimum of 30 g water vapour at 30°C.*
   d. *True.*
   e. *True. HME requires 5–20 minutes before it reaches its optimal ability to humidify dry gases.*

Chapter 10

Noninvasive monitoring

Clinical observation provides vital information regarding the patient. Observations gained from the use of the various monitors should augment that information; skin perfusion, capillary refill, cyanosis, pallor, skin temperature and turgor, chest movement and heart auscultation are just a few examples. The equipment used to monitor the patient is becoming more sophisticated. It is vital that the clinician using these monitors is aware of their limitations and the potential causes of error. Errors can be due to patient, equipment and/or sampling factors.

Monitoring equipment can be invasive or noninvasive. The latter is discussed in this chapter, whereas the former is discussed in Chapter 11.

Integrated monitoring

It was common to see the anaesthetic machine adorned with discrete, bulky monitoring devices. Significant advances in information technology have allowed an integrated monitoring approach to occur. Plug-in

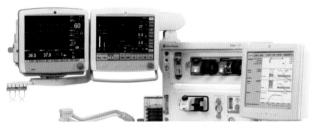

Fig. 10.1 GE integrated patient and machine monitoring mounted on Aisys CS² anaesthetic machine.

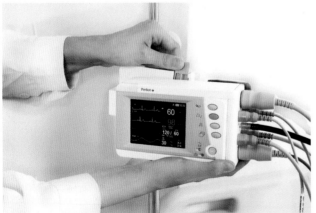

Fig. 10.2 Portable and compact Penlon AnaVue EMS monitor. (Courtesy Penlon, Abingdon, UK.)

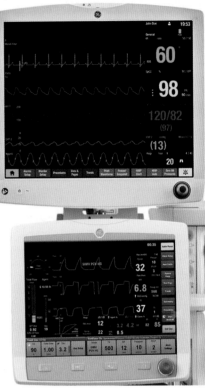

Fig. 10.3 Colour-coded values and waveforms displayed on the GE Aisys CS² monitor. (Courtesy GE, Hatfield, Hertfordshire, UK.)

monitoring modules feed a single visual display on which selected values and waveforms can be arranged and colour-coded (Figs. 10.1–10.3).

Although some would argue that such monitoring systems are complex and potentially confusing, their benefits in terms of flexibility and ergonomics are undisputed. Although there have been attempts to use wire-free devices using Bluetooth or wireless internet, it has not been widely accepted yet.

Electrocardiogram (ECG)

This monitors the electrical activity of the heart with electrical potentials of 0.5–2 mV at the skin surface. It is useful in determining the heart rate, ischaemia, the presence of arrhythmias and conduction defects. It should be emphasized that it gives no assessment of cardiac output.

The bipolar leads (I, II, III, AVR, AVL and AVF) measure voltage difference between two electrodes. The unipolar leads (V1–V6) measure voltage at different electrodes relative to a zero point.

Components

1. Skin electrodes detect the electrical activity of the heart (Fig. 10.4). Silver and silver chloride form a stable electrode combination. Both are held in a cup and separated from the skin by a foam pad soaked in conducting gel. Changes in potential difference at the skin lead to polarization of the silver/silver chloride electrode.
2. Colour-coded cables transmit the polarization signal from electrodes to the monitor. Cables are available in 3- and 5-lead versions as snap or grabber design and with a variety of lengths. All the cables of a particular set should have the same length to minimize the effect of electromagnetic interference.
3. The ECG signal is then boosted using an amplifier. The amplifier covers a frequency range of 0.05–150 Hz. It also filters out some of the frequencies considered to be noise. The amplifier has ECG filters that are used to remove the noise/artefacts from ECG and produce a 'clean' signal.
4. An oscilloscope displays the amplified ECG signal. A high-resolution monochrome or colour monitor is used.

Mechanism of action

1. Proper attachment of ECG electrodes involves cleaning the skin, gently abrading the stratum corneum and ensuring adequate contact using conductive gel. Skin impedance varies at different sites and it is thought to be higher in females. The electrodes are best positioned on bony prominences to reduce artefacts from respiration.

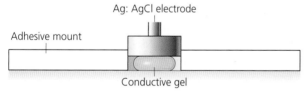

Fig. 10.4 An electrocardiogram electrode.

2. Modern ECG monitors use multiple filters for signal processing. The filters used should be capable of removing the unwanted frequencies, leaving the signal intact (Fig. 10.5). Two types of filters are used for this purpose:
   a. *high-pass filters* attenuate the frequency components of a signal below a certain frequency. They help to remove lower frequency noise from the signal; they block lower frequencies and let higher frequency content pass. For example, the respiratory component of an ECG can be removed by turning on a 1-Hz high-pass filter on the amplifier. The filter will centre the signal around the zero isoline.
   b. *low-pass filters* attenuate the frequency components of a signal above a certain frequency. They block higher frequencies and let lower frequency content pass. They are useful for removing noise from higher-frequency signals. So an amplifier with a 35-Hz low-pass filter will remove/attenuate signals above 35 Hz and help to 'clean' the ECG signal. They reduce interference from diathermy, muscle shivering, spasms and other movement artefacts.
3. The ECG monitor can have two modes:
   a. the *monitoring mode* has a limited frequency response of 0.5–40 Hz. Filters are used to narrow the bandwidth to reduce environmental artefacts. The high-frequency filters reduce distortions from muscle movement and mains current and electromagnetic interference from other equipment. The low-frequency filters help provide a stable baseline by reducing respiratory and body movement artefacts.
   b. the *diagnostic mode* has a wider frequency response of 0.05–150 Hz. The high-frequency limit allows the assessment of the ST segment, QRS morphology and tachyarrhythmias. The low-frequency limit allows representation of P- and T-wave morphology and ST-segment analysis.

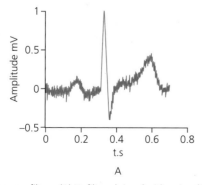
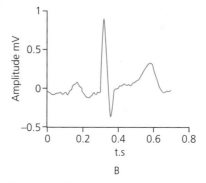

Fig. 10.5 Electrocardiogram filters. (A) Unfiltered signal with noise. (B) Filtered 'clean' signal.

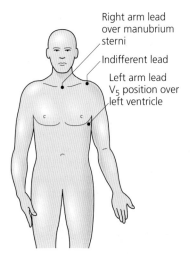

Right arm lead over manubrium sterni

Indifferent lead

Left arm lead V$_5$ position over left ventricle

Fig. 10.6 The CM5 electrocardiogram lead configuration.

4. There are many ECG electrode configurations. Usually during anaesthesia, three skin electrodes are used (right arm, left arm and indifferent leads). The three limb leads used include two that are 'active' and one that is 'inactive' (earth). Sometimes five electrodes are used. Lead II is ideal for detecting arrhythmias but only 35% of ischaemic changes. CM5 configuration is able to detect 66%–75% of ST-segment changes due to left ventricular ischaemia. In CM5, the right-arm electrode is positioned on the manubrium (chest lead from manubrium), the left-arm electrode is on V5 position (fifth interspace in the left anterior axillary line) and the indifferent lead is on the left shoulder or any convenient position (Fig. 10.6).

5. The CB5 configuration is useful during thoracic anaesthesia. The right-arm electrode is positioned over the centre of the right scapula and the left-arm electrode is over V5.

6. A display speed of 25 mm/s and a sensitivity of 1 mV/cm are standard in the United Kingdom.

Problems in practice and safety features

1. Incorrect placement of the ECG electrodes in relation to the heart is a common error, leading to false information.

2. Electrical interference can be a 50-Hz (in the United Kingdom) mains line interference because of capacitance or inductive coupling effect. Any electrical device powered by alternating current (AC) can act as one plate of a capacitor and the patient acts as the other plate. Interference can also be because of high-frequency current interference from diathermy. Most modern monitors have the facilities to avoid interference. Shielding of cables and leads, differential amplifiers and electronic filters all help to produce an interference-free monitoring system. Differential amplifiers measure the difference between the potential from two different sources. If interference is common to the two input terminals (e.g. mains frequency), it can be eliminated as only the differences between the two terminals is amplified. This is called *common mode rejection ratio (CMRR)*. Amplifiers used in ECG monitoring should have a high CMRR of 100,000:1 to 1,000,000:1, which is a measurement of capability to reject the noise. They should also have a high input impedance (about 10 MΩ) to minimize the current taken from the electrodes. Table 10.1 shows the various types and sources of interference and how to reduce the interference.

3. Muscular activity, such as shivering, can produce artefacts. Positioning the electrodes over bony prominences and the use of low-pass filters can reduce these artefacts.

4. High and low ventricular rate alarms and an audible indicator of ventricular rate are standard on most designs. More advanced monitors have the facility to monitor the ST segment (Fig. 10.7). Continuous monitoring and measurement of the height of the ST segment allows early diagnosis of ischaemic changes.

5. Absence of or improperly positioned patient diathermy plate can cause burns at the site of ECG skin electrodes. This is because of the passage of the diathermy current via the electrodes, causing a relatively high current density.

ECG

- Silver and silver chloride skin electrodes detect the electrical activity of the heart, 0.5–2 mV at the skin surface.
- The signal is boosted by an amplifier and displayed by an oscilloscope.
- The ECG monitor can have two modes: the monitoring mode (frequency range 0.5–40 Hz) and the diagnostic mode (frequency range 0.05–150 Hz).
- CM5 configuration is used to monitor left ventricular ischaemia.
- Electrical interference can be due to either diathermy or mains frequency.
- Differential amplifiers are used to reduce interference (common mode rejection).

Table 10.1 ECG signal interference		
Type of interference	**Sources of interference**	**How to reduce interference**
Electromagnetic induction	Any electrical cable or light	Use long ECG and twisted leads (rejecting the induced signal as common mode) Use selective filters in amplifiers
Electrostatic induction and capacitance coupling	Stray capacitances between table, lights, monitors, patients and electrical cables	ECG leads are surrounded by copper screens
Radiofrequency interference (>150 Hz)	Diathermy enters the system by: mains supply direct application by probe radio transmission via probe and wire	High-frequency filters clean up signal before entering input Filtering power supply of amplifiers Double screen electronic components of amplifiers and earth outer screen Newer machines operate at higher frequencies

ECG, Electrocardiogram.

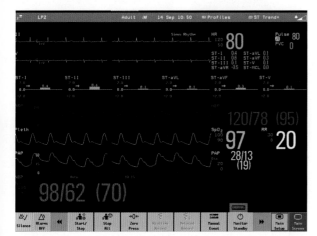

Fig. 10.7 Electrocardiogram and ST-segment monitoring. (Courtesy Philips Healthcare, Guildford, UK.)

Arterial blood pressure

Oscillometry is the commonest method used to measure arterial blood pressure noninvasively during anaesthesia. The systolic, diastolic and mean arterial pressures and pulse rate are measured, calculated and displayed. These devices give reliable trend information about the blood pressure. They are less reliable in circumstances where a sudden change in blood pressure is anticipated or where a minimal change in blood pressure is clinically relevant. The term 'device for indirect noninvasive automated mean arterial pressure' is used for such devices.

Components

1. A cuff with a tube is used for inflation and deflation. Some designs have an extra tube for transmitting pressure fluctuations to the pressure transducer.
2. The case where the microprocessor, pressure transducer and a solenoid valve that controls the deflation of the arm cuff are housed. It contains the display and a timing mechanism, which adjusts the frequency of measurements. Alarm limits can be set for both high and low values.

Mechanism of action

1. The microprocessor is set to control the sequence of inflation and deflation.
2. The cuff is inflated to a pressure above the previous systolic pressure, then it is deflated incrementally. The return of blood flow causes oscillation in cuff pressure (Fig. 10.8).
3. The transducer senses the pressure changes, which are interpreted by the microprocessor. This transducer has an accuracy of ±2%.
4. The output signal from the transducer passes through a filter to an amplifier that amplifies the oscillations. The output from the amplifier passes to the microprocessor through the analogue digital converter (ADC). The microprocessor controls the pneumatic pump for inflation of the cuff and the solenoid valve for deflation of the cuff.
5. The systolic pressure corresponds to the onset of rapidly increasing oscillations. The mean arterial blood pressure corresponds to the maximum oscillation at the lowest cuff pressure.

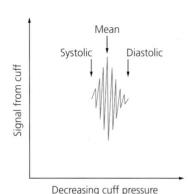

Fig. 10.8 Diagram showing how oscillations in cuff pressure correspond to mean, systolic and diastolic pressures.

Table 10.2 A guide to the correct blood pressure cuff size

Width (cm)	Patient
3	Neonate
5	Infant
6	Child
9	Small adult
12	Standard adult
15	Large adult

6. The diastolic pressure corresponds to the onset of rapidly decreasing oscillations. In addition, it is mathematically computed from the systolic and mean pressure values (mean blood pressure = diastolic blood pressure + 1/3 pulse pressure).
7. The cuff must be of the correct size (Table 10.2). It should cover at least two-thirds of the upper arm. The width of the cuff's bladder should be 40% of the mid-circumference of the limb. The middle of the cuff's bladder should be positioned over the brachial artery.
8. Some designs have the ability to apply venous stasis to facilitate intravenous cannulation.

Problems in practice and safety features

1. For the device to measure the arterial blood pressure accurately, it should have a fast cuff inflation and a slow cuff deflation (at a rate of 3 mmHg/s or 2 mmHg/beat). The former is to avoid venous congestion, and the latter provides enough time to detect the arterial pulsation.
2. If the cuff is too small, the blood pressure is over-read, whereas it is under-read if the cuff is too large. The error is greater with too small than too large a cuff.
3. The systolic pressure is over-read at low pressures (systolic pressure less than 60 mmHg) and under-read at high systolic pressures.
4. Atrial fibrillation and other arrhythmias affect performance.
5. External pressure on the cuff or its tubing can cause inaccuracies.
6. Frequently repeated cuff inflations can cause ulnar nerve palsy and petechial haemorrhage of the skin under the cuff.

The Finapres (**fin**ger arterial **pres**sure) device uses a combination of oscillometry and a servo control unit. The volume of blood in the finger varies with the cardiac cycle. A small cuff placed around the finger is

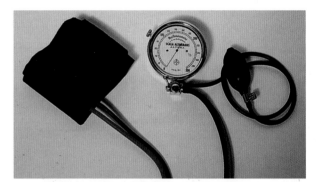

Fig. 10.9 The Von Recklinghausen oscillotonometer.

used to keep the blood volume of the finger constant. An infrared photo-plethysmograph detects changes in the volume of blood within the finger with each cardiac cycle. A controller system alters the pressure in the cuff accordingly to keep the volume of blood in the finger constant. The applied pressure waveform correlates with the arterial blood volume and, therefore, with the arterial blood pressure. This applied pressure is then displayed continuously, in real time, as the arterial blood pressure waveform.

THE VON RECKLINGHAUSEN OSCILLOTONOMETER

During the premicroprocessor era, the *Von Recklinghausen oscillotonometer* was widely used (Fig. 10.9).

Components

1. It has two cuffs: the upper, occluding cuff (5-cm wide) overlaps a lower, sensing cuff (10-cm wide). An inflation bulb is attached.

2. The case contains:
   a. two bellows: one connected to the atmosphere and the other connected to the lower sensing cuff
   b. a mechanical amplification system
   c. the oscillating needle and dial
   d. the control lever
   e. the release valve.

Mechanism of action

1. With the control lever at rest, air is pumped into both cuffs and the air-tight case of the instrument using the inflation bulb to a pressure exceeding systolic arterial pressure. By operating the control lever, the lower sensing cuff is isolated and the pressure in the upper cuff and instrument case is allowed to decrease slowly through an adjustable leak controlled by the release valve. As systolic pressure is reached, pulsation of the artery under the lower cuff results in pressure oscillations within the cuff and its bellows. The pressure oscillations are transmitted via a mechanical amplification system to the needle. As the pressure in the upper cuff decreases below diastolic pressure, the pulsation ceases.
2. The mean pressure is at the point of maximum oscillation.
3. This method is reliable at low pressures. It is useful to measure trends in blood pressure.

Problems in practice and safety features

1. In order for the device to operate accurately, the cuffs must be correctly positioned and attached to their respective tubes.
2. The diastolic pressure is not measured accurately with this device.

Arterial blood pressure
- Oscillometry is the method used.
- Mean arterial pressure corresponds to maximum oscillation.
- A cuff with a tube(s) is connected to a transducer and a microprocessor.
- Accurate within the normal range of blood pressure.
- Arrhythmias and external pressure affect the performance.

PULSE OXIMETRY

This is a noninvasive measurement of the arterial blood oxygen saturation at the level of the arterioles. A continuous display of the oxygenation (plethysmographic oxygen saturation [SpO_2]) is achieved by a simple, accurate and rapid method (Fig. 10.10).

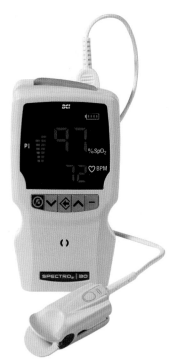

Fig. 10.10 Smiths Medical handheld Spectro oximeter. (Courtesy Smiths Medical, Ashford, Kent, UK.)

Pulse oximetry has proved to be a powerful monitoring tool in the operating theatre, recovery wards, intensive care units, general wards and during the transport of critically ill patients. It is considered to be the greatest recent technical advance in monitoring. It enables the detection of arterial hypoxaemia, allowing treatment before tissue damage occurs.

Components

1. A probe is positioned on the finger, toe, ear lobe or nose (Fig. 10.11). Two light-emitting diodes (LEDs) produce beams at red and infrared frequencies (660 nm and 940 nm, respectively) on one side, and there is a sensitive photodetector on the other side. The LEDs operate in sequence at a rate of about 30 times/s (Fig. 10.12).
2. The case houses the microprocessor. There is a display of the oxygen saturation, pulse rate and a plethysmographic waveform of the pulse. Alarm limits can be set for a low saturation value and for both high and low pulse rates.

Mechanism of action

1. The oxygen saturation is estimated by measuring the transmission of light through a pulsatile vascular tissue bed (e.g. finger). This is based on Beer's law

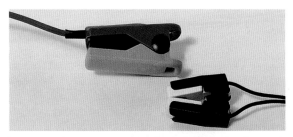

Fig. 10.11 Pulse oximeter probes. Finger probe *(top)* and ear probe *(bottom)*.

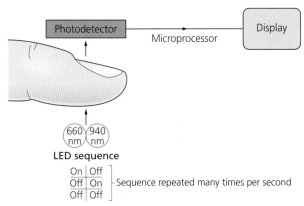

Fig. 10.12 Working principles of the pulse oximeter. The light-emitting diodes *(LEDs)* operate in sequence, and when both are off, the photodetector measures the background level of ambient light.

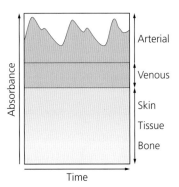

Fig. 10.13 Schematic representation of the contribution of various body components to the absorbance of light.

(the relation between the light absorbed and the concentration of solute in the solution) and Lambert's law (relation between absorption of light and the thickness of the absorbing layer).

2. The amount of light transmitted depends on many factors. The light absorbed by nonpulsatile tissues (e.g. skin, soft tissues, bone and venous blood) is constant (direct current [DC]). The nonconstant absorption (AC) is the result of arterial blood pulsations (Fig. 10.13). The sensitive photodetector generates a voltage proportional to the transmitted light. The AC component of the wave is about 1%–5% of the total signal.

3. The high frequency of the LEDs allows the absorption to be sampled many times during each pulse beat. This is used to enable running averages of saturation to be calculated many times per second. This decreases the 'noise' (e.g. movement) effect on the signal.

4. The microprocessor is programmed to mathematically analyse both the DC and AC components at 660 and 940 nm, calculating the ratio of absorption at these two frequencies (R:IR ratio). The result is related to the arterial saturation. The absorption of oxyhaemoglobin

and deoxyhaemoglobin at these two wavelengths is very different. This allows these two wavelengths to provide good sensitivity. One of the isobestic points of oxyhaemoglobin and deoxyhaemoglobin is 805 nm. The OFF part allows a baseline measurement for any changes in ambient light.

5. A more recent design uses multiple wavelengths to eradicate false readings from carboxyhaemoglobin and methaemoglobinaemia. Advanced oximeters use more than seven light wavelengths. This has enabled the measurement of haemoglobin value, oxygen content and carboxyhaemoglobin and methaemoglobin concentrations.

6. A variable pitch beep provides an audible signal of changes in saturation.

Problems in practice and safety features

1. It is accurate (±2%) in the 70%–100% range. Below the saturation of 70%, readings are extrapolated. Pulse oximeter accuracy is highest at saturations of 90%–100%, intermediate at 80%–90%, and lowest below 80%.

2. The absolute measurement of oxygen saturation may vary from one probe to another but with accurate trends. This is due to the variability of the centre wavelength of the LEDs.

3. Carbon monoxide poisoning (including smoking), coloured nail varnish, intravenous injections of certain dyes (e.g. methylene blue, indocyanine green) and drugs responsible for the production of methaemoglobinaemia are all sources of error (Table 10.3).

4. Hypoperfusion and severe peripheral vasoconstriction affect the performance of the pulse oximeter. This is because the AC signal sensed is about 1%–5% of the DC signal when the pulse volume is normal. This makes it less accurate during vasoconstriction when the AC component is reduced.

Table 10.3 Sources of error in pulse oximetry

HbF	No significant clinical change (absorption spectrum is similar to the adult Hb over the range of wavelengths used)
MetHb	False low reading
CoHb	False high reading
SulphHb	Not a clinical problem
Bilirubin	Not a clinical problem
Dark skin	No effect
Methylene blue	False low reading
Indocyanine green	False low reading
Nail varnish	May cause false low reading

Pulse oximetry
- Consists of a probe with two LEDs and a photodetector.
- A microprocessor analyses the signal.
- Accurate within the clinical range.
- Inaccurate readings in carbon monoxide poisoning, the presence of dyes and methaemoglobinaemia.
- Hypoperfusion and severe vasoconstriction affect the reading.

 Exam tip: It is important to have a good understanding of the physical principles used in pulse oximetry. Also know its limitations and the factors that can affect its accuracy.

5. The device monitors the oxygen saturation with no direct information regarding oxygen delivery to the tissues.
6. Pulse oximeters average their readings every 10–20 seconds. They cannot detect acute desaturation. The response time to desaturation is longer with the finger probe (more than 60 seconds), whereas the ear probe has a response time of 10–15 seconds.
7. Excessive movement or malposition of the probe is a source of error. Newer designs such as the Masimo oximeter claim more stability despite motion. External fluorescent light can be a source of interference.
8. Inaccurate measurement can be caused by venous pulsation. This can be because of high airway pressures, the Valsalva manoeuvre or other consequences of impaired venous return. Pulse oximeters assume that any pulsatile absorption is caused by arterial blood pulsation only.
9. The site of the application should be checked at regular intervals as the probe can cause pressure sores with continuous use. Some manufacturers recommend changing the site of application every 2 hours especially in patients with impaired microcirculation. Burns in infants have been reported.
10. Pulse oximetry only gives information about a patient's oxygenation. It does not give any indication of a patient's ability to eliminate carbon dioxide.

Masimo

Masimo is a company that offers a suite of innovative monitoring options. The pulse oximetry is based on signal extraction technology, which allows the saturation of the venous blood to be ignored. Two wavelengths of light are used (as per conventional pulse oximetry), but through signal processing techniques (parallel engines and adaptive filters), a more accurate assessment of the true arterial oxygen saturation can be achieved. This is also true for moving patients or patients with poor peripheral circulation, where conventional pulse oximetry often fails.

A more advanced version of the pulse oximeter uses 'rainbow pulse co-oximetry', whereby more than seven wavelengths of light continuously and noninvasively measure haemoglobin (SpHb), carboxyhaemoglobin (SpCO), methaemoglobin (SpMet), oxygen saturation (SpO$_2$), pulse rate, perfusion index (PI) and pleth variability index (PVI) (Fig. 10.14).

The Sed Line (Masimo, Basingstoke, UK) monitors brain function and the effects of anaesthesia and sedation. By monitoring four channels of bilateral electroencephalogram (EEG) waveforms via adhesive electrodes applied to the forehead, a continuous display can be produced on a combined monitor (Fig. 10.15).

1. The EEG information is displayed as: 'Patient State Index', which is related to the depth of anaesthesia.
2. 'Density Spectral Array', which represents activity in both sides of the brain.

O3 (Masimo, Basingstoke, UK) regional oximetry is also available and offers an alternative to conventional pulse oximetry for monitoring cerebral oxygenation.

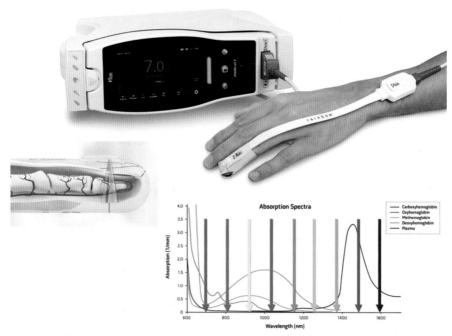

Fig. 10.14 Masimo oximetry with rainbow technology.

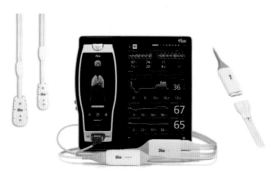

Fig. 10.15 The SedLine monitor and electrode.

> **Technical terms used in measuring end-tidal CO_2**
> - *Capnograph* is the device that records and shows the graphical display of waveform of CO_2 (measured in kPa or mmHg). It displays the value of CO_2 at the end of expiration, which is known as end-tidal CO_2.
> - *Capnogram* is the graphical plot of CO_2 partial pressure (or percentage) versus time.
> - *Capnometer* is the device that only shows numerical concentration of CO_2 without a waveform.

End-tidal carbon dioxide analysers (capnographs)

Gases with molecules that contain at least two dissimilar atoms absorb radiation in the infrared region of the spectrum. Using this property, both inspired and exhaled carbon dioxide concentration can be measured directly and continuously throughout the respiratory cycle (Fig. 10.16).

The end-tidal CO_2 is less than alveolar CO_2 because the end-tidal CO_2 is always diluted with alveolar dead space gas from unperfused alveoli. These alveoli do not take part in gas exchange and so contain no CO_2. Alveolar CO_2 is less than arterial CO_2 as the blood from unventilated alveoli and lung parenchyma (both have higher CO_2 contents) mixes with the blood from ventilated alveoli. In healthy adults with normal lungs, end-tidal CO_2 is 0.3–0.6 kPa less than arterial CO_2. This difference is reduced if the lungs are ventilated with large tidal volumes. The Greek root *kapnos*, meaning 'smoke', give us the term *capnography* (CO_2 can be thought as the 'smoke' of cellular metabolism).

End-tidal CO_2 < alveolar CO_2 < $PaCO_2$

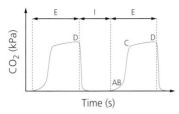

Fig. 10.16 Diagram of an end-tidal carbon dioxide waveform. *A–B* represents the emptying of the upper dead space of the airways. As this has not undergone gas exchange, the CO_2 concentration is zero. *B–C* represents the gas mixture from the upper airways and the CO_2-rich alveolar gas. The CO_2 concentration rises continuously. *C–D* represents the alveolar gas and is described as the 'alveolar plateau'. The curve rises very slowly. D is the end-tidal CO_2 partial pressure where the highest possible concentration of exhaled CO_2 is achieved at the end of expiration. It represents the final portion of gas that was involved in the gas exchange in the alveoli. Under certain conditions (see text) it represents a reliable index of the arterial CO_2 partial pressure. *D–A* represents inspiration where the fresh gas contains no CO_2. *E*, Expiration; *I*, inspiration.

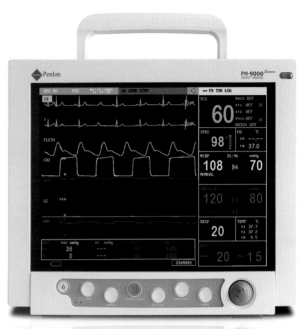

Fig. 10.18 The Penlon PM9000 Express, which measures end-tidal CO_2, oximetry and inhalational agent concentration using a side-stream method. (Courtesy Penlon Ltd, Abingdon, UK.)

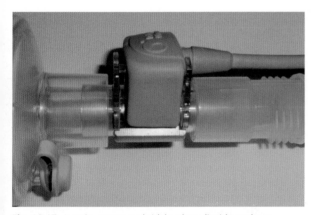

Fig. 10.17 A main-stream end-tidal carbon dioxide analyser.

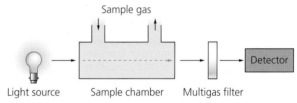

Fig. 10.19 Components of a gas analyser using an infrared light source suitable for end-tidal carbon dioxide measurement. The reference chamber has been omitted for the sake of clarity.

In reality, the devices used cannot determine the different phases of respiration but simply report the minimum and maximum CO_2 concentrations during each respiratory cycle.

Components

1. The sampling chamber can either be positioned within the patient's gas stream (main-stream version [Fig. 10.17]) or connected to the distal end of the breathing system via a sampling tube (side-stream version [Fig. 10.18]).
2. A photodetector measures light reaching it from a light source at the correct infrared wavelength (using optical filters) after passing through two chambers. One acts as a reference, whereas the other one is the sampling chamber (Fig. 10.19).

Mechanism of action

1. Carbon dioxide absorbs the infrared radiation particularly at a wavelength of 4.3 μm.
2. The amount of infrared radiation absorbed is proportional to the number of carbon dioxide molecules (partial pressure of carbon dioxide) present in the chamber.
3. The remaining infrared radiation falls on the thermopile detector, which in turn produces heat. The heat is measured by a temperature sensor and is proportional to the partial pressure of carbon dioxide gas present in the mixture in the sample chamber. This produces an electrical output. This means that the amount of gas present is inversely proportional to the

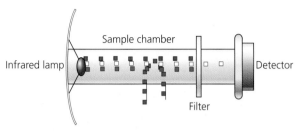

Fig. 10.20 Principles of infrared detector: due to the large amount of infrared absorption in the sample chamber by the carbon dioxide, little infrared finally reaches the detector.

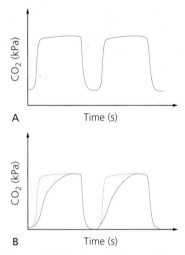

Fig. 10.21 (A) An end-tidal carbon dioxide waveform that does not return to the baseline during inspiration, indicating that rebreathing is occurring. (B) An end-tidal carbon dioxide waveform that illustrates the sloping plateau seen in patients with chronic obstructive airways disease. The normal waveform is superimposed *(dotted line).*

amount of infrared light present at the detector in the sample chamber (Fig. 10.20).

4. In the same way, a beam of light passes through the reference chamber, which contains room air. The absorption detected from the sample chamber is compared to that in the reference chamber. This allows the calculation of carbon dioxide values.

5. The inspired and exhaled carbon dioxide forms a square wave with a zero baseline unless there is rebreathing (Fig. 10.21A).

6. A microprocessor-controlled infrared lamp is used. This produces a stable infrared source with a constant output. The current is measured with a current-sensing resistor, the voltage across, which is proportional to the current flowing through it. The supply to the light source is controlled by the feedback from the sensing resistor, maintaining a constant current of 150 mA.

7. Using the rise and fall of the carbon dioxide during the respiratory cycle, monitors are designed to measure the respiratory rate.

8. Alarm limits can be set for both high and low values.

9. To avoid drift, the monitor should be calibrated regularly with known concentrations of CO_2 to ensure accurate measurement.

Photoacoustic spectroscopy: In these infrared absorption devices, the sample gas is irradiated with pulsatile infrared radiation of a suitable wavelength. The periodic expansion and contraction produces a pressure fluctuation of audible frequency that can be detected by a microphone. The advantages of photoacoustic spectrometry over conventional infrared absorption spectrometry are as follows:

1. The photoacoustic technique is extremely stable, and its calibration remains constant over much longer periods of time.

2. The very fast rise and fall times give a much more accurate representation of any change in CO_2 concentration.

Carbon dioxide analysers can be either side-stream or main-stream analysers.

SIDE-STREAM ANALYSERS

1. This consists of a 1.2-mm internal diameter tube that samples the gases (both inspired and exhaled) at a constant rate, e.g. 150–200 mL/min, with modern monitors using flow rates as low as 50 mL/min. The tube is connected to a lightweight adapter near the patient's end of the breathing system (usually with a pneumotachograph for spirometry) with a small increase in the dead space. It delivers the gases to the sample chamber. The tube is made of Teflon so it is impermeable to carbon dioxide and does not react with anaesthetic agents.

2. As the gases are humid, there is a moisture trap with an exhaust port, allowing gas to be vented to the atmosphere or returned to the breathing system.

3. In order to accurately measure end-tidal carbon dioxide, the sampling tube should be positioned as close as possible to the patient's trachea.

4. A variable time delay before the sample is presented to the sample chamber is expected. The *transit time* delay depends on the length (which should be as short as possible, e.g. 2 m) and diameter of the sampling tube and the sampling rate. A delay of less than 3.8 seconds is acceptable. The *rise time* delay is the time for the analyser to respond to the signal and depends upon the size of the sample chamber and the gas flow.

5. Other gases and vapours can be analysed from the same sample.

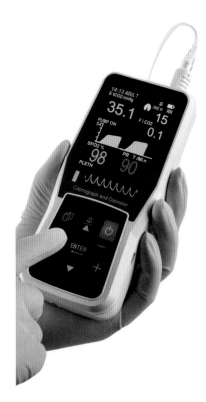

Fig. 10.22 The PC-900B portable capnograph and oximeter. (Courtesy Proact Medical, Corby, UK.)

6. Portable handheld side-stream analysers are available (Fig. 10.22). They can be used during patient transport and in out-of-hospital situations.

MAIN-STREAM ANALYSER

1. The sample chamber is positioned within the patient's gas stream, increasing the dead space. In order to prevent water vapour condensation on its windows, it is heated to about 41°C.
2. Since there is no need for a sampling tube, there is no transport time delay in gas delivery to the sample chamber.
3. Other gases and vapours are not measured simultaneously.

See Table 10.4 for a comparison of side-stream and main-stream analysers.

Uses (Table 10.5)

In addition to its use as an indicator for the level of ventilation (hypo-, normo- or hyperventilation), end-tidal carbon dioxide measurement is useful:

1. To diagnose oesophageal intubation (no or very little carbon dioxide is detected). Following manual ventilation or the ingestion of carbonated drinks, some carbon dioxide might be present in the stomach. Characteristically, this may result in up to 5–6 waveforms with an abnormal shape and decreasing in amplitude.
2. As a disconnection alarm for a ventilator or breathing system. There is sudden absence of the end-tidal carbon dioxide.
3. To diagnose lung embolism as a sudden decrease in end-tidal carbon dioxide, assuming that the arterial blood pressure remains stable.
4. To diagnose malignant hyperpyrexia as a gradual increase in end-tidal carbon dioxide.

Table 10.4 Comparison of various qualities between side-stream and main-stream analysers

	Side stream	Main stream
Disconnection possible	Yes	Yes
Sampling catheter leak common	Yes	No
Calibration gas required	Yes	No
Sensor damage common	No	Some
Multiple gas analysis possible	Yes	No
Use on nonintubated patients	Yes	No

Table 10.5 Summary of the uses of end-tidal CO_2

Increased end-tidal CO_2	Decreased end-tidal CO_2
Hypoventilation	Hyperventilation
Rebreathing	Pulmonary embolism
Sepsis	Hypoperfusion
Malignant hyperpyrexia	Hypometabolism
Hyperthermia	Hypothermia
Skeletal muscle activity	Hypovolaemia
Hypermetabolism	Hypotension

Problems in practice and safety features

1. In patients with chronic obstructive airways disease, the waveform shows a sloping trace and does not accurately reflect the end-tidal carbon dioxide (see Fig. 10.21B). An ascending plateau usually indicates impairment of the ventilation:perfusion ratio because of uneven emptying of the alveoli.

2. During paediatric anaesthesia, it can be difficult to produce and interpret end-tidal carbon dioxide because of the high respiratory rates and small tidal volumes. The patient's tidal breath can be diluted with fresh gas.

3. During a prolonged expiration or end-expiratory pause, the gas flow exiting the trachea approaches zero. The sampling line may aspirate gas from the trachea and the inspiratory limb, causing ripples on the expired CO_2 trace (cardiogenic oscillations). They appear during the alveolar plateau in synchrony with the heartbeat. It is thought to be due to mechanical agitation of deep lung regions that expel CO_2-rich gas. Such fluctuations can be smoothed over by increasing lung volume using positive end expiratory pressure (PEEP).

4. Dilution of the end-tidal carbon dioxide can occur whenever there are loose connections and system leaks.

5. Nitrous oxide (may be present in the sample for analysis) absorbs infrared light with an absorption spectrum partly overlapping that of carbon dioxide (Fig. 10.23). This causes inaccuracy of the detector, with nitrous oxide being interpreted as carbon dioxide. By careful choice of the wavelength using special filters, this can be avoided. This is not a problem in most modern analysers.

6. Collision broadening or pressure broadening is a cause of error. The absorption of carbon dioxide is increased because of the presence of nitrous oxide or nitrogen. Calibration with a gas mixture that contains the same background gases as the sample solves this problem.

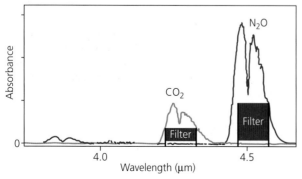

Fig. 10.23 Carbon dioxide and nitrous oxide infrared absorption spectrum.

End-tidal carbon dioxide measurement

- Uses the principle of infrared absorption by carbon dioxide.
- The infrared radiation falls on a temperature sensor, producing an electrical output.
- Photoacoustic spectroscopy with a microphone can also be used.
- Sampling can be either side stream or main stream.
- It reflects accurately the arterial carbon dioxide partial pressure in healthy individuals. End-tidal CO_2 < alveolar CO_2 < arterial CO_2.
- It is used to monitor the level of ventilation, affirm tracheal intubation as a disconnection alarm and to diagnose lung embolization and malignant hyperpyrexia.
- Nitrous oxide can distort the analysis in some designs.

 Exam tip: A good understanding of the physical principles of capnography is essential. What information can be gained from monitoring the end-tidal CO_2? Knowledge of the more common capnograph waveforms is required.

Oxygen concentration analysers

It is fundamental to monitor oxygen concentration in the gas mixture delivered to the patient during general anaesthesia. The fractional inspired oxygen concentration (FiO_2) is measured using a galvanic, polarographic or paramagnetic method (Fig. 10.24). The galvanic and polarographic analysers have a slow response time (20–30 seconds) because they are dependent on membrane diffusion. The paramagnetic analyser has a rapid response time. The paramagnetic analyser is currently more widely used. These analysers measure the oxygen partial pressure, displayed as a percentage.

PARAMAGNETIC (PAULING) OXYGEN ANALYSERS

Components

1. Two chambers are separated by a sensitive pressure transducer. The gas sample containing oxygen is delivered to the measuring chamber. The reference (room air) is delivered to the other chamber. This is accomplished via a sampling tube.

2. An electromagnet is rapidly switched on and off (a frequency of about 100–110 Hz), creating a changing magnetic field to which the gases are subjected. The electromagnet is designed to have its poles in close proximity, forming a narrow gap.

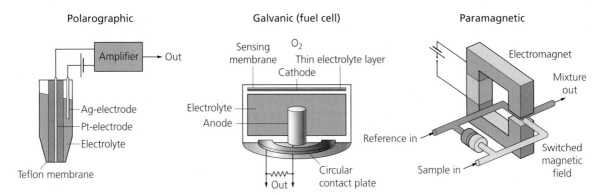

Fig. 10.24 Different types of oxygen analysers.

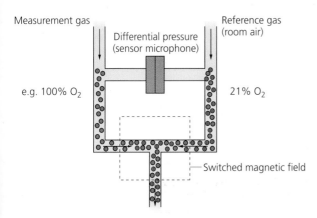

Fig. 10.25 Paramagnetic oxygen analyser.

Mechanism of action (Fig. 10.25)

1. Oxygen is attracted to the magnetic field (paramagnetism) because of the fact that it has two electrons in unpaired orbits. Most of the gases used in anaesthesia are repelled by the magnetic field (diamagnetism).
2. The magnetic field causes the oxygen molecules to be attracted and agitated. This leads to changes in pressure on both sides of the transducer. The pressure difference (about 20–50 µbar) across the transducer is proportional to the oxygen partial pressure difference between the sample and reference gases. The transducer converts this pressure force to an electrical signal that is displayed as oxygen partial pressure or is converted to a reading in volume percentage.
3. They are very accurate and highly sensitive. The analyser should function continuously without any service breaks.
4. The modern paramagnetic oxygen analysers have a rapid response making it possible to analyse the inspired and expired oxygen concentration on a breath-to-breath basis. The older designs of oxygen analysers had a slow response time (nearly 1 minute).
5. The audible alarms can be set for low and high concentration limits.

The old version of the paramagnetic analyser consists of a container with two spheres filled with nitrogen (a weak diamagnetic gas). The spheres are suspended by a wire, allowing them to rotate in a nonuniform magnetic field.

When the sample enters the container, it is attracted by the magnetic field, causing the spheres to rotate. The degree of rotation depends on the number of oxygen molecules present in the sample. The rotation of the spheres displaces a mirror attached to the wire and a light deflected from the mirror falls on a calibrated screen for measuring oxygen concentration.

THE GALVANIC OXYGEN ANALYSER (HERSCH FUEL CELL)

1. It generates a current proportional to the partial pressure of oxygen (so acting as a battery requiring oxygen for the current to flow). It does not require an external power source.
2. It consists of a noble metal cathode and a lead anode in a potassium chloride electrolyte solution. An oxygen-permeable membrane separates the cell from the gases in the breathing system.
3. The oxygen molecules diffuse through the membrane and electrolyte solution to the gold cathode (see Fig. 10.24), generating an electrical current proportional to the partial pressure of oxygen.
4. At the cathode: $O_2 + 4e \rightarrow 4(OH)^-$
   At the anode: $Pb + 2(OH) \rightarrow PbO + H_2O + 2e^-$
5. Calibration is achieved using 100% oxygen and room air (21% oxygen).
6. It reads either the inspiratory or expiratory oxygen concentration. It is usually positioned at the common gas outlet of the anaesthetic machine.
7. Water vapour does not affect its performance.

8. It is depleted by continuous exposure to oxygen because of exhaustion of the cell, so limiting its lifespan to about 1 year.
9. The fuel cell has a slow response time of about 20 seconds with an accuracy of ±3%.

POLAROGRAPHIC (CLARK ELECTRODE) OXYGEN ANALYSERS

1. They have similar principles to the galvanic analysers (see Fig. 10.23). A platinum cathode and a silver anode in an electrolyte solution are used. The electrodes are polarized by a 600–800 mV power source. An oxygen-permeable Teflon membrane separates the cell from the sample.
2. The number of oxygen molecules that traverse the membrane is proportional to its partial pressure in the sample. An electrical current is produced when the cathode donates electrons that are accepted by the anode. For every molecule of oxygen, four electrons are supplied, making the current produced proportional to the oxygen partial pressure in the sample.
3. They give only one reading, which is the average of inspiratory and expiratory concentrations.
4. Their life expectancy is limited (about 3 years) because of the deterioration of the membrane.

Problems in practice and safety features

1. Regular calibration of the analysers is vital.
2. Paramagnetic analysers are affected by water vapour; therefore a water trap is incorporated in their design.
3. The galvanic and the polarographic cells have limited lifespans and need regular service.
4. The fuel cell and the polarographic electrode have slow response times of about 20–30 seconds with an accuracy of ±3%.
5. The positioning of the oxygen analyser is debatable. It has been recommended that slow responding analysers are positioned on the inspiratory limb of the breathing system and fast responding analysers are positioned as close as possible to the patient.

Oxygen analysers
- Paramagnetic, galvanic and polarographic cells are used. The former is more widely used.
- The galvanic and polarographic analysers have a slow response time because of membrane diffusion. The paramagnetic analyser has a rapid response time.
- Oxygen is attracted by the magnetic field whereas the gases or vapours are repelled.
- The paramagnetic cell measures the inspired and ex-pired oxygen concentration simultaneously on a breath-by-breath basis.

 Exam tip: There is a need to have a good understanding of the various methods used to measure oxygen concentration. Knowledge is also needed of which method is usually used as an oxygen concentration analyser in an anaesthetic machine.

Nitrous oxide and inhalational agent concentration analysers

Modern vaporizers are capable of delivering accurate concentrations of the anaesthetic agent(s) with different flows. It is important to monitor the inspired and end-tidal concentrations of the agents. This is of vital importance in the circle system as the exhaled inhalational agent is recirculated and added to the fresh gas flow. In addition, because of the low flow, the inhalational agent concentration the patient is receiving is different from the setting of the vaporizer.

Modern analysers can measure the concentration of all the agents available, halothane, enflurane, isoflurane, sevoflurane and desflurane, on a breath-by-breath basis (Fig. 10.26) using infrared.

Components

1. A sampling tube from an adapter within the breathing system delivers gas to the analyser.
2. A sample chamber to which gas for analysis is delivered.
3. It has an infrared light source.
4. Optical filters are used.
5. It has a photodetector.

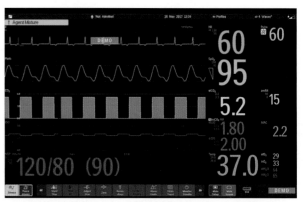

Fig. 10.26 Inspired (Fi) and end-tidal (ET) values are displayed for carbon dioxide, oxygen, nitrous oxide and isoflurane (ISO). (Courtesy Philips Healthcare, Guildford, UK.)

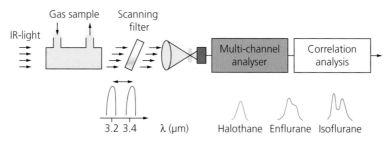

Fig. 10.27 Mechanism of action of an infrared *(IR)* anaesthetic agent monitor with automatic agent identification properties. Agents absorb IR light differently over a wavelength band of 3.2–3.4 mm. The monitor can therefore identify the agent in use automatically by analysing its unique absorbance pattern.

Mechanism of action

1. Infrared absorption analysers are used (Fig. 10.27). The sampled gas enters a chamber where it is exposed to infrared light. A photodetector measures the light, reaching it across the correct infrared wavelength band. Absorption of the infrared light is proportional to the vapour concentration. The electrical signal is then analysed and processed to give a measurement of the agent concentration.
2. Optical filters are used to select the desired wavelengths. Different analyser designs use different wavelengths for anaesthetic agent analysis. An infrared light of a wavelength of 4.6 μm is used for N_2O. For the inhalational agents, higher wavelengths are used, between 8 and 9 μm. This is to avoid interference from methane and alcohol that happen at the lower 3.3-μm band.
3. Modern sensors can automatically identify and measure concentrations of up to three agents present in a mixture and produce a warning message to the user. Five sensors are used to produce a spectral shape where the five outputs are compared and the shape produced represents the spectral signal of the agent present in the sample. This is compared with the spectral shapes stored in the memory of the sensor and used to identify the agent. Currently, it is possible to detect and measure the concentrations of halothane, enflurane, isoflurane, sevoflurane and desflurane (Figs. 10.28 and 10.29).
4. The amplitude of the spectral shape represents the amount of vapour present in the mixture. The amplitude is inversely proportional to the amount of agent present. The output of the infrared lamp is kept constant with a constant supply of current. Optical filters are used to filter the desirable wavelengths. Because of the autodetection, individual calibration for each agent is not necessary.
5. A reference beam is incorporated. This allows the detector software to calculate how much energy has been absorbed by the sample at each wavelength and therefore the concentration of agent in the sample.

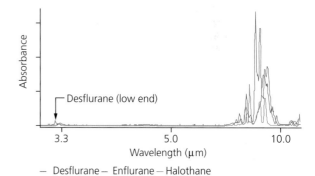

Fig. 10.28 Inhalational agents infrared absorption spectrum.

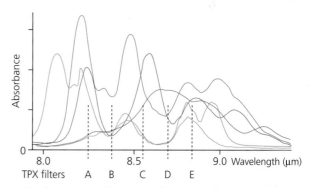

Fig. 10.29 Agent identification and measurement: to measure and identify the agents, all five sensors are used to produce a spectral shape. When the detectors at all five outputs are compared, *A, B, C, D* and *E*, a spectral shape is produced, representing the spectral signal of the agent present in the sample.

6. The sample gas can be returned to the breathing system, making the analysers suitable for use with the circle breathing system.
7. No individual calibration for each agent is necessary.
8. Water vapour has no effect on the performance and accuracy of the analyser.

PIEZOELECTRIC QUARTZ CRYSTAL OSCILLATION

Piezoelectric quartz crystal oscillation can be used to measure the concentration of inhalational agents. A lipophilic-coated piezoelectric quartz crystal undergoes changes in natural resonant frequency when exposed to the lipid-soluble inhalational agents. This change in frequency is directly proportional to the partial pressure of agent. Such a technique lacks agent specificity and sensitivity to water vapour.

Other methods less commonly used for measuring inhalational agent concentration are:

1. *Raman spectroscopy:* the anaesthetic gas sample is illuminated by an intense argon laser. Some light energy is simply reflected, but some energy stimulates the sample molecules, causing them to scatter light of a different wavelength from that of the incident light energy (Raman scattering). This scattered light is detected at right angles to the laser beam, and the difference in energy level between the incident and reflected light is measured. All molecules in the gas/volatile phase can be identified by their characteristic spectrum of (Raman) scattering.
2. *Ultraviolet absorption:* in the case of halothane, with similar principles to infrared absorption but using ultraviolet absorption.

Problems in practice and safety features

1. Some designs of infrared light absorption analysers are not agent specific. These must be programmed by the user for the specific agent being administered. Incorrect programming results in erroneous measurements.
2. Alarms can be set for inspired and exhaled inhalational agent concentration.

Inhalational agent concentration analysers

- A sample of gas is used to measure the concentration of inhalational agent using infrared light absorption.
- By selecting light of the correct wavelengths, the inspired and expired concentrations of the agent(s) can be measured.
- An infrared light of a wavelength of 4.6 μm is used for N_2O. For other inhalational agents, higher wavelengths are used, between 8 and 9 μm.
- Ultraviolet absorption, mass spectrometry and quartz crystal oscillation are other methods of measuring the inhalational agents' concentration.

MASS SPECTROMETER

This can be used to identify and measure, on a breath-to-breath basis, the concentrations of the gases and vapours used during anaesthesia. The principle of action is to charge the particles of the sample (bombard them with an electron beam) and then separate the components into a spectrum according to their specific mass:charge ratios, so each has its own 'fingerprint'.

The creation and manipulation of the ions are done in a high vacuum (10^{-5} mmHg) to avoid interference by outside air and to minimize random collisions among the ions and the residual gas. The relative abundance of ions at certain specific mass:charge ratios is determined and is related to the fractional composition of the original gas mixture.

A permanent magnet is used to separate the ion beam into its component ion spectra. Because of the high expense, multiplexed mass spectrometer systems are used with several patient sampling locations on a time-shared basis.

Table 10.6 summarizes the methods used in gas and in vapour analysis.

Table 10.6 The various methods used in gas and vapour analysis				
Technology	**O_2**	**CO_2**	**N_2O**	**Inhalational agent**
Infrared		✓	✓	✓
Paramagnetic	✓			
Polarography	✓			
Fuel cell	✓			
Mass spectrometry	✓	✓	✓	✓
Raman spectroscopy	✓	✓	✓	✓
Piezoelectric resonance				✓

Wright respirometer

This compact and light (weighs less than 150 g) respirometer is used to measure the tidal volume and minute volume (Fig. 10.30).

Components

1. The respirometer consists of an inlet and an outlet.
2. A rotating vane surrounded by angled slits (Fig. 10.31). The vane is attached to a pointer.
3. Buttons on the side of the respirometer to turn the device on and off and reset the pointer to the zero position.

Mechanism of action

1. The Wright respirometer is a one-way system. It allows the measurement of the tidal volume if the flow of the gases is in one direction only. The correct direction for gas flow is indicated by an arrow.
2. The slits surrounding the vane are to create a circular flow in order to rotate the vane. The vane does 150 revolutions for each litre of gas passing through. This causes the pointer to rotate a round the respirometer display.
3. The outer display is calibrated at 100 mL per division. The small inner display is calibrated at 1 L per division.
4. It is usually positioned on the expiratory side of the breathing system, which is at a lower pressure than the inspiratory side. This minimizes the loss of gas volume due to leaks and expansion of the tubing.
5. For clinical use, the respirometer reads accurately the tidal volume and minute volume ($\pm 5\%$–10%) within the range of 4–24 L/min. A minimum flow of 2 L/min is required for the respirometer to function accurately.
6. To improve accuracy, the respirometer should be positioned as close to the patient's trachea as possible.
7. The resistance to breathing is very low, at about 2 cm H_2O at 100 L/min.
8. A paediatric version exists with a capability of accurate tidal volume measurements between 15 and 200 mL.
9. A more accurate version of the Wright respirometer uses light reflection to measure the tidal volume. The mechanical causes of inaccuracies (friction and inertia) and the accumulation of water vapour are avoided. Other designs use a semiconductive device that is sensitive to changes in magnetic field. Tidal volume and minute volume can be measured by converting these changes electronically. An alarm system can also be added.

Problems in practice and safety features

1. The Wright respirometer tends to over-read at high flow rates and under-read at low flows.
2. Water condensation from the expired gases causes the pointer to stick, thus preventing it from rotating freely.

Wright respirometer
- Rotating vane attached to a pointer.
- Fitted on the expiratory limb to measure the tidal and minute volume with an accuracy of $\pm 5\%$–10%.
- The flow is unidirectional.
- It over-reads at high flows and under-reads at low flows.

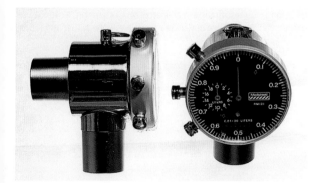

Fig. 10.30 A Wright respirometer. An *arrow* on the side of the casing indicates the direction of gas flow.

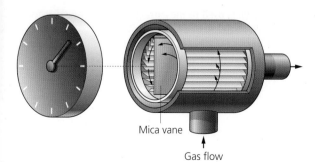

Mica vane

Gas flow

Fig. 10.31 Mechanism of action of the Wright respirometer.

Pneumotachograph

Pneumotachograph measures gas flow. From this, gas volume can be calculated. It is a constant orifice (or resistance), variable pressure flowmeter.

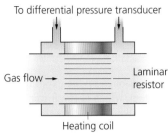

Fig. 10.32 A pneumotachograph. See text for details.

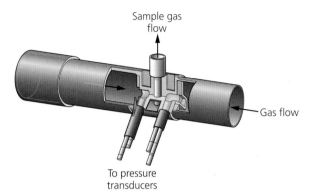

Fig. 10.33 Combined pneumotachograph and Pitot tube. (Courtesy GE Healthcare, Hatfield, UK.)

Components

1. A tube with a fixed resistance. The resistance can be a bundle of parallel tubes (Fig. 10.32).
2. Two sensitive pressure transducers on either side of the resistance.

Mechanism of action

1. The principle of its function is sensing the change in pressure across a fixed resistance through which gas flow is laminar.
2. The pressure change is only a few millimetres of water and is linearly proportional, over a certain range, to the flow rate of gas passing through the resistance.
3. The tidal volumes can be summated over a period of a minute to give the minute volume.
4. It can measure flows in both inspiration and expiration (i.e. bidirectional).

Problems in practice and safety features

Water vapour condensation at the resistance will encourage the formation of turbulent flow, affecting the accuracy of the measurement. This can be avoided by heating the parallel tubes.

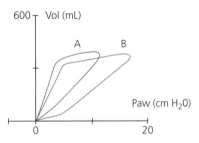

Fig. 10.34 Volume pressure loops in a patient (A) before and (B) during CO_2 insufflation in a laparoscopic operation. Note the decrease in compliance and increase in airway pressure (Paw).

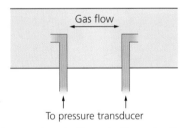

Fig. 10.35 Cross section of a Pitot tube flowmeter. The two ports are facing in opposite directions within the gas flow.

Combined pneumotachograph and Pitot tube

This combination (Fig. 10.33) is designed to improve accuracy and calculate and measure the compliance, airway pressures, gas flow, volume/pressure (Fig. 10.34) and flow/volume loops. Modern devices can be used accurately even in neonates and infants.

THE PITOT TUBE

Components

1. It has two pressure ports: one facing the direction of gas flow, the other facing perpendicular to the gas flow. This is used to measure gas flow in one direction only.
2. In order to measure bidirectional flows (inspiration and expiration), two pressure ports face in opposite directions within the gas flow (Fig. 10.35).
3. These pressure ports are connected to pressure transducers.

Mechanism of action

The pressure difference between the ports is proportional to the square of the flow rate.

Problems in practice and safety features

The effects of the density and viscosity of the gas(es) can alter the accuracy. This can be compensated for by continuous gas composition analysis via a sampling tube.

Factors affecting the readings in pneumotachograph

- **Location:** should be placed between the breathing system Y-piece and the tracheal tube.
- **Gas composition:** nominal values of gas composition need to be known with sensors calibrated accordingly.
- **Gas temperature:** a knowledge of gas temperatures is required. Usually, the sensors' software provides default values for a typical patient.
- **Humidity:** moisture can affect measurement and generation of pressure drop. Have the pressure ports directed upwards to prevent fluid from draining into them.
- **Apparatus dead space:** sensors need to have a minimum dead space; <10 mL for the adult flow sensors and <1 mL for the neonatal sensors.
- **Operating range of flow sensor:** sensors are designed to function accurately with a very wide range of tidal volumes, I:E ratios, frequencies and flow ranges.
- **Inter-sensor variability:** individual sensors can have different performances. There should be no need for individual device calibration of the flow/pressure characteristics.

The effects of the density and viscosity of the gas(es) can alter the accuracy. This can be compensated for by continuous gas composition analysis via a sampling tube.

Pneumotachograph

- A bidirectional device to measure the flow rate and tidal and minute volumes.
- A laminar flow across a fixed resistance causes changes in pressure, which are measured by transducers.
- Condensation at the resistance can cause turbulent flow and inaccuracies.
- Improved accuracy is achieved by adding a Pitot tube(s) and continuous gas composition analysis.

Ventilator alarms

It is mandatory to use a ventilator alarm during intermittent positive pressure ventilation (IPPV) to guard against patient disconnection, leaks, obstruction or malfunction. These can be pressure- and/or volume-monitoring alarms. Clinical observation, end-tidal carbon dioxide concentration, airway pressure and pulse oximetry are also ventilator monitors.

PRESSURE MONITORING ALARM

Such devices were widely used in conjunction with the Manley ventilator (see Chapter 8). Although such devices are not commonly used in the current practice, it is important to understand its principles.

Components

1. The case where the pressure alarm limits are set, an automatic on/off switch. A light flashes with each ventilator cycle (Fig. 10.36).
2. The alarm is pressurized by a sensing tube, connecting it to the inspiratory limb of the ventilator system.

Mechanism of action

1. In this alarm, the peak inspiratory pressure is usually measured and monitored during controlled ventilation.
2. A decrease in peak inspiratory pressure activates the alarm. This indicates that the ventilator is unable to achieve the preset threshold pressure in the breathing system. Causes can be disconnection, gas leak or inadequate fresh gas flow.
3. An increase in the peak inspiratory pressure usually indicates an obstruction.
4. The low-pressure alarm can be set to 7 cm H_2O, 7 cm H_2O plus time delay or 13 cm H_2O. The high-pressure alarm is set at 60 cm H_2O.

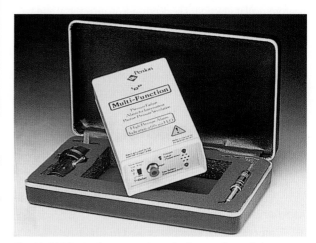

Fig. 10.36 The Penlon pressure monitoring ventilator alarm.

Problems in practice and safety features

Disconnection of the breathing system with partial obstruction of the alarm sensing tube may lead to a condition where the alarm is not activated despite inadequate ventilation.

VOLUME MONITORING ALARM

The expired gas volume can be measured and monitored. Gas volume can be measured either directly using a respirometer or indirectly by integration of the gas flow (pneumotachograph).

These alarms are usually inserted in the expiratory limb with a continuous display of tidal and minute volume. The alarm limits are set for a minimum and maximum tidal and/or minute volume.

> *Ventilator alarms*
> - They can be pressure- and/or volume-monitoring alarms.
> - They detect disconnection (low pressure) or obstruction (high pressure) in the ventilator breathing system.
> - The pressure alarms are fitted on the inspiratory limb, whereas the volume alarms are fitted on the expiratory limb of the breathing system.
> - Regular servicing is required.

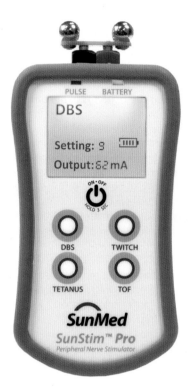

Fig. 10.37 The SunStim Pro peripheral nerve stimulator (Courtesy Blue Box Medical, Southampton, UK.)

Peripheral nerve stimulators and neuromuscular blockade monitoring

These devices are used to monitor transmission across the neuromuscular junction. The depth, adequate reversal and type of neuromuscular blockade can be established (Fig. 10.37).

Components

1. Two surface electrodes (small ECG electrodes) are positioned over the nerve and connected via the leads to the nerve stimulator.
2. Alternatively skin contact can be made via ball electrodes that are mounted on the nerve stimulator casing.
3. The case consists of an on/off switch, facility to deliver a twitch, train-of-four ([TOF] at 2 Hz) and tetanus (50 Hz). The stimulator is battery operated.

Mechanism of action

1. A supramaximal stimulus is used to stimulate a peripheral nerve. This ensures that all the motor fibres of the nerve are depolarized. The response of the muscle(s) supplied by the nerve is observed. A current of 15–40 mA is used for the ulnar nerve (a current of 50–60 mA may have to be used in obese patients).
2. This device should be battery powered and capable of delivering a constant current. It is the current magnitude that determines whether the nerve depolarizes or not, so delivering a constant current is more important than delivering a constant voltage as the skin resistance is variable (Ohm's law).
3. The muscle contraction can be observed visually, palpated, measured using a force transducer, or the electrical activity can be measured (electromyogram [EMG]).
4. The duration of the stimulus is less than 0.2–0.3 ms. The stimulus should have a monophasic square wave shape to avoid repetitive nerve firing.
5. Superficial, accessible peripheral nerves are most commonly used for monitoring purposes, e.g. ulnar nerve at the wrist, common peroneal nerve at the neck of the fibula, posterior tibial nerve at the ankle and the facial nerve.
6. The negative electrode is positioned directly over the most superficial part of the nerve. The positive

electrode is positioned along the proximal course of the nerve to avoid direct muscle stimulation.

7. Consider the ulnar nerve at the wrist. Two electrodes are positioned over the nerve, with the negative electrode placed distally and the positive electrode positioned about 2 cm proximally. Successful ulnar nerve stimulation causes the contraction of the adductor pollicis brevis muscle.

More advanced devices offer continuous monitoring of the transmission across the neuromuscular junction (Fig. 10.38). A graphical and numerical display of the TOF (Fig. 10.39) and the trend provide optimal monitoring. Skin electrodes are used. A reference measurement should be made where the device calculates the supramaximal current needed before the muscle relaxant is given. The device can be used to locate nerves and plexuses with a much lower current (e.g. a maximum of 5.0 mA) during regional anaesthesia. In this mode, a short stimulus can be used, e.g. 40 ms, to reduce the patient's discomfort.

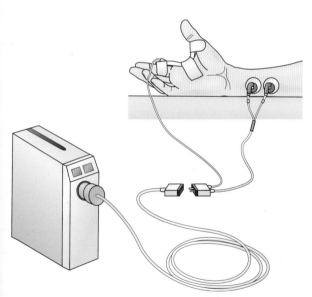

Fig. 10.38 Continuous neuromuscular transmission.

NEUROMUSCULAR TRANSMISSION MONITORING

There are various methods for monitoring the neuromuscular transmission using a nerve stimulator: twitch, tetanic stimulation, TOF, post-tetanic facilitation and double-burst stimulation (Fig. 10.40).

1. *Twitch:* a short duration (0.1–0.2 ms) square wave stimulus of a frequency of 0.1–1 Hz (one stimulus every 10 seconds to one stimulus every 1 second) is applied to a peripheral nerve. When used on its own, it is of limited use. It is the least precise method of assessing partial neuromuscular block.

2. *Tetanic stimulation:* a tetanus of 50–100 Hz is used to detect any residual neuromuscular block. Fade will be apparent even with normal response to a twitch. Tetanus is usually applied to anaesthetized patients because of the discomfort caused.

3. *TOF:* used to monitor the degree of the neuromuscular block clinically. The ratio of the fourth to the first twitch is called the TOF ratio:
   a. four twitches of 2 Hz each applied over 2 seconds. A gap of 10 seconds between each TOF
   b. as the muscle relaxant is administered, fade is noticed first, followed by the disappearance of the fourth twitch. This is followed by the disappearance of the third then the second and last by the first twitch
   c. on recovery, the first twitch appears first then the second followed by the third and fourth; reversal of the neuromuscular block is easier if the second twitch is visible
   d. for upper abdominal surgery, at least three twitches must be absent to achieve adequate surgical conditions
   e. the TOF ratio can be estimated using visible or tactile means. Electrical recording of the response is more accurate.

4. *Post-tetanic facilitation or potentiation:* this is used to assess more profound degrees of neuromuscular block.

5. *Double-burst stimulation* (Fig. 10.41): this allows a more accurate visual assessment than TOF for residual neuromuscular blockade. Two short bursts of 50 Hz tetanus are applied with a 750-ms interval. Each burst comprises two or three square wave impulses lasting for 0.2 ms.

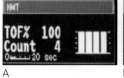 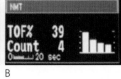 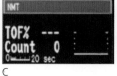 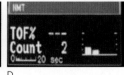 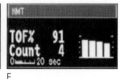

A   B   C   D   E

Fig. 10.39 Continuous monitoring and display of the neuromuscular transmission. (A) Reference measurement before administering the muscle relaxant, (B) fade with a lower train-of-four *(TOF)* percent as the muscle relaxant started to function, (C) complete paralysis, (D) gradual recovery of neuromuscular transmission and (E) near full recovery.

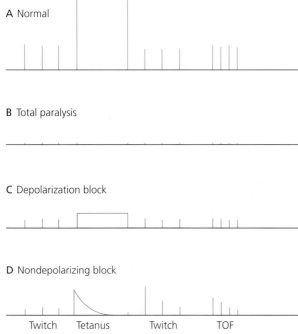

A Normal

B Total paralysis

C Depolarization block

D Nondepolarizing block

Twitch   Tetanus   Twitch   TOF

Fig. 10.40 Effects of a single twitch, tetanus and train-of-four *(TOF)* assessed by a force transducer recording contraction of the adductor pollicis muscle.

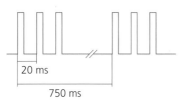

20 ms

750 ms

Fig. 10.41 The pattern of double-burst stimulation. Three impulses of 50 Hz tetanus, at 20-ms intervals, every 750 ms is shown.

Problems in practice and safety features

As the muscles of the hand are small in comparison with the diaphragm (the main respiratory muscle), monitoring the neuromuscular block peripherally does not reflect the true picture of the depth of the diaphragmatic block. The smaller the muscle is, the more sensitive it is to a muscle relaxant.

Peripheral nerve stimulators

- Used to ensure adequate reversal and to monitor the depth and the type of the block.
- Supramaximal stimulus is used to stimulate the nerve.
- The contraction of the muscle is observed visually, palpated or measured by a pressure transducer.
- The ulnar, facial, posterior tibial and the common peroneal nerves are often used.

Bispectral index (BIS) analysis

The BIS monitor is a device to monitor the electrical activity and the level of sedation in the brain and to assess the risk of awareness while under sedation/anaesthesia. In addition, it allows titration of hypnotics based on individual requirements to reduce underdosing and overdosing. BIS has been shown to correlate with measures of sedation/hypnosis, awareness and recall end points likely to be reflected in the cortical EEG. It can provide a continuous and consistent measure of sedation/hypnosis induced by most of the widely used sedative-hypnotic agents. Although BIS can measure the hypnotic components, it is less sensitive to the analgesic/opiate components of an anaesthetic.

Components

1. The display has the following features:
   a. BIS (as a single value or trend) (Fig. 10.42)
   b. facial EMG (in decibels)
   c. EEG suppression measured
   d. signal quality index (SQI), which indicates the amount of interference from EMG.
2. A forehead sensor with four numbered electrodes (elements) and a smart chip. The sensor uses small tines, which part the outer layers of the skin, and a hydrogel to make electrical contact. It is designed to lower the impedance and to optimize the quality of the signal (Figs. 10.43 and 10.44).
3. A smaller paediatric sensor with three electrodes is available. It has a flexible design to adjust to various head sizes and contours (Fig. 10.45).

Mechanism of action

1. Bispectral analysis is a statistical method that quantifies the level of synchronization of the underlying frequencies in the signal.

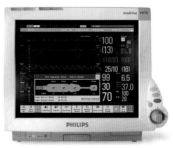

Fig. 10.42 Bispectral index value as part of patient monitoring. (Courtesy Philips Healthcare, Guildford, UK.)

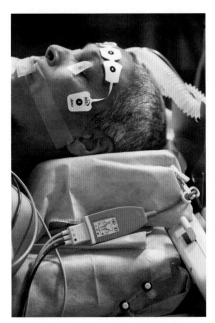

Fig. 10.43 Adult bispectral index electrode. (Courtesy Philips Healthcare, Guildford, UK.)

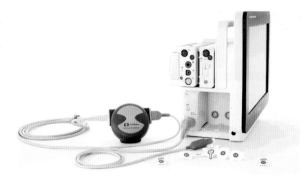

Fig. 10.44 Adult bispectral index electrode and monitor. (Courtesy Philips Healthcare, Guildford, UK.)

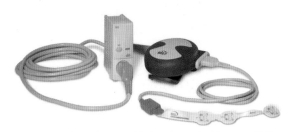

Fig. 10.45 Paediatric bispectral index electrode. (Courtesy Philips Healthcare, Guildford, UK.)

2. BIS is a value derived mathematically using information from EEG power and frequency as well as bispectral information. Along with the traditional amplitude and frequency variables, it provides a more complete description of complex EEG patterns. BIS is widely used to monitor the hypnotic component of anaesthesia, especially when neuromuscular blockers and/or total intravenous anaesthesia (TIVA) are used.

3. BIS is an empirical, statistically derived measurement. It uses a linear, dimensionless scale from 0 to 100. The lower the value, the greater the hypnotic effect. A value of 100 represents an awake EEG, whereas zero represents complete electrical silence (cortical suppression). BIS values of 65–85 are recommended for sedation, whereas values of 40–60 are recommended for general anaesthesia. At BIS values of less than 40, cortical suppression becomes discernible in raw EEG as a burst suppression pattern (Fig. 10.46).

4. BIS is also sensitive to changes in EMG activity. When neuromuscular blockers are used, this can decrease the value of BIS due to the absence of EMG activity. The lack of EMG activity does not equate to sedation or anaesthesia.

5. BIS measures the state of the brain, not the concentration of a particular drug. So a low value for BIS indicates hypnosis irrespective of how it was produced.

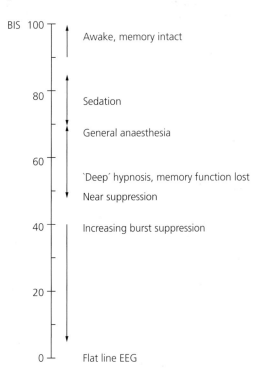

Fig. 10.46 Bispectral index *(BIS)* values scale. *EEG,* Electroencephalogram.

6. It has been shown that return of consciousness occurs consistently when the BIS is above 60 and, interestingly, at the same time, changes in blood pressure and heart rate are poor predictors for response.

7. The facial EMG (in decibels) is displayed to inform the user of possible interference affecting the BIS value.

8. The sensor is applied on the forehead at an angle. It can be placed on either the right or the left side of the head. Element *number 1* is placed at the centre of the forehead, 5 cm above the nose. Element *number 4* is positioned just above and adjacent to the eyebrow. Element *number 2* is positioned between *number 1* and *number 4*. Element *number 3* is positioned on either temple between the corner of the eye and the hairline. The sensor will not function beyond the hairline. Each element should be pressed for 5 seconds with the fingertip.

9. Cerebral ischaemia from any cause can result in a decrease in the BIS value if severe enough to cause a global EEG slowing or outright suppression.

10. BIS is being 'incorporated' as an additional monitoring module that can be added to the existing modular patient monitors such as Datex-Ohmeda S/5, Philips Viridia or GE Marquette Solar 8000 M. In addition to its use in the operating theatre, BIS has also been used in the intensive care setting to assess the level of sedation in mechanically ventilated patients.

Problems and safety features

1. Hypothermia of less than 33°C results in a decrease in BIS levels as the brain processes slow. In such situations, e.g. during cardiac bypass procedures, BIS reflects the synergistic effects of hypothermia and hypnotic drugs. A rapid rise in BIS usually occurs during rewarming.

2. Interference from non-EEG electrical signals such as EMG. High-frequency facial EMG activity may be present in sedated, spontaneously breathing patients and during awakening, causing BIS to increase in conjunction with higher EMG. Significant EMG interference can lead to a faulty high BIS despite the patient being still unresponsive. EEG signals are considered to exist in the 0.5–30-Hz band whereas EMG signals exist in the 30–300-Hz band. Separation is not absolute and low-frequency EMG signals can occur in the conventional EEG band range. The more recent BIS XP is less affected by EMG. However, care must be taken in interpreting the BIS when muscle relaxants are used due to the complete absence of EMG activity lowering the BIS score.

3. BIS cannot be used to monitor hypnosis during ketamine anaesthesia. This is due to ketamine being a dissociative anaesthetic with excitatory effects on the EEG.

4. Sedative concentrations of nitrous oxide (up to 70%) do not appear to affect BIS.

5. There are conflicting data regarding opioid dose–response and interaction of opioids with hypnotics on BIS.

6. Currently, there are insufficient data to evaluate the use of BIS in patients with neurological diseases.

7. When the SQI value goes below 50%, the BIS is not stored in the trend memory. The BIS value on the monitor appears in 'reverse video' to indicate this.

8. Interference from surgical diathermy. A recent version, BIS XP, is better protected from the diathermy.

9. As with any other monitor, the use of BIS does not obviate the need for critical clinical judgement.

BIS

- Monitors the electrical activity in the brain.
- Uses a linear dimensionless scale from 0 to 100. The lower the value, the greater the hypnotic effect. General anaesthesia is at 40–60.
- Interference can be from diathermy or EMG.
- Changes in body temperature and cerebral ischaemia can affect the value.

Entropy of the EEG

This is a more recent technique used to measure the depth of sedation/anaesthesia by measuring the 'regularity' or the amount of disorder of the EEG signal. High levels of entropy during anaesthesia show that the patient is awake, and low levels correlate with deep unconsciousness.

The EEG signal is recorded using electrodes applied to the forehead and side of the head, as with the BIS. The device uses Fourier transformation to calculate the frequencies of voltages for each given time sample (epoch). This is then converted into a normalized frequency spectrum (by squaring the transformed components) for the selected frequency range.

State entropy (SE) index is calculated from a low-frequency range (under 32 Hz), corresponding predominantly to EEG activity.

Response entropy (RE) index uses a higher frequency range (up to 47 Hz) and includes EMG activity from frontalis muscle.

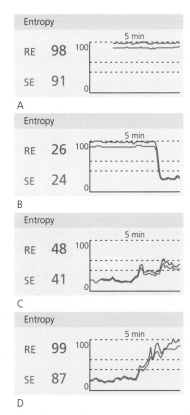

A

B

C

D

Fig. 10.47 Entropy of electroencephalogram. (A) Awake state. Note the difference between the two entropies, indicating muscle activity on the face. (B) Immediately after induction of anaesthesia. (C) Maintenance of anaesthesia. (D) Recovery from anaesthesia. *RE,* Response entropy; *SE,* state entropy.

The concept of *Shannon entropy* is then applied to normalize the entropy values to between 0 (total regularity) and 1 (total irregularity).

The commercially available M-entropy module (GE Healthcare) converts the entropy scale of 0 to 1 into a scale of 0 to 100 (similar to the BIS scale). The conversion is not exactly linear to give greater resolution at the most important area to monitor 'depth of anaesthesia', which is between 0.5 and 1.0.

Both RE and SE are displayed with the RE ranges from 100 to 0 and the SE ranges from a maximum of 91 to 0 (Fig. 10.47). In practice, 0 corresponds to a very 'deep' level of anaesthesia, and values close to 100 correspond to the awake patient. Like BIS, values between 40 and 60 represent clinically desirable depths of anaesthesia. At this level, the SE and RE indexes should be similar if not identical.

As the patient awakens, an increase in the difference between the SE and RE values is seen due to a diminishing effect of drugs on the central nervous system (CNS) and an increasing contribution from frontalis EMG.

> **Entropy of EEG**
> - The 'regularity' or the amount of disorder of the EEG signal is used to measure the depth of sedation/anaesthesia.
> - During anaesthesia, low levels correlate with deep unconsciousness.
> - SE index corresponds predominantly to EEG activity.
> - RE index includes EMG activity from the frontalis muscle.

SUGGESTED FURTHER READING

Kodali, B.S., 2013. Capnography outside the operating rooms. Anesthesiology 118 (1), 192–201.

McGrath, C.D., Hunter, J.M., 2006. Monitoring of neuromuscular block. Contin. Educ. Anaesth. Crit. Care Pain 6 (1), 7–12.

Medicines and Healthcare Products Regulatory Agency (MHRA), 2012. Top tips for pulse oximetry. Available from: http://webarchive.nationalarchives.gov.uk/201 41205150130/http://www.mhra.gov.uk/home/groups/dts-iac/documents/publication/con103021.pdf.

National Institute of Health and Care Excellence, 2012. Depth of anaesthesia monitors – Bispectral Index (BIS), E-Entropy and Narcotrend-Compact M. NICE diagnostics guidance [DG6]. Available from: http://www.nice.org.uk/guidance/dg6.

Pandit, J.J., Cook, T.M. (Eds.), 2014. Accidental awareness during general anaesthesia in the United Kingdom and Ireland. National Audit Project 5. Available from: http://www.nationalauditprojects.org.uk/NAP5report.

Patel, S., Souter, M., 2008. Equipment-related electrocardiographic artifacts: causes, characteristics, consequences, and correction. Anesthesiology 108, 138–148.

Pulse Oximeter Accuracy and Limitations: FDA Safety Communication, 2021. Available from: Pulse Oximeter Accuracy and Limitations: FDA Safety Communication | FDA.

Tosh, W., Patteril, M., 2016. Cerebral oximetry. Br. J. Anaesth. Educ. 16 (12), 417–421.

SELF-ASSESSMENT QUESTIONS

Please check your eBook for additional self-assessment

MCQs

In the following lists, which of the statements (a) to (e) are true?

1. **Concerning capnography**
   a. Capnography is a more useful indicator of ventilator disconnection and oesophageal intubation than pulse oximetry.
   b. Capnography typically works on the absorption of CO_2 in the ultraviolet region of the spectrum.
   c. In side-stream analysers, a delay in measurement of less than 38 seconds is acceptable.
   d. The main-stream analyser type can measure other gases simultaneously.
   e. In patients with chronic obstructive airway disease, the waveform can show a sloping trace instead of the square shape wave.

2. **Concerning oxygen concentration measurement**
   a. An infrared absorption technique is used.
   b. Paramagnetic analysers are commonly used because oxygen is repelled by the magnetic field.
   c. The galvanic (fuel cell) analyser has a slow response time of about 20 seconds and a lifespan of about 1 year.
   d. The fast responding analysers should be positioned as near the patient as possible.
   e. Paramagnetic analysers can provide breath-to-breath measurement.

3. **Pulse oximetry**
   a. The probe consists of two emitting diodes producing beams at red and infrared frequencies.
   b. Accurately reflects the ability of the patient to eliminate CO_2.
   c. The measurements are accurate within the clinical range of 70%–100%.
   d. Carbon monoxide in the blood causes a false under-reading.
   e. The site of the probe has to be checked frequently.

4. **Arterial blood pressure**
   a. Mean blood pressure is the systolic pressure plus one-third of the pulse pressure.
   b. Too small a cuff causes a false high pressure.
   c. Oscillotonometry is widely used to measure blood pressure.
   d. The Finapres technique uses ultraviolet light absorption to measure the blood pressure.
   e. A slow cuff inflation followed by a fast deflation are needed to improve the accuracy of a noninvasive blood pressure technique.

5. **Pneumotachograph**
   a. It is a fixed orifice variable pressure flowmeter.
   b. It consists of two sensitive pressure transducers positioned on either side of a resistance.
   c. It is capable of flowing in one direction only.
   d. A Pitot tube can be added to improve accuracy.
   e. Humidity and water vapour condensation have no effect on its accuracy.

6. **Polarographic oxygen electrode**
   a. It can measure oxygen partial pressure in a blood or gas sample.
   b. The electrode acts as a battery requiring no power source.
   c. Oxygen molecules pass from the sample to the potassium chloride solution across a semipermeable membrane.
   d. It uses a silver cathode and a platinum anode.
   e. The amount of electrical current generated is proportional to the oxygen partial pressure.

7. **Wright respirometer**
   a. It is best positioned on the inspiratory limb of the ventilator breathing system.
   b. It is a bidirectional device.
   c. It is accurate for clinical use.
   d. It over-reads at high flow rates and under-reads at low flow rates.
   e. It can measure both tidal volume and minute volume.

8. Paramagnetic gases include
   a. Oxygen.
   b. Sevoflurane.
   c. Nitrous oxide.
   d. Carbon dioxide.
   e. Halothane.

9. Oxygen in a gas mixture can be measured by
   a. Fuel cell.
   b. Ultraviolet absorption.
   c. Mass spectrometer.
   d. Clark oxygen (polarographic) electrode.
   e. Infrared absorption.

10. The concentrations of volatile agents can be measured using
    a. Fuel cell.
    b. Piezoelectric crystal.
    c. Ultraviolet spectroscopy.
    d. Infrared spectroscopy.
    e. Clark electrode.

11. A patient with healthy lungs and a $PaCO_2$ of 40 mmHg will have which of the following percentages of CO_2 in the end-expiratory mixture?
    a. 4%.
    b. 5%.
    c. 2%.
    d. 1%.
    e. 7%.

12. Bispectral index (BIS) monitor
    a. It uses a linear dimensionless scale from 0 to 100 Hz.
    b. Hypothermia can increase the BIS value.
    c. The BIS value is not accurate during ketamine anaesthesia.
    d. Interference can occur due to electromyogram (EMG) or diathermy.
    e. BIS can measure the drug concentration of a particular drug.

13. Concerning electrocardiogram (ECG)
    a. The monitoring mode of ECG has a wider frequency response range than the diagnostic mode.
    b. The electrical potentials have a range of 0.5–2 V.
    c. Interference due to electrostatic induction can be reduced by surrounding ECG leads with copper screens.
    d. Silver and silver chloride electrodes are used.
    e. It is standard in the United Kingdom to use a display speed of 25 cm/s and a sensitivity of 1 mV/cm.

14. Infrared spectrometry
    a. CO_2 absorbs infrared radiation mainly at a wavelength of 4.3 mm.
    b. Photoacoustic spectrometry is more stable than the conventional infrared spectrometry.
    c. Sampling catheter leak is a potential problem with the side-stream analysers.
    d. A wavelength of 4.6 μm is used for nitrous oxide measurement.
    e. A wavelength of 3.3 μm is used to measure the concentration of inhalational agents.

Single best answer

15. Regarding the minimum monitoring required for anaesthesia
    a. Renders bed-side clinical signs obsolete.
    b. ECG monitoring is essential.
    c. Modern ECG monitoring is immune from artefacts.
    d. Noninvasive blood pressure requires two cuffs and a minimum cycle time of 1 minute.
    e. National Institute for Health and Clinical Excellence guidelines forbid temperature monitoring.

Answers

1. Concerning capnography
   a. *True. Capnography gives a fast warning in cases of disconnection or oesophageal intubation. The end-tidal CO_2 will decrease sharply and suddenly. The pulse oximeter will be very slow in detecting disconnection or oesophageal intubation as the arterial oxygen saturation will remain normal for longer periods especially if the patient was preoxygenated.*
   b. *False. CO_2 is absorbed in the infrared region.*
   c. *False. In side-stream analysers, a delay of less than 3.8 seconds is acceptable. The length of the sampling tubing should be as short as possible, e.g. 2 m, with an internal diameter of 1.2 mm and a sampling rate of about 150 mL/min.*
   d. *False. Only CO_2 can be measured by the main-stream analyser. CO_2, N_2O and inhalational agents can be measured simultaneously with a side-stream analyser.*
   e. *True. In patients with chronic obstructive airway disease, the alveoli empty at different rates because of the differing time constants in different regions of the lung with various degrees of altered compliance and airway resistance.*

2. Concerning oxygen concentration measurement
   a. *False. Oxygen does not absorb infrared radiation. Only molecules with two differing atoms can absorb infrared radiation.*
   b. *False. Oxygen is attracted by the magnetic field because it has two electrons in unpaired orbits.*
   c. *True. The fuel cell is depleted by continuous exposure to oxygen due to the exhaustion of the cell, giving it a lifespan of about 1 year.*
   d. *True. Although the positioning of the oxygen analyser is still debatable, it has been recommended that the fast responding ones are positioned as close to the patient as possible. The slow responding analysers are positioned on the inspiratory limb of the breathing system.*
   e. *True. Modern paramagnetic analysers have a rapid response, allowing them to provide breath-to-breath measurement. Older versions have a 1-minute response time.*

3. Pulse oximetry
   a. *True. The probe uses light-emitting diodes (LEDs) that emit light at red (660 nm) and infrared (940 nm) frequencies. The LEDs operate in sequence with an 'off' period when the photodetector measures the background level of ambient light. This sequence happens at a rate of about 30 times/s.*
   b. *False. Pulse oximetry is a measurement of the arterial oxygen saturation.*
   c. *True. Readings below 70% are extrapolated by the manufacturers.*
   d. *False. Using a pulse oximeter, carbon monoxide causes a false high reading of the arterial oxygen saturation.*
   e. *True. The probe can cause pressure sores with continuous use so its site should be checked at regular intervals. Some recommend changing the site every 2 hours.*

4. Arterial blood pressure
   a. *False. The mean blood pressure is the diastolic pressure plus one-third of the pulse pressure (systolic pressure – diastolic pressure).*
   b. *True. The opposite is also correct.*
   c. *True. Most of the noninvasive blood pressure measuring devices use oscillometry as the basis for measuring blood pressure. Return of the blood flow during deflation causes pressure changes in the cuff. The transducer senses the pressure changes, which are interpreted by the microprocessor.*
   d. *False. The Finapres uses oscillometry, and a servo control unit is used.*
   e. *False. Slow cuff inflation leads to venous congestion and inaccuracy. A fast cuff deflation might miss the oscillations caused by the return of blood flow (i.e. systolic pressure). A fast inflation and slow deflation of the cuff is needed. A deflation rate of 3 mmHg/s or 2 mmHg/beat is adequate.*

5. Pneumotachograph
   a. *True. The pneumotachograph consists of a tube with a fixed resistance, usually as a bundle of parallel tubes, and is therefore a 'fixed orifice' device. As the fluid (gas or liquid) passes across the resistance, the pressure across the resistance changes, therefore it is a 'variable pressure' flowmeter.*
   b. *True. The two pressure transducers measure the pressures on either side of the resistance. The pressure changes are proportional to the flow rate across the resistance.*

c. *False. It can measure flows in both directions, i.e. it is bidirectional.*

d. *True. The combined design improves accuracy and allows the measurement and calculation of other parameters: compliance, airway pressure, gas flow, volume/pressure and flow/volume loops.*

e. *False. A laminar flow is required for the pneumotachograph to measure accurately. Water vapour condensation at the site of the resistance leads to the formation of turbulent flow, thus reducing the accuracy of the measurement.*

6. Polarographic oxygen electrode

a. *True. The polarographic (Clark) electrode analysers can be used to measure oxygen partial pressure in a gas sample (e.g. on an anaesthetic machine giving an average inspiratory and expiratory concentration) or in blood in a blood gas analyser.*

b. *False. A power source of about 700 mV is needed in a polarographic analyser. The galvanic analyser (fuel cell) acts as a battery requiring no power source.*

c. *True. The oxygen molecules pass across a Teflon semipermeable membrane at a rate proportional to their partial pressure in the sample into the sodium chloride solution. The performance of the electrode is affected as the membrane deteriorates or perforates.*

d. *False. The opposite is correct: the anode is made of silver, and the cathode is made of platinum.*

e. *True. When the oxygen molecules pass across the membrane, very small electrical currents are generated as electrons move from the cathode to the anode.*

7. Wright respirometer

a. *False. The Wright respirometer is best positioned on the expiratory limb of the ventilator breathing system. This minimizes the loss of gas volume due to leaks and expansion of the tubing on the inspiratory limb.*

b. *False. It is a unidirectional device allowing the measurement of the tidal volume if the flow of gases is in one direction only. An arrow on the device indicates the correct direction of the gas flow.*

c. *True. It is suitable for routine clinical use with an accuracy of ±5%–10% within a range of flows of 4–24 L/min.*

d. *True. Over-reading at high flows and under-reading at low flows is due to the effect of inertia on the rotating vane. Using a Wright respirometer based on light reflection or the use of a semiconductive device sensitive to changes in magnetic field instead of the mechanical components improves the accuracy.*

e. *True. The Wright respirometer can measure the volume per breath, and if the measurement is continued for 1 minute, the minute volume can be measured as well.*

8. Paramagnetic gases include

a. *True. Oxygen is attracted by the magnetic field because it has two electrons in unpaired orbits, causing it to possess paramagnetic properties.*

b. *False.*

c. *False.*

d. *False.*

e. *False.*

9. Oxygen in a gas mixture can be measured by

a. *True. The oxygen molecules diffuse through a membrane and electrolyte solution to reach the cathode. This generates a current proportional to the partial pressure of oxygen in the mixture.*

b. *False. Oxygen does not absorb ultraviolet radiation. Halothane absorbs ultraviolet radiation.*

c. *True. Mass spectrometry can be used for the measurement of any gas. It separates the gases according to their molecular weight. The sample is ionized and then the ions are separated. Mass spectrometry allows rapid simultaneous breath-to-breath measurement of oxygen concentration.*

d. *True. Although polarographic analysers are used mainly to measure oxygen partial pressure in a blood sample in blood gas analysers, they can also be used to measure the partial pressure in a gas sample. See Question 6 above.*

e. *False. Gases that absorb infrared radiation have molecules with two different atoms (e.g. carbon and oxygen in CO_2). An oxygen molecule has two similar atoms.*

10. The concentrations of volatile agents can be measured using

a. *False. The fuel cell is used to measure the oxygen concentration.*

b. *True. A piezoelectric quartz crystal with a lipophilic coat undergoes changes in natural frequency when exposed to a lipid-soluble inhalational agent. It lacks agent specificity. It is not widely used in current anaesthetic practice.*

c. *True. Halothane can absorb ultraviolet radiation. It is not used in current anaesthetic practice.*

d. *True. Infrared radiation is absorbed by all the gases with dissimilar atoms in the molecule. Infrared analysers can be either side stream or main stream.*

e. *False. The Clark polarographic electrode is used to measure oxygen concentration.*

11. A patient with healthy lungs and a $PaCO_2$ of 40 mmHg will have which of the following percentages of CO_2 in the end-expiratory mixture?
    a. False.
    b. True. *In a patient with healthy lungs, the end-tidal CO_2 concentration is a true reflection of the arterial CO_2. A $PaCO_2$ of 40 mmHg (5.3 kPa) is therefore equivalent to an end-tidal CO_2 of about 5 kPa. One atmospheric pressure is 760 mmHg or 101.33 kPa. That makes the end-tidal CO_2 percentage about 5%.*
    c. False.
    d. False.
    e. False.

12. BIS monitor
    a. False. *BIS uses a linear dimensionless scale of 0–100 without any units. The lower the BIS value, the greater the hypnotic effect. General anaesthesia is between 40 and 60.*
    b. False. *Hypothermia below 33°C decreases the BIS value as the electrical activity in the brain is decreased by the low temperature.*
    c. True. *The BIS value is not accurate during ketamine anaesthesia. Ketamine is a dissociative anaesthetic with excitatory effects on the electroencephalogram.*
    d. True. *Newer versions have better protection from diathermy and EMG.*
    e. False. *BIS monitors the electrical activity in the brain and not the concentration of a particular drug.*

13. Concerning ECG
    a. False. *The monitoring mode has a limited frequency response of 0.5–40 Hz, whereas the diagnostic mode has a much wider range of 0.05–100 Hz.*
    b. False. *The electrical activity of the heart has an electrical potential range of 0.5–2 mV.*
    c. True. *Surrounding the ECG leads with copper screens reduces interference due to electrostatic induction and capacitance coupling.*
    d. True. *Silver and silver chloride form a stable electrode combination. They are held in a cup and separated from the skin by a foam pad soaked in conducting gel.*
    e. False. *The standard in the United Kingdom is to use a display speed of 25 mm/s and a sensitivity of 1 mV/cm.*

14. Infrared spectrometry
    a. False. *CO_2 absorbs infrared radiation mainly at a wavelength of 4.3 μm.*
    b. True. *Photoacoustic spectrometry is more stable than the conventional infrared spectrometry. Its calibration remains constant over much longer periods of time.*
    c. True. *This is not the case with the main-stream analysers.*
    d. True. *Optical filters are used to select the desired wavelengths to avoid interference from other vapours or gases.*
    e. False. *For the inhalational agents, higher wavelengths are used, such as 8–9 μm, to avoid interference from methane and alcohol (at 3.3 μm).*

15. *b.*

Chapter 11

Invasive monitoring

Invasive arterial pressure monitoring

Invasive arterial pressure monitoring provides beat-to-beat real-time information with sustained accuracy.

Components

1. An indwelling Teflon arterial cannula (20-G or 22-G) is used (Fig. 11.1). The cannula has parallel walls to minimize the effect on blood flow to the distal parts of the limb. Cannulation can be achieved by directly threading the cannula (either by direct insertion method or a transfixation technique) or by using a modified Seldinger technique with a guidewire to assist in the insertion as in some designs (Fig. 11.2).
2. A column of bubble-free 0.9% normal saline at a pressure of 300 mmHg incorporates a flushing device.
3. Via the fluid column, the cannula is connected to a transducer (Figs. 11.3 and 11.4). This in turn is connected to an amplifier and oscilloscope. A strain gauge variable resistor transducer is used.

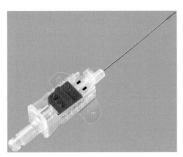

Fig. 11.1 BD Flowswitch arterial cannula. Note the on–off switch valve. (Courtesy BD Medical.)

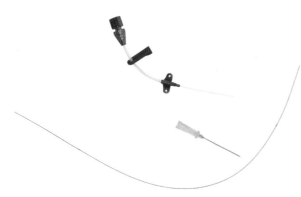

Fig. 11.2 Arrow arterial cannula with its introducer and guidewire. (Image courtesy Teleflex Incorporated. © [2021] Teleflex Incorporated. All rights reserved.)

4. The diaphragm (a very thin membrane) acts as an interface between the transducer and the fluid column.
5. The pressure transducer is a device that changes either electrical resistance or capacitance in response to changes in pressure on a solid-state device. The moving part of the transducer is very small and has little mass.

Mechanism of action

1. The saline column moves back and forth with the arterial pulsation, causing the diaphragm to move. This causes changes in the resistance and current flow through the wires of the transducer.
2. The transducer is connected to a Wheatstone bridge circuit (Fig. 11.5). This is an electrical circuit for the precise comparison of resistors. It uses a null-deflection system consisting of a very sensitive galvanometer and four resistors in two parallel branches: two constant resistors, a variable resistor and the unknown resistor. Changes in resistance and current are measured, electronically converted and displayed as systolic, diastolic and mean arterial pressures. The Wheatstone bridge circuit is ideal for measuring the small changes in resistance found in strain gauges. Most pressure transducers contain four strain gauges that form the four resistors of the Wheatstone bridge.
3. The flushing device allows 3–4 mL/h of saline to flush the cannula. This is to prevent clotting and backflow through the catheter. Manual flushing of the system is also possible when indicated.
4. The radial artery is the most commonly used artery because the ulnar artery is the dominant artery in the hand. The ulnar artery is connected to the radial artery through the palmar arch in 95% of patients. The brachial, femoral, ulnar or dorsalis pedis arteries are used occasionally.
5. The information gained from invasive arterial pressure monitoring includes heart rate, pulse pressure, the presence of a respiratory swing, left ventricular (LV) contractility, vascular tone (systematic vascular resistance [SVR]) and stroke volume.

The arterial pressure waveform (Fig. 11.6)

1. This can be characterized as a complex sine wave that is the summation of a series of simple sine waves of different amplitudes and frequencies.
2. The fundamental frequency (or first harmonic) is equal to the heart rate, so a heart rate of 60 beats/min = 1 beat/s or 1 cycle/s or 1 Hz. The first 10 harmonics of the fundamental frequency contribute to the waveform.

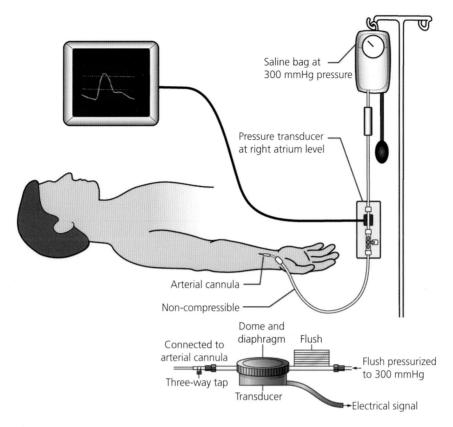

Saline bag at
300 mmHg pressure

Pressure transducer
at right atrium level

Arterial cannula

Non-compressible

Connected to
arterial cannula

Dome and
diaphragm

Flush

Three-way tap

Transducer

Flush pressurized
to 300 mmHg

Electrical signal

Fig. 11.3 Components of a pressure measuring system.

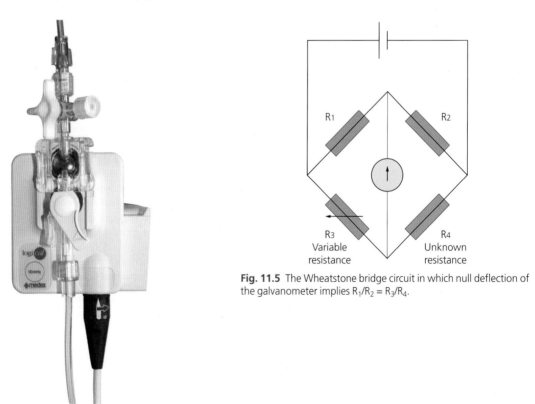

Fig. 11.4 Medex integrated pressure transducer. Note the flushing device just distal to the transducer. (Courtesy Smiths Medical, Ashford, Kent, UK.)

R1

R2

R3
Variable
resistance

R4
Unknown
resistance

Fig. 11.5 The Wheatstone bridge circuit in which null deflection of the galvanometer implies $R_1/R_2 = R_3/R_4$.

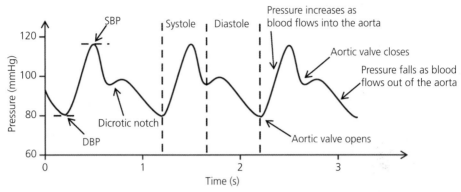

Fig. 11.6 Arterial pressure waveform showing systolic and diastolic pressures and other components. *DBP,* Diastolic blood pressure; *SBP,* systolic blood pressure.

3. The system used to measure arterial blood pressure should be capable of responding to a frequency range of 0.5–40 Hz in order to display the arterial waveform correctly.
4. The dicrotic notch in the arterial pressure waveform represents changes in pressure because of vibrations caused by the closure of the aortic valve.
5. The rate of rise of the upstroke part of the wave (dP/dt) reflects the myocardial contractility. A slow rise upstroke might indicate a need for inotropic support. A positive response to the inotropic support will show a steeper upstroke. The maximum upward slope of the arterial waveform during systole is related to the speed of ventricular ejection.
6. The position of the dicrotic notch on the downstroke of the wave reflects the peripheral vascular resistance. In vasodilated patients, e.g. following an epidural block or in septic patients, the dicrotic notch is positioned lower on the curve. The notch is higher in vasoconstricted patients.
7. The downstroke slope indicates resistance to outflow. A slow fall is seen in vasoconstriction.
8. The stroke volume can be estimated by measuring the area from the beginning of the upstroke to the dicrotic notch. Multiply that by the heart rate, and the cardiac output can be estimated.
9. Systolic time indicates the myocardial oxygen demand. Diastolic time indicates myocardial oxygen supply.
10. Mean blood pressure is the average pressure throughout the cardiac cycle. As systole is shorter than diastole, the mean arterial pressure (MAP) is slightly less than the value halfway between systolic and diastolic pressures. An estimate of MAP can be obtained by adding a third of the pulse pressure (systolic pressure – diastolic pressure) to the diastolic pressure. MAP can also be determined by integrating a pressure signal over the duration of one cycle, divided by time.

The natural frequency

The natural frequency of an object is that frequency at which it vibrates/oscillates after being moved or strummed. In the case of the pressure monitoring system, it is the frequency at which the monitoring system itself resonates and amplifies the signal by up to 20%–40%. This determines the frequency response of the monitoring system. Therefore it is important for the monitoring system to have a significantly different frequency from the patient's pulse rate. The natural frequency should be at least 10 times the fundamental frequency, which is the patient's pulse rate. The natural frequency of the measuring system is much higher than the fundamental or primary frequency of the arterial waveform, which is 1–2 Hz, corresponding to a pulse rate of 60–120 beats/min. The maximum pulse rate a patient could have might be 180–240 beats/min or 3–4 Hz. Therefore the monitoring system should have a natural frequency of at least 40 Hz. Stiffer (low compliance) tubing or a shorter length of tubing (less mass) produces higher natural frequencies. This results in the system requiring a much higher pulse rate before amplification.

The natural frequency of the monitoring system is:

1. directly related to the catheter diameter
2. inversely related to the square root of the system compliance
3. inversely related to the square root of the length of the tubing
4. inversely related to the square root of the density of the fluid in the system.

Problems in practice and safety features

1. The arterial pressure waveform should be displayed (Fig. 11.7) in order to detect damping or resonance. The monitoring system should be able to apply an optimal damping value of 0.64.
   a. *Damping* is caused by dissipation of stored energy. Anything that takes energy out of the system results in a progressive diminution of amplitude of oscillations. Increased damping lowers the systolic and elevates the diastolic pressures with loss of detail in the waveform. Damping can be caused by an air bubble (air is more compressible in comparison to the saline column), clot or a highly compliant, soft transducer diaphragm and tube.
   b. *Resonance* occurs when the frequency of the driving force coincides with the resonant frequency of the system. If the natural frequency is less than 40 Hz, it falls within the range of the blood pressure and a sine wave will be superimposed on the blood pressure wave. Increased resonance elevates the systolic and lowers the diastolic pressures. The mean pressure should stay unchanged. Resonance can be due to a stiff, noncompliant diaphragm and tube. It is worse with tachycardia.
2. To determine the optimum damping of the system, a square wave test (fast flush test) is used (Fig. 11.8). The system is flushed by applying a pressure of 300 mmHg (compress and release the flush button or pull the lever located near the transducer). This results in a square waveform followed by oscillations:

   a. in an *optimally damped* system, there will be two or three oscillations before settling to zero
   b. an *overdamped* system settles to zero without any oscillations
   c. an *underdamped* system oscillates for more than three to four cycles before settling to zero.
3. The transducer should be positioned at the level of the right atrium as a reference point that is at the level of the midaxillary line. Raising or lowering the transducer above or below the level of the right atrium gives error readings equivalent to 7.5 mmHg for each 10 cm.
4. Ischaemia distal to the cannula is rare but should be monitored for. Multiple attempts at insertion and haematoma formation increase the risk of ischaemia.
5. Arterial thrombosis occurs in 20%–25% of cases with very rare adverse effects such as ischaemia or necrosis of the hand. Cannulae in place for less than 24 hours very rarely cause thrombosis.
6. The arterial pressure wave narrows and increases in amplitude in peripheral vessels. This makes the systolic pressure higher in the dorsalis pedis than in the radial artery. When compared to the aorta, peripheral arteries contain less elastic fibres, so they are stiffer and less compliant. The arterial distensibility determines the amplitude and contour of the pressure waveform. In addition, the narrowing and bifurcation of arteries leads to impedance of forward blood flow, which results in backward reflection of the pressure wave.
7. There is a risk of bleeding due to disconnection.
8. An arterial cannula should be clearly labelled. This alerts staff to what could be fatal errors. Inadvertent air injection results in air embolus. Inadvertent drug injection causes distal vascular occlusion and necrosis.
9. Local infection is thought to be less than 20%. Systemic infection is thought to be less than 5%. This is more common in patients with an arterial cannula for more than 4 days with a traumatic insertion.
10. Arterial cannulae should not be inserted in sites with evidence of infection and trauma or through a vascular prosthesis.
11. Periodic checks, calibrations and rezeroing are carried out to prevent baseline drift of the transducer electrical circuits. Zero calibration eliminates the effect of atmospheric pressure on the measured pressure. This ensures that the monitor indicates zero pressure in the absence of applied pressure, so eliminating the *offset drift* (zero drift). To eliminate the *gradient drift*, calibration at a higher pressure is necessary. The transducer is connected to an aneroid manometer using a sterile tubing through a three-way stopcock, and the manometer pressure is raised

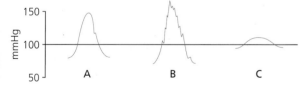

Fig. 11.7 Arterial pressure waveform. (A) Correct, optimally damped waveform. (B) Underdamped waveform. (C) Overdamped waveform.

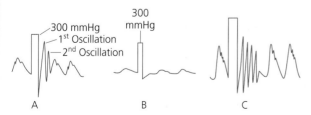

Fig. 11.8 The square wave test (fast flush test). (A) Optimally damped system. (B) Overdamped system. (C) Underdamped system.

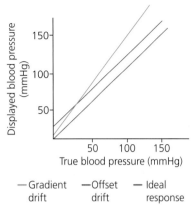

Fig. 11.9 Calibration of invasive pressure monitor.

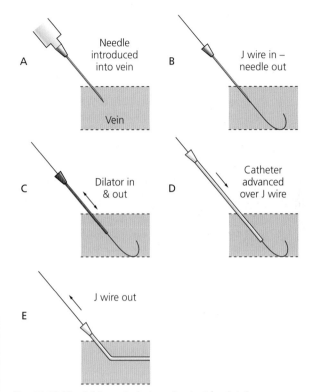

Fig. 11.10 The Seldinger technique. See text for details.

to 100 and 200 mmHg. The monitor display should read the same pressure as is applied to the transducer (Fig. 11.9).

Invasive arterial blood pressure
- Consists of an arterial cannula, a saline-based fluid column, a flushing device, a transducer, an amplifier and an oscilloscope.
- In addition to blood pressure, other parameters can be measured and estimated such as myocardial contractility, vascular tone and stroke volume.
- The waveform should be displayed to detect any resonance or damping.
- The measuring system should be able to cover a frequency range of 0.5–40 Hz.
- The monitoring system should be able to apply an optimal damping value of 0.64.

 Exam tip: Invasive arterial pressure is a very popular topic in exams. Know and understand the components of an invasive pressure system, how it works, factors that can affect its accuracy and the different waveforms. To be able to draw and explain a Wheatstone bridge circuit is also important.

Central venous catheterization and pressure

The central venous pressure (CVP) is the filling pressure of the right atrium. It can be measured directly using a central venous catheter. The catheter can also be used to administer fluids, blood, drugs, parenteral nutrition

and sample blood. Specialized catheters can be used for haemofiltration, haemodialysis (see Chapter 13, Haemofiltration) and transvenous pacemaker placement.

The tip of the catheter is usually positioned in the superior vena cava at the entrance to the right atrium. The internal jugular, subclavian and basilic veins are possible routes for central venous catheterization. The subclavian route is associated with the highest rate of complications but is convenient for the patient and for the nursing care.

The *Seldinger technique* is the common and standard method used for central venous catheterization (Fig. 11.10) regardless of catheter type. The procedure should be done under sterile conditions:

1. Introduce the cannula or needle into the vein using the appropriate landmark technique or an ultrasound-locating device.
2. A J-shaped soft tip guidewire is introduced through the needle (and syringe in some designs) into the vein. The needle can then be removed. The J-shaped tip is designed to minimize trauma to the vessels' endothelium.
3. After a small incision in the skin has been made, a dilator is introduced over the guidewire to make a track through the skin and subcutaneous tissues and is then withdrawn.

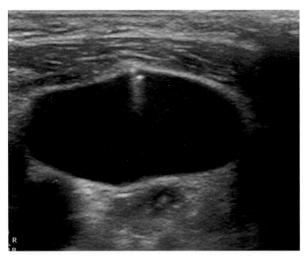

Fig. 11.11 Ultrasound image showing a needle in the internal jugular vein. The carotid artery is at the left lower corner.

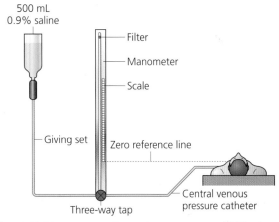

Fig. 11.12 Measurement of central venous pressure (CVP) using a manometer. The manometer's fluid level falls until the height of the fluid column above the zero reference point is equal to the CVP.

4. The catheter is then railroaded over the guidewire into its final position before the guidewire is withdrawn.
5. Blood should be aspirated easily from all ports, which should then be flushed with saline. All the port sites that are not intended for immediate use are sealed. A port should never be left open to air during insertion because of the risk of air embolism.
6. The catheter is secured onto the skin and covered with a sterile dressing.
7. A chest X-ray is performed to ensure correct positioning of the catheter and to detect pneumothorax and/or haemothorax.
8. The use of ultrasound guidance should be routinely considered for the insertion of central venous catheters (Fig. 11.11). Evidence shows that its use during internal jugular venous catheterization reduces the number of mechanical complications, the number of catheter-placement failures and the time required for insertion.

The CVP is read using either a pressure transducer or a water manometer.

PRESSURE TRANSDUCER

1. A similar measuring system to that used for invasive arterial pressure monitoring (catheter, saline column, transducer, diaphragm, flushing device and oscilloscope system). The transducer is positioned at the level of the right atrium.
2. A measuring system of limited frequency range is adequate because of the shape of the waveform and the values of the CVP.

FLUID MANOMETER (Fig. 11.12)

1. A giving set with either normal saline or 5% dextrose is connected to the vertical manometer via a three-way tap. The latter is also connected to the central venous catheter.
2. The manometer has a spirit-level side arm positioned at the level of the right atrium (zero reference point). The upper end of the column is open to air via a filter. This filter must stay dry to maintain direct connection with the atmosphere.
3. The vertical manometer is filled to about the 20-cm mark. By opening the three-way tap to the patient, a swing of the column should be seen with respiration. The CVP is read in cm H_2O when the fluid level stabilizes.
4. The manometer uses a balance of forces: downward pressure of the fluid (determined by density and height) against pressure of the central venous system (caused by hydrostatic and recoil forces).

In both techniques, the monitoring system has to be zeroed at the level of the right atrium (usually at the midaxillary line). This eliminates the effect of hydrostatic pressure on the CVP value.

CATHETERS

Different types of catheters are used for central venous cannulation and CVP measurement. They differ in their lumen size, length, number of lumens, the presence or absence of a subcutaneous cuff and the material they are made of. The vast majority of catheters are designed to be

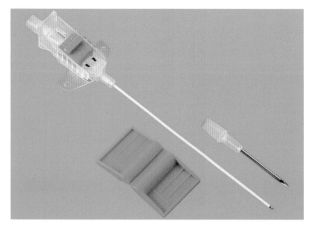

Fig. 11.13 Argon cannula over a needle central line. (Courtesy Argon Medical Devices.)

inserted using the Seldinger technique, although some are designed as 'long' intravenous cannulae (cannula over a needle) (Fig. 11.13).

Antimicrobial-coated catheters have been designed to reduce the incidence of catheter-related bloodstream infection. These can be either antiseptic coated (e.g. chlorhexidine/silver sulfadiazine, benzalkonium chloride, platinum/silver) or antibiotic coated (e.g. minocycline/rifampin) on either the internal or external surface or both. The antibiotic-coated central lines are thought to be more effective in reducing the incidence of line infection (Fig. 11.14). Chlorhexidine impregnated foam discs (e.g. Biopatch) can also be used to surround the skin entry site of the vascular device as part of the line dressing. This is also thought to reduce the incidence of line infection.

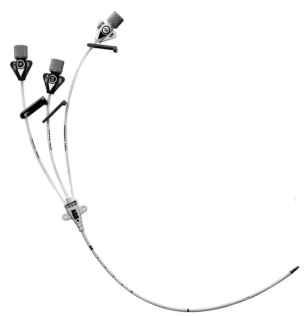

Fig. 11.14 Chlorhexidine-impregnated triple lumen central venous catheter. The inside and outside of the catheter and the hubs are impregnated with chlorhexidine. (Image courtesy Teleflex Incorporated. © [2021] Teleflex Incorporated. All rights reserved.)

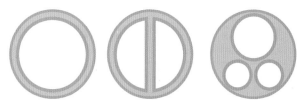

Fig. 11.15 Central vascular catheter lumens: single, double and triple.

Multilumen catheter

1. The catheter has two or more lumens of different sizes (Fig. 11.15), e.g. 16G and 18G (Fig. 11.16). Paediatric sizes also exist (Fig. 11.17).
2. The different lumens should be flushed with saline before insertion.
3. Single and double lumen versions exist.
4. Simultaneous administration of drugs and CVP monitoring is possible. It does not allow the insertion of a pulmonary artery (PA) catheter.
5. These catheters are made of polyurethane. This provides good tensile strength, allowing larger lumens for smaller internal diameter.

Long central catheters/peripherally inserted central catheters (PICC)

1. These catheters, usually around 60 cm in length, are designed to be inserted through an introducing

peel-away sheath via an upper arm vein, usually the basilic (Fig. 11.18).
2. They are used when a central catheter is required in situations when it is unnecessary or undesirable to gain access via the internal jugular or the subclavian veins. Most PICCs are sited for long-term cancer chemotherapy or antibiotic treatment, for example treating osteomyelitis or endocarditis.
3. They are made of soft flexible polyurethane or silicone. Single (4 Fr), double (5 Fr) and triple (5 or 6 Fr) versions exist. Some designs are suitable for power injection needed for contrast during computed tomography scans.

Hickman catheters

1. These central catheters are made of polyurethane or silicone and are usually inserted into the internal

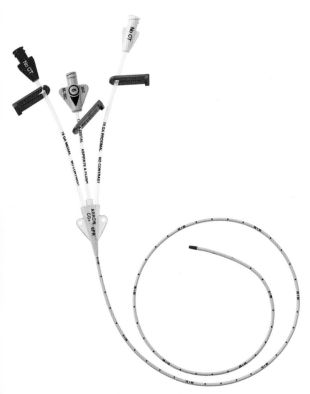

Fig. 11.16 Adult Arrow triple lumen central vascular catheter. (Image courtesy Teleflex Incorporated. © [2021] Teleflex Incorporated. All rights reserved.)

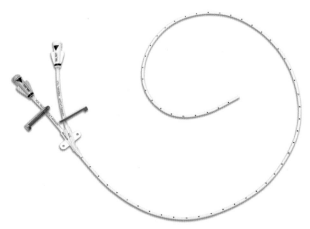

Fig. 11.18 Double lumen peripherally inserted central catheter line. (Image courtesy Teleflex Incorporated. © [2021] Teleflex Incorporated. All rights reserved.)

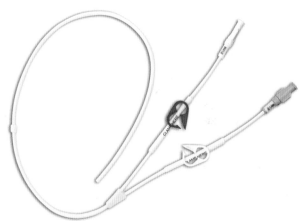

Fig. 11.19 A double lumen long-term Hickman catheter. Note the Dacron cuff. (Courtesy Vygon (UK) Ltd. © Vygon (UK) Ltd.)

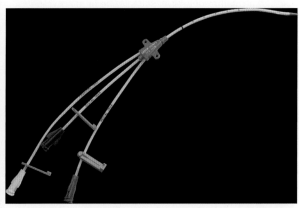

Fig. 11.17 A paediatric triple lumen catheter. (Courtesy Vygon (UK) Ltd. © Vygon (UK) Ltd.)

jugular or subclavian vein. The catheter can have one, two or three lumens (Fig. 11.19).

2. The proximal end is tunnelled under the skin for a distance of about 10 cm.

3. A Dacron cuff is positioned 3–4 cm from the site of entry under the skin. It induces a fibroblastic reaction to anchor the catheter in place (Fig. 11.20). The cuff also reduces the risk of infection as it stops the spread of infection from the site of entry to the skin. Some catheters also have a silver-impregnated cuff that acts as an antimicrobial barrier.

4. They are used for long-term chemotherapy, parenteral nutrition, blood sampling or as a readily available venous access, especially in children requiring frequent anaesthetics during cancer treatment.

5. These lines are designed to remain in situ for several months unless they become infected but require some degree of daily maintenance.

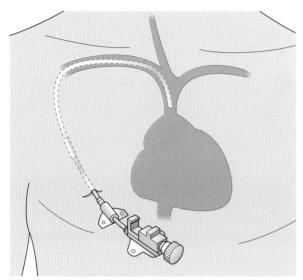

Fig. 11.20 Final position of a tunnelled Hickman catheter. (Reproduced with permission from Viggo-Spectramed, a division of BOC Healthcare, Manchester, UK.)

Dialysis catheters

These are large-calibre catheters designed to allow high flow rates of at least 300 mL/min. They are made of silicone or polyurethane. Most of them are dual lumen with staggered end and side holes to prevent admixture of blood at the inflow and outflow portions, so reducing recirculation.

Problems in practice and safety features

1. Inaccurate readings can be due to catheter blockage, catheter inserted too far or using the wrong zero level.
2. Pneumo and/or haemothorax (with an incidence of 2%–10% with subclavian vein catheterization and 1%–2% with internal jugular catheterization), accidental arterial puncture and associated trauma to the arteries (carotid, subclavian and brachial) with potential arteriovenous fistula formation, air embolism, haematoma and tracheal puncture are complications of insertion.
3. Sepsis and infection are common complications with an incidence of 2.8%–20%. *Staphylococcus aureus* and *Enterococcus* are the most common organisms.

Guidelines for reduction in sepsis and infection rates with the use of central venous catheters

- Education and training of staff who insert and maintain the catheters.
- Use the maximum sterile barrier precautions during central venous catheter insertion.
- Use of >0.5% chlorhexidine preparation with alcohol preparations for skin antisepsis. If there is a contraindication to chlorhexidine, tincture of iodine, an iodophor or 70% alcohol can be used as alternative. Antiseptics should be allowed to dry according to the manufacturer's recommendation prior to placing the catheter.
- Use a subclavian site rather than a jugular or a femoral site in adult patients to minimize infection risk for non-tunnelled central vascular catheter (CVC) placement.
- Use ultrasound guidance to place central venous catheters (if this technology is available) to reduce the number of cannulation attempts and mechanical complications. Ultrasound guidance should only be used by those fully trained in its technique.
- Use a CVC with the minimum number of ports or lumens essential for the management of the patient.
- Promptly remove any intravascular catheter that is no longer essential.
- When adherence to aseptic technique cannot be ensured (i.e. catheters inserted during a medical emergency), replace the catheter as soon as possible, i.e. within 48 hours.
- Use either sterile gauze or sterile, transparent, semipermeable dressing to cover the catheter site.
- Use a chlorhexidine/silver sulfadiazine or minocycline/rifampin-impregnated CVC in patients whose catheter is expected to remain in place >5 days.

(From Centers for Disease Control, 2011. Guidelines for the prevention of intravascular catheter-related infections.)

4. A false passage may be created if the guidewire or dilator is advanced against resistance. The insertion should be smooth.
5. There may be cardiac complications such as self-limiting arrhythmias due to the irritation caused by the guidewire or catheter. Gradual withdrawal of the device is usually adequate to restore normal rhythm. More serious but unusual complications such as venous or cardiac perforation can be lethal.
6. Catheter-related venous thrombosis is thought to be up to 40% depending on the site, the duration of placement, the technique and the condition of the patient.

7. Microshock may occur. A central venous catheter presents a direct pathway to the heart muscle. Faulty electrical equipment can produce minute electrical currents (less than 1 ampere), which can travel via this route to the myocardium. This can produce ventricular fibrillation (VF) if the tip of the catheter is in direct contact with the myocardium (see Chapter 14). This very small current does not cause any adverse effects if applied to the body surface, but if passed directly to the heart, the current density will be high enough to cause VF, hence the name microshock.

> ### Central venous catheterization and pressure
> - There are different routes of insertion, e.g. the internal jugular, subclavian and basilic veins.
> - The Seldinger technique is the most commonly used.
> - The catheters differ in size, length, number of lumens and material.
> - A pressure transducer or water manometer is used to measure CVP.
> - Sepsis and infection are common.
> - Antibiotic- and/or antiseptic-coated catheters can reduce the incidence of infections.

Invasive electrocardiogram (ECG)

In addition to using skin electrodes to record ECG, other more invasive methods can be used (Fig. 11.21). The following methods can be used:

1. Oesophageal ECG can be recorded by using oesophageal electrodes that are incorporated into an oesophageal stethoscope and temperature probe. It has

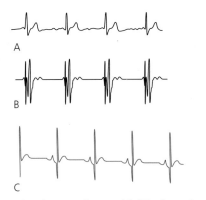

Fig. 11.21 Invasive electrocardiogram. (A) Skin electrodes. (B) Oesophageal. (C) Intracardiac.

been found to be useful in detecting atrial arrhythmias. As it is positioned near the posterior aspect of the left ventricle, it can be helpful in detecting posterior wall ischaemia.

2. Intracardiac ECG with electrodes are inserted using a multipurpose PA flotation catheter. There are three atrial and two ventricular electrodes. In addition to ECG recording, these electrodes can be used in atrial or atrioventricular (AV) pacing. Such ECG recording has great diagnostic capabilities and can be part of an implantable defibrillator. It is used for loci that cannot be assessed by body surface electrodes, such as the bundle of His or ventricular septal activity.

3. Tracheal ECG uses two electrodes embedded into a tracheal tube. It is useful in diagnosing atrial arrhythmias especially in children.

Cardiac output

Cardiac output monitoring (the measurement of flow, rather than pressure) has been the subject of a lot of technical development over the last few decades. It is helpful to consider the history of this development briefly.

The PA catheter was developed in the 1970s and was the only bedside piece of equipment available to measure cardiac output. It gained widespread acceptance in the intensive care and anaesthetic community. However, it lost favour due to its technically demanding insertion. Also some papers appeared in journals during the late 1980s and mid 1990s associating its use with an increased mortality in patients. This finding has now been refuted; however, the PA catheter remains challenging to insert in some circumstances. Indeed thermodilution remains the gold standard method for measuring the cardiac output at the bedside.

As a result, there was a strong move to adopt less invasive technologies and develop them to replace the PA catheter.

The following techniques exist to provide measurement of cardiac output. Some use a combination of these, for example, LiDCO, which uses lithium indicator dilution to calibrate its arterial waveform analysis software. Detailed discussion of each is beyond the scope of this book, and the reader is referred to the further reading section.

1. Arterial waveform analysis either via direct arterial cannulation or 'simulated' via a plethysmographic trace (such as that obtained with the pulse oximeter). Some devices need to be calibrated (either internally or externally), and some need no calibration:
   a. pulse contour analysis
   b. conservation of mass

c. PRAM Vytech MostCare (pressure recording analytical method)
d. pleth variability index (Masimo PVI).
2. Aortic velocimetry using:
   a. Doppler frequency shift (oesophageal and suprasternal Doppler)
   b. electrical velocimetry (EV; Aesculon and Icon).
3. Formal echocardiography:
   a. transoesophageal
   b. transthoracic.
4. Transthoracic impedance.
5. Pulmonary gas clearance.
6. Indicator dilution:
   a. thermal dilution
   b. lithium dilution
   c. dye dilution.
7. EV is the technique that noninvasively measures rate-of-change of electrical conductivity of blood in the aorta using four standard ECG surface electrodes.

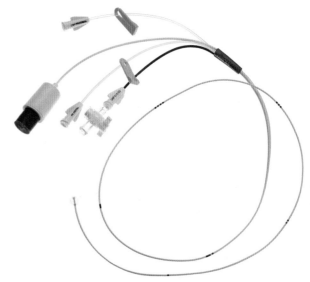

Fig. 11.22 Arrow balloon-tipped, flow-guided pulmonary artery catheter. (Image courtesy Teleflex Incorporated. © [2021] Teleflex Incorporated. All rights reserved.)

Balloon-tipped, flow-guided PA catheter

PA catheters are usually inserted via the right internal jugular or left subclavian veins via an 8-Fr introducer. They are floated through the right atrium and ventricle into the PA.

> **Indications for using a PA catheter**
> - Ischaemic and valvular heart disease, cardiogenic shock, left and/or right ventricle failure.
> - Sepsis and septic shock.
> - Adult respiratory distress syndrome.
> - Oliguria and unexplained hypotension.
> - Perioperative monitoring, e.g. coronary artery bypass graft (CABG), major vascular surgery.

Components

PA catheters are available in sizes 5–8G and are usually 110 cm in length (Fig. 11.22). They have up to five lumens and are marked at 10-cm intervals:

1. The distal lumen ends in the PA. It is used to measure PA and pulmonary capillary wedge (PCW) pressures and to sample mixed venous blood.
2. The proximal lumen should ideally open in the right atrium, being positioned about 30 cm from the tip of the catheter. It can be used to continuously monitor the CVP, to administer the injectate, to measure the cardiac output (by thermodilution) or to infuse fluids. Depending on the design, a second proximal lumen may be present, which is usually dedicated to infusions of drugs.
3. Another lumen contains two insulated wires leading to a thermistor that is about 3.7 cm from the catheter tip. Proximally it is connected to a cardiac output computer.
4. The balloon inflation lumen is used to inflate the balloon, which is situated at the catheter tip.

Up to 1.5 mL of air is needed. When the balloon is inflated, the catheter floats with the blood flow into a PA branch (Fig. 11.23).

Mechanism of action

1. Before insertion, flush all the lines and test the balloon with 1–1.5 mL of air.
2. The most distal lumen of the catheter is connected to a transducer pressure measuring system for continuous monitoring as the catheter is advanced. As the catheter passes via the superior vena cava to the right atrium, low pressure waves (mean of 3–8 mmHg normally) are displayed (Fig. 11.24). The distance from the internal jugular or the subclavian vein to the right atrium is about 15–20 cm.
3. The balloon is inflated, enabling the blood flow to carry the catheter tip through the tricuspid valve into

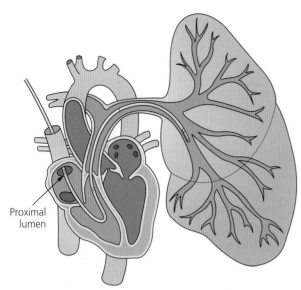

Proximal
lumen

Fig. 11.23 Position of the pulmonary artery catheter tip in a pulmonary artery branch. The desired position of the proximal lumen in the right atrium is indicated by an *arrow*.

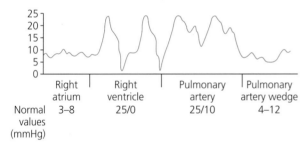

	Right atrium	Right ventricle	Pulmonary artery	Pulmonary artery wedge
Normal values (mmHg)	3–8	25/0	25/10	4–12

Fig. 11.24 Diagrammatic representation of the pressure waveforms seen as a pulmonary artery flotation catheter is advanced until it wedges in a branch of the pulmonary artery.

the right ventricle. Tall right ventricular (RV) pressure waves (15–25 mmHg systolic and 0–10 mmHg diastolic) are displayed.

4. As the balloon tip floats through the pulmonary valve into the PA, the pressure waveform changes with higher diastolic pressure (10–20 mmHg) but similar systolic pressures. The dicrotic notch, caused by the closure of the pulmonary valve, can be noted. The distance from the right ventricle to the PA should be less than 10 cm, unless there is cardiomegaly.

5. The balloon is fully inflated, enabling the blood flow to carry the tip of the catheter into a PA branch where it wedges. This is shown as a damped pressure waveform (PCWP), mean pressure of 4–12 mmHg). This reflects the left atrial filling pressure. The balloon should then be deflated so the catheter floats back

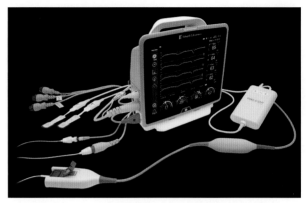

Fig. 11.25 Edwards Lifesciences HemoSphere cardiac output monitor with its other connectors such as tissue oxygen saturation and continuous noninvasive arterial blood pressure monitoring. (From Edwards, Edwards Lifesciences, ForeSight, ForeSight Elite, HemoSphere, Swan and Swan-Ganz are trademarks of Edwards Lifesciences Corporation. Edwards Lifesciences LLC, Irvine, CA, USA.)

into the PA. The balloon should be kept deflated until another PCWP reading is required.

6. The cardiac output is measured using thermodilution. Traditionally, 10 mL of cold injectate is bolused upstream via the proximal lumen. The thermistor (in the PA) measures the change in temperature of the blood downstream. A temperature–time curve is displayed from which the computer can calculate the cardiac output (Fig. 11.25). The volume of injectate should be known accurately and the whole volume injected quickly. Usually the mean of three readings is taken.

7. Increasingly popular designs that automatically display 'continuous' cardiac output also exist (Fig. 11.25). These use a heating filament that is wrapped around the catheter, from 14 to 25 cm from the tip, to heat up passing blood periodically. The small change in blood temperature is measured by the thermistor 4 cm from the tip, in the PA.

8. Some designs have the facility to continuously monitor the mixed venous oxygen saturation using fibreoptic technology (Figs. 11.26 and 11.27). Cardiac pacing capability is present in some designs.

Information gained from PA catheter

The responses to fluid challenges and therapeutic regimens (vasodilators and/or inotropic agents) are monitored in preference to isolated individual readings. The following can be measured: CVP, RV pressure, PA pressure, PCWP, cardiac output, cardiac index, stroke volume, stroke volume index, LV and RV stroke work index, SVR, pulmonary vascular resistance, mixed venous oximetry

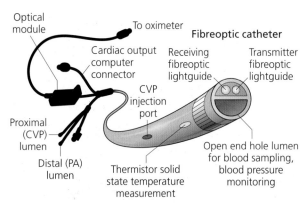

Fig. 11.26 Mechanism of action of the Abbott Oximetrix pulmonary artery catheter. This uses fibreoptic technology to measure mixed venous oxygen saturation (SvO_2). *CVP,* Central venous pressure; *PA,* pulmonary artery.

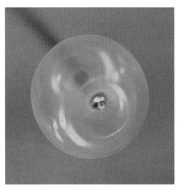

Fig. 11.27 The Abbott Oximetrix pulmonary artery catheter tip.

(SvO_2), blood temperature and degree of shunt. Oxygen delivery and consumption can also be calculated.

Problems in practice and safety features

The overall patient morbidity of using such catheters is 0.4%.

1. There are also the complications due to central venous cannulation (as stated previously).
2. Complications due to catheter passage and advancement. These include arrhythmias (ventricular ectopics, ventricular tachycardia and others), heart block, knotting/kinking (common in low-flow states and patients with large hearts; a 'rule of thumb' is that the catheter should not be advanced more than 10–15 cm without a change in the pressure waveform), valvular damage and perforation of PA vessel.
3. Complications due to the presence in the PA. These include thrombosis (can be reduced by the use of heparin-bonded catheters), PA rupture (more common in the elderly, may present as haemoptysis and is often fatal), infection, balloon rupture, pulmonary infarction, valve damage and arrhythmias.

4. In certain conditions, the PCWP does not accurately reflect LV filling pressure. Such conditions include mitral stenosis and regurgitation, left atrial myxoma, ball valve thrombus, pulmonary veno-occlusive disease, total anomalous pulmonary venous drainage, cardiac tamponade and acute RV dilatation resulting from RV infarction, massive pulmonary embolism and acute severe tricuspid regurgitation.
5. Catheter whip can occur because of the coursing of the pulmonary catheter through the right heart. Cardiac contractions can produce 'shock transients' or 'whip' artefacts. Negative deflections due to a whip artefact may lead to an underestimation of PA pressures.

Balloon-tipped, flow-guided pulmonary artery catheter

- Inserted via a large central vein into the right atrium, right ventricle, PA and branch with contiguous pressure monitoring.
- Used to measure LV filling pressure in addition to other parameters.
- Complications are due to central venous cannulation, the passage of the catheter through different structures and the presence of the catheter in the circulation.
- PCWP does not accurately reflect LV filling pressure in certain conditions.

 Exam tip: You need to be able to draw the pressure waveforms during an insertion of a balloon-tipped, flow-guided PA catheter as it moves from one chamber to another. In addition, the knowledge of the physiological measurements (both direct and derived) gained from such a catheter is important.

Oesophageal Doppler haemodynamic measurement

An estimate of cardiac output can be quickly obtained using the minimally invasive oesophageal Doppler. Patient response to therapeutic manoeuvres (e.g. fluid challenge) can also be rapidly assessed. The technique has the advantage of the smooth muscle tone of the oesophagus acting as a natural means of maintaining the probe in position for repeated measurements. In addition, the oesophagus is in close anatomical proximity to the aorta so that signal interference from bone, soft tissue and lung is minimized. Over the past three decades, the oesophageal Doppler has evolved from an experimental technique to a relatively simple bedside procedure, with the latest models

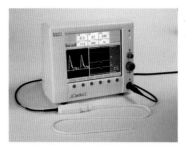

Fig. 11.28 The CardioQ oesophageal Doppler machine and attached probe (foreground).

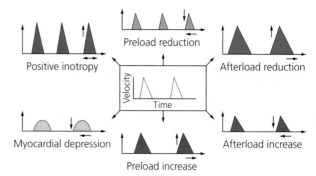

Fig. 11.29 Changes in oesophageal Doppler waveform associated with a variety of clinical situations. (Courtesy Dr. M. Singer.)

incorporating both Doppler and echo-ultrasound in a single probe.

The measurement of cardiac output using the oesophageal Doppler method correlates well with that obtained from a PA catheter. Oesophageal Doppler ultrasonography has been used for intravascular volume optimization in both the perioperative period and in the critical care setting. Its use in cardiac, general and orthopaedic surgery has been associated with a reduction in morbidity and hospital stay. Because of the mild discomfort associated with placing the probe and maintaining it in a fixed position, patients require adequate sedation.

Components

1. A monitor housing that contains the following:
   a. a screen for visual verification of correct signal measurement (Fig. 11.28)
   b. technology that enables beat-to-beat calculation of the stroke volume and cardiac output.
2. An insulated, thin, latex-free silicone oesophageal probe contains a Doppler transducer angled at 45 degrees (Fig. 11.28). The probe has a diameter of 6 mm with an internal spring coil to ensure flexibility and rigidity. A paediatric probe is available for children >3 kg.

Mechanism of action

1. The device relies on the Doppler principle. There is an increase in observed frequency of a signal when the signal source approaches the observer and a decrease when the source moves away.
2. The changes in the frequency of the transmitted ultrasound result from the encounter of the wavefront with moving red blood cells. If the transmitted sound waves encounter a group of red cells moving towards the source, they are reflected back at a frequency higher than that at which they were sent, producing a *positive Doppler shift*. The opposite effect occurs when a given frequency sent into tissues encounters red cells moving away. The result is the return of a frequency lower than that transmitted, resulting in a *negative Doppler*

shift. Analysis of the reflected frequencies allows determination of velocity of flow.

3. The lubricated probe is inserted via the mouth with the bevel of the tip facing up at the back of the patient's throat into the distal oesophagus to a depth of about 35–40 cm from the teeth.
4. The probe is rotated and slowly pulled back while listening to the audible signal. The ideal probe tip location is at the level between the fifth and sixth thoracic vertebrae because, at that level, the descending aorta is adjacent and parallel to the distal oesophagus. This location is achieved by superficially landmarking the distance to the third sternocostal junction anteriorly. A correctly positioned probe can measure the blood flow in this major vessel using a high ultrasound frequency of 4 MHz.
5. The Doppler signal waveform is analysed, and the stroke volume and total cardiac output are computed using the Doppler equation and a normogram, which corrects for variations found with differing patient age, sex and body surface area.

The Doppler equation

$$v = \frac{cf_d}{2f_T\cos\theta}$$

where:
v is the flow velocity
c is the speed of sound in body tissue (1540 m/s)
f_d is the Doppler frequency shift
$\cos\theta$ is the cosine of the angle between the sound beam and the blood flow (45 degrees)
f_T is the frequency of transmitted ultrasound (Hz).

---

6. The parameters obtained from analysis of the Doppler signal waveform allow the operator to gain an assessment of cardiac output, stroke volume, volaemic status, SVR and myocardial function (Fig. 11.29).

Problems in practice and safety features

1. The probe is fully insulated and safe when diathermy is being used.
2. The probe cannot easily be held in the correct position for long periods. Frequent repositioning may be necessary if continuous monitoring is required.
3. Oesophageal Doppler measurement can only be used in an adequately sedated, intubated patient. Its use in awake patients has been described using local anaesthesia. A suprasternal probe is also available and can be used in awake patients.
4. Insertion of the probe is not recommended in patients with pharyngo-oesophageal pathology (e.g. oesophageal varices).
5. The role of the oesophageal Doppler in children is still being evaluated.

Oesophageal Doppler
- Minimally invasive and rapid estimate of cardiac output using the Doppler principle.
- Insulated Doppler probe lies in the distal oesophagus emitting a high ultrasound frequency of 4 MHz.
- Continuous monitoring is possible, although frequent probe repositioning is a problem.

LiDCOrapid

LiDCOrapid (LiDCO, London, UK) is a cardiac output monitor that uses arterial pressure waveform analysis software to generate a 'nominal' cardiac output value. Because it does not require calibration, it can be quickly set up and the effects of fluids or inotropes assessed (Fig. 11.30).

Components

1. The monitor housing contains:
   a. screen displaying real-time cardiac output parameters

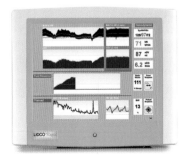

Fig. 11.30 The LiDCOrapid cardiac output monitor.

b. software technology for computing the cardiac output and other parameters
c. electrical connection feeding the arterial waveform from the patient's bedside invasive pressure monitor.

Mechanism of action

1. The patient's existing invasive blood pressure trace is fed by a cable into the LiDCOrapid. From this, the software algorithm generates a nominal stroke volume and cardiac output.
2. The LiDCOrapid displays the following parameters: heart rate, pressures (MAP, systolic and diastolic), stroke volume and cardiac output.
3. Dynamic preload parameters can also be generated by the software to assess the stroke volume response to a fluid challenge.

Problems in practice and safety features

The performance of the software may be compromised in the following patient groups:
1. Patients with aortic valve regurgitation.
2. Patients being treated with an intra-aortic balloon pump or cardiac arrhythmias that will disrupt the usual arterial waveform pattern.
3. Patients with highly damped peripheral arterial lines or with pronounced peripheral arterial vasoconstriction.
4. The LiDCOplus (LiDCO, London, UK) can be calibrated using a single-point lithium indicator dilution process. This offers more accurate cardiac output measurement.

Temperature probes

Monitoring a patient's temperature during surgery is a common and routine procedure. Different types of thermometers are available.

THERMISTOR

Components

1. It has a small bead of a temperature-dependent semiconductor.
2. It has a Wheatstone bridge circuit.

Mechanism of action

1. The thermistor has electrical resistance, which changes nonlinearly with temperature. The response is made linear electronically. This property allows them to accurately measure temperature to an order of 0.1°C.

2. It can be made in very small sizes and is relatively cheap to manufacture.
3. It is mounted in a plastic or stainless steel probe, making it mechanically robust, and it can be chemically sterilized.
4. It is used in PA catheters to measure cardiac output.
5. In the negative thermal conductivity thermistors, such as cobalt oxide, copper oxide and manganese oxide, the electrical resistance decreases as the temperature increases. In the positive thermal conductivity thermistors, such as barium titanate, the electrical resistance increases with the temperature.

Problems in practice and safety features

Thermistors need to be stabilized as they age.

INFRARED TYMPANIC THERMOMETER

Components

1. A small probe with a disposable and transparent cover is inserted into the external auditory meatus.
2. The detector (which consists of a series of thermocouples called a *thermopile*).

Mechanism of action

1. The detector receives infrared radiation from the tympanic membrane.
2. The infrared signal detected is converted into an electrical signal that is processed to measure accurately the core temperature within 3 seconds.
3. The rate of radiation by an object is proportional to temperature to the fourth power.

Problems in practice and safety features

1. Noncontinuous intermittent readings.
2. The probe has to be accurately aimed at the tympanic membrane. False low readings from the sides of the ear canal can be a problem.
3. Wax in the ear can affect the accuracy.

THERMOCOUPLES

These are devices that make use of the principle that two different metals in contact generate a voltage, which is temperature dependent (Fig. 11.31).

Components

1. It uses two strips of dissimilar metals (0.4–2 mm diameter) of different specific heats and in contact

from both ends. Usually copper–constantan (copper with 40% nickel) junctions are used.
2. It has a galvanometer.

Mechanism of action

1. One junction is used as the measuring junction, whereas the other one is the reference. The latter is kept at a constant temperature.
2. The metals expand and contract to different degrees with change in temperature producing an electrical potential that is compared to a reference junction. The current produced is directly proportional to the temperature difference between the two junctions, i.e. there is a linear relationship between voltage and temperature.
3. The voltage produced is called the Seebeck effect or thermoelectric effect.
4. The measuring junction produces a potential of 40 μV/°C. This potential is measured by an amplifier.
5. They are stable and accurate to 0.1°C.
6. If multiple thermocouples are linked in series, they constitute a thermopile. This is done to improve their sensitivity.

Body core temperature can be measured using different sites:

1. *Rectal* temperature does not accurately reflect the core temperature in anaesthetized patients. During an operation, changes in temperature are relatively rapid and the rectal temperature lags behind.
2. *Oesophageal* temperature accurately reflects the core temperature with the probe positioned in the lower oesophagus (at the level of the left atrium). Here the probe is not affected by the cooler tracheal temperature (Fig. 11.32).

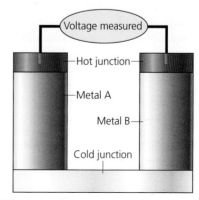

Fig. 11.31 Thermocouple.

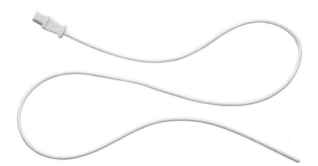

Fig. 11.32 Oesophageal/rectal temperature probe. (Courtesy Smiths Medical, Ashford, Kent, UK.)

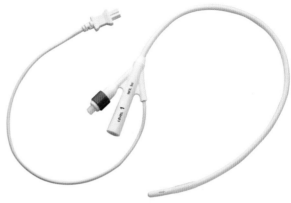

Fig. 11.35 Smiths Medical bladder catheter with a temperature probe. (Courtesy Smiths Medical, Ashford, Kent, UK.)

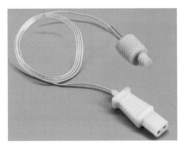

Fig. 11.33 Tympanic membrane temperature probe. (Courtesy Smiths Medical, Ashford, Kent, UK.)

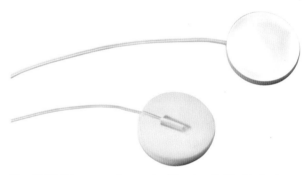

Fig. 11.36 Skin temperature probe. (Courtesy Smiths Medical, Ashford, Kent, UK.)

5. *Skin* temperature, when measured with the core temperature, can be useful in determining the volaemic status of the patient (Fig. 11.36).

The axilla is the best location for monitoring muscle temperature, making it most suitable for detecting malignant hyperthermia.

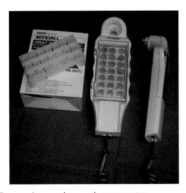

Fig. 11.34 Tympanic membrane thermometer.

3. *Tympanic membrane* temperature is closely associated with brain temperature. It accurately reflects core temperature compared with lower oesophageal temperature. Thermocouple and thermistor probes as well as the infrared probe can be used (Figs. 11.33 and 11.34).
4. *Bladder* temperature correlates well with the core temperature when urine output is normal (Fig. 11.35).

Temperature probes
- They can be thermistors, thermocouples or infrared thermometers.
- Core and skin temperatures can be measured.
- Core temperature can be measured from the rectum, oesophagus, tympanic membrane or the bladder.

Exam tip: It is important to know the various methods and routes used to measure the temperature in the operating theatre.

SUGGESTED FURTHER READING

Centers for Disease Control and Prevention, 2011. Guidelines for the Prevention of Intravascular Catheter-related Infections. Available from: https://www.cdc.gov/infectioncontrol/pdf/guidelines/bsi-guidelines-H.pdf.

Centers for Disease Control and Prevention, 2017. Update. Available from: https://www.cdc.gov/infectioncontrol/guidelines/bsi/updates.html.

The Joint Commission, 2013. CVC Insertion Bundles. Available from: https://www.jointcommission.org/assets/1/6/CLABSI_Toolkit_Tool_3-18_CVC_Insertion_Bundles.pdf.

MHRA, 2019. Blood pressure measurement devices. Available from: https://assets.publishing.service.gov.uk/government/uploads/system/uploads/attachment_data/file/841944/BP_monitoring_2019_v2.2.pdf.

National Institute for Health and Clinical Excellence, 2008/2016. Hypothermia: prevention and management in adults having surgery. Available from: https://www.nice.org.uk/guidance/cg65/evidence.

Saugel, B., Kouz, K., Scheeren, T.W.L., et al., 2021. Cardiac output estimation using pulse wave analysis-physiology, algorithms, and technologies: a narrative review. Br. J. Anaesth. 126 (1), 67–76.

SELF-ASSESSMENT QUESTIONS

Please check your eBook for additional self-assessment

MCQs

In the following lists, which of the statements (a) to (e) are true?

1. Thermometers

a. The electrical resistance of a thermistor changes nonlinearly with temperature.
b. Thermocouples are used in measuring cardiac output using the thermodilution method.
c. The Seebeck effect is used to measure the temperature with thermocouples.
d. Thermometers can be used to measure core and peripheral temperatures at the same time.
e. A galvanometer is used to measure the potential in a thermocouple.

2. Concerning direct arterial blood pressure measurement

a. A 16-G radial artery cannula is suitable.
b. The position of the dicrotic notch in the waveform can reflect the vascular tone.
c. The monitoring system should be capable of responding to a frequency range of up to 40 Hz.
d. Increased damping of the waveform causes an increase in systolic pressure and a decrease in diastolic pressure.
e. Air bubbles produce an overdamped waveform.

3. Balloon-tipped, flow-guided pulmonary artery (PA) catheter

a. They can have up to five separate lumens.
b. They measure the cardiac output using the Doppler technique.
c. The balloon should be left wedged and inflated in order to get a continuous reading of the left ventricular filling pressure.
d. Mixed venous blood oxygen saturation can be measured.
e. They use a thermocouple at the tip to measure the temperature of the blood.

4. If the mean arterial blood pressure is 100 mmHg, pulmonary capillary wedge pressure is 10 mmHg, mean PA pressure is 15 mmHg, cardiac output is 5 L/min and central venous pressure (CVP) is 5 mmHg, which of the following statements are correct?

a. The unit for vascular resistance is dyne s^{-1} cm^5.
b. The pulmonary vascular resistance is about 800.
c. The peripheral vascular resistance is about 1500.
d. The patient has pulmonary hypertension.
e. The patient has normal peripheral vascular resistance.

5. Concerning central venous pressure and cannulation

a. 10 mmHg is equivalent to 7.5 cm H_2O.
b. During cannulation, the left internal jugular vein is the approach of choice since the heart lies mainly in the left side of the chest.
c. Subclavian vein cannulation has a higher incidence of pneumothorax than the internal jugular vein.
d. The J-shaped end of the guidewire is inserted first.
e. The Dacron cuff used in a Hickman's line is to anchor the catheter only.

6. In an invasive pressure measurement system, which of the following is/are correct

a. A clot causes high systolic and low diastolic pressures.
b. A transducer diaphragm with very low compliance causes low systolic and high diastolic pressures.
c. A soft wide lumen catheter causes low systolic and high diastolic pressures.
d. An air bubble causes low systolic and diastolic pressures.
e. A short and narrow lumen catheter is ideal.

7. Concerning the oesophageal Doppler

a. The ideal probe location is at the level between the fifth and sixth thoracic vertebrae.
b. It emits a pulsed ultrasound wave of 4 Hz.

c. Red cells moving towards the ultrasound source reflect the sound back at a frequency lower than that at which it was sent, producing a positive Doppler shift.

d. The oesophageal probe tip is located at a depth of about 40 cm.

e. The angle between the ultrasound beam and blood flow is 75 degrees.

Single best answer

8. **Direct arterial pressure monitoring**
   a. A minimum of a 16G cannula should be used.
   b. Bubbles of air in the transducer aid accuracy.
   c. The first 10 harmonics of the fundamental frequency can be ignored.
   d. The system needs to respond to a frequency range of 0.5–40 Hz.
   e. Vasoconstriction lowers the position of the dicrotic notch.

Answers

1. Thermometers
   a. *True. The response is nonlinear but can be made linear electronically.*
   b. *False. Thermistors are used in measuring the cardiac output by thermodilution. Thermocouples are not used in measuring the cardiac output by thermodilution.*
   c. *True. The Seebeck effect is when the electrical potential produced at the junction of two dissimilar metals is dependent on the temperature of the junction. This is the principle used in thermocouples.*
   d. *True. The gradient between the core and peripheral temperatures is useful in assessing the degree of skin perfusion and the circulatory volume. For example, hypovolaemia causes a decrease in skin perfusion, which reduces the peripheral temperature and thus increases the gradient. The normal gradient is about 2–4°C.*
   e. *True. The galvanometer is placed between the junctions of the thermocouple, the reference and the measuring junctions. This allows the current to be measured. Changes in current are calibrated to measure the temperature difference between the two junctions.*

2. Concerning direct arterial blood pressure measurement
   a. *False. A 16-G cannula is far too big to be inserted into an artery. A 20- or 22-G cannula is usually used, allowing adequate blood flow to pass by the cannula distally.*

   b. *True. The position of the dicrotic notch (which represents the closure of the aortic valve) is on the downstroke curve. A high dicrotic notch can be seen in vasoconstricted patients with high peripheral vascular resistance. A low dicrotic notch can be seen in vasodilated patients (e.g. patients with epidurals or sepsis).*
   c. *True. The addition of the shape of the dicrotic notch to an already simple waveform makes a maximum frequency of 40 Hz adequate for such a monitoring system. Because of the complicated waveform of the electrocardiogram, the monitoring system requires a much wider range of frequencies (maximum of 100 Hz).*
   d. *False. Increased damping leads to a decrease in systolic pressure and an increase in diastolic pressure. Decreased damping causes the opposite. The mean pressure remains the same.*
   e. *True. This is due to the difference in the compressibility of the two media: air and saline. Air is more compressible in contrast to the saline column.*

3. Balloon-tipped, flow-guided PA catheter
   a. *True. The most distal lumen is in the PA. There are one or two proximal lumens in the right atrium: one lumen carries the insulated wires leading to the thermistor proximal to the tip of the catheter, and another lumen is used to inflate the balloon at the tip of the catheter.*

b. *False. The cardiac output is measured by thermodilution. A 'cold' injectate (e.g. saline) is injected via the proximal lumen. The changes in blood temperature are measured by the thermistor in the PA. A temperature–time curve is displayed from which the cardiac output can be calculated.*

c. *False. Leaving the balloon wedged and inflated is dangerous and should not be done. This is due to the risk of ischaemia to the distal parts of the lungs supplied by the PA or its branches.*

d. *True. Using fibreoptics, the mixed venous oxygen saturation can be measured on some designs. This allows the calculation of oxygen extraction by the tissues.*

e. *False. A thermistor is used to measure the temperature of the blood. Thermistors are made to very small sizes.*

4. If the mean arterial blood pressure is 100 mmHg, pulmonary capillary wedge pressure is 10 mmHg, mean PA pressure is 15 mmHg, cardiac output is 5 L/min and CVP is 5 mmHg, which of the following statements are correct?

a. *False. The unit for vascular resistance is dyne s cm^{-5}.*

b. *False. The pulmonary vascular resistance = mean pulmonary artery pressure – left atrial pressure × 80/cardiac output (15 – 10 × 80/5 = 80 dyne s cm^{-5}).*

c. *True. The peripheral vascular resistance = mean arterial pressure – right atrial pressure × 80/cardiac output (100 – 5 × 80/5 = 1520 dyne s cm^{-5}.*

d. *False. The normal mean PA pressure is about 15 mmHg (systolic pressure of about 25 and a diastolic pressure of about 10 mmHg) and pulmonary vascular resistance is 80–120 dyne s cm^{-5}.*

e. *True. The normal peripheral vascular resistance is 1000–1500 dyne s cm^{-5}.*

5. Concerning central venous pressure and cannulation

a. *False. 10 cm H_2O is equivalent to 7.5 mmHg or 1 kPa.*

b. *False. The right internal jugular is usually preferred first as the internal jugular, the brachiocephalic veins and the superior vena cava are nearly in a straight line.*

c. *True. The higher incidence of pneumothorax with the subclavian approach makes the internal jugular the preferred vein.*

d. *True. The J-shaped end of the guidewire is inserted first because it is atraumatic and soft.*

e. *False. In addition to anchoring the catheter, the cuff also reduces the risk of infection by stopping the spread of infection from the site of skin entry. Some catheters have a silver-impregnated cuff that acts as an antimicrobial barrier.*

6. In an invasive pressure measurement system, which of the following is/are correct?

a. *False. A clot will cause damping of the system as pressure changes are not accurately transmitted. The systolic pressure is decreased and the diastolic pressure is increased.*

b. *False. A too rigid diaphragm will cause the system to resonate. This leads to high systolic and low diastolic pressures.*

c. *True. A soft, wide lumen catheter will increase the damping of the system (see 6a).*

d. *False. An air bubble will increase the damping of the system (see 6a).*

e. *True. A catheter that is short and narrow allows transmission of pressure changes accurately. For clinical use, a maximum length of 2 m is acceptable.*

7. Concerning the oesophageal Doppler

a. *True. The ideal probe tip location is at the level between the fifth and sixth thoracic vertebrae. At that level, the descending aorta is adjacent and parallel to the distal oesophagus. This location is achieved by superficially landmarking the distance to the third sternocostal junction anteriorly.*

b. *False. The frequency used is 4 MHz.*

c. *False. Red cells moving towards the ultrasound source reflect the sound back at a frequency higher than that at which they were sent, producing a positive Doppler shift. The opposite produces a negative Doppler shift.*

d. *True. The tip of the probe is positioned in the distal oesophagus at about a 40-cm depth.*

e. *False. The angle between the ultrasound beam and blood flow is 45 degrees.*

8. *d.*

Chapter 12

Pumps, pain management and regional anaesthesia

Patient-controlled analgesia (PCA)

PCA represents one of the most significant advances in the treatment of postoperative pain. Improved technology enables pumps to accurately deliver boluses of opioid when a demand button is activated by the patient.

It is the patient who determines the plasma concentration of the opioid, this being a balance between the dose required to control the pain and that which causes side effects. The plasma concentration of the opioid is maintained at a relatively constant level with the dose requirements being generally smaller. Patient-controlled epidural analgesia (PCEA) also exists and uses similar principles.

Components

1. It has a pump with an accuracy of at least ±5% of the programmed dose (Fig. 12.1).
2. The remote demand button is connected to the pump and activated by the patient.
3. It has an antisiphon and backflow valve.

Mechanism of action

1. Different modes of analgesic administration can be employed:
   a. patient-controlled, on-demand bolus administration
   b. continuous background infusion and patient-controlled bolus administration.
2. The initial programming of the pump must be for the individual patient. The mode of administration, the amount of analgesic administered per bolus, the 'lock-out' time (i.e. the time period during which the patient is prevented from receiving another bolus despite activating the demand button), the duration of the administration of the bolus and the maximum amount of analgesic permitted per unit time are all variable settings on a PCA device.

3. Some designs have the capability to be used as a PCA pump for a particular variable duration then switching automatically to a continuous infusion as programmed or vice versa.
4. The history of the drug administration including the total dose of the analgesic, the number of boluses and the number of successful and failed attempts can be displayed.
5. The devices have memory capabilities so they retain their programming during syringe changing.
6. Tamper-resistant features are included.
7. Some designs have a safety measure where an accidental triggering of the device is usually prevented by the need for the patient to make two successive presses on the hand control within 1 second.
8. PCA devices operate on mains power sources or battery.
9. Different routes of administration can be used for PCA, e.g. intravenous, intramuscular, subcutaneous or epidural routes.
10. Alarms are included for malfunction, occlusion and disconnection.
11. Ambulatory PCA pumps are available, allowing patient's mobilization during use (Fig. 12.2).

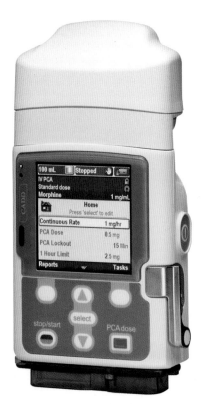

Fig. 12.2 CADD Solis portable patent-controlled analgesia pump. (Courtesy Smiths Medical, Ashford, Kent, UK.)

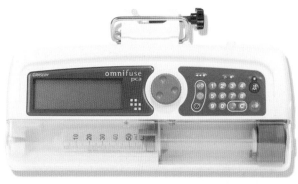

Fig. 12.1 The Graseby Omnifuse patient-controlled analgesia pump.

Problems in practice and safety features

1. The ability of the patient to cooperate and understand is essential.
2. Availability of trained staff to programme the device and monitor the patient is vital.
3. In the PCA mode, the patient may awaken in severe pain because no boluses were administered during sleep.
4. Some PCA devices require special giving sets and syringes.
5. Technical errors can be fatal due to the potential for opiate overdose.

Patient-controlled analgesia

- The patient has the ability to administer the opioid as required.
- The device is programmed by the anaesthetist.
- Different modes of administration.
- Tamper-resistant designs are featured.
- Ambulatory designs are available.
- Technical errors can be fatal.

SYRINGE PUMPS

These are programmable pumps that can be adjusted to give variable rates of infusion and also bolus administration (Fig. 12.3). They are used to maintain continuous infusions of analgesics (or other drugs).

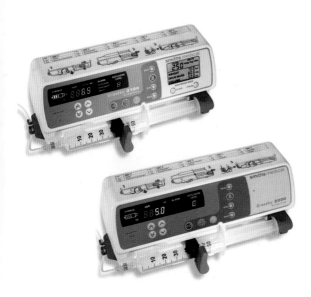

Fig. 12.3 Graseby syringe pumps. (Courtesy Smiths Medical, Ashford, Kent, UK.)

The type of flow is pulsatile continuous delivery, and their accuracy is within ±2%–5%. Some designs can accept a variety of different size syringes. The power source can be battery and/or main power sources.

Problems in practice and safety features

1. It is important to ensure the infusion is unidirectional with no free flow. Antisiphon valves are usually used to achieve this. An alarm is activated if there is a crack in the syringe, allowing air to enter.
2. The syringe should be securely clamped to the pump. Inadvertent free flow can occur if the syringe barrel or plunger is not engaged firmly in the pump mechanism.
3. Syringe drivers should not be positioned above the level of the patient. If the pump is more than 100 cm above the patient, a gravitational pressure can be generated that overcomes the friction between a nonsecured plunger and barrel.
4. Some pumps have a 'back-off' function that prevents the pump from administering a bolus following an obstruction due to increased pressure in the system.
5. An antireflux valve should be inserted in any other line that is connected to the infusion line. Antireflux valves prevent backflow up the secondary (and usually lower pressure) line, should a distal occlusion occur. They would then avoid a subsequent inadvertent bolus.
6. Newer, smart infusion pumps are designed to alert the user when there is a risk of an adverse drug interaction or when the user sets the pump's parameters outside of specified safety limits. This is done via programmable dose and infusion rate limits.
7. In order to change the rate or to give a bolus, there is a need for two distinct or simultaneous actions.

VOLUMETRIC PUMPS

These are programmable pumps designed to be used with specific giving set tubing (Fig. 12.4). They are more suitable for infusions where accuracy of total volume is more important than precise flow rate. Their accuracy is generally within ±5%–10%. Volumetric pump accuracy is sensitive to the internal diameter of the giving set tubing. Various mechanisms of action exist. Peristaltic, cassette and reservoir systems are commonly used.

The power source can be battery and/or main power sources.

TARGET-CONTROLLED INFUSION PUMPS

These pumps have advanced software technology where the age and the weight of the patient are entered in addition to the drug's desired plasma concentration. They are mainly used with a propofol and remifentanil infusion technique. The software is capable of estimating the plasma and effect (brain) concentrations, allowing the anaesthetist to adjust the infusion rate accordingly.

Elastomeric pumps

These light, portable and disposable pumps allow continuous infusions of local anaesthetic solutions. Continuous incisional infiltration or nerve blocks can be used, so allowing the delivery of continuous analgesia (Fig. 12.5).

Components

1. A small balloon-like pump is filled with local anaesthetic. Variable volumes of 100–600 mL are available.

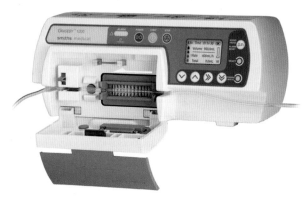

Fig. 12.4 Graseby 1200 volumetric pump. (Courtesy Smiths Medical, Ashford, Kent, UK.)

2. Specially designed catheters have lengths of 7–30 cm and of different gauges.
3. It has a bacterial filter and a flow restrictor.

Mechanism of action

1. The balloon deflates slowly and spontaneously, delivering a set amount of local anaesthetic solution per hour. Rates of 2–14 mL/h can be programmed.
2. Catheters are designed with multiple orifices, allowing the infusion of local anaesthetic solution over a large area.
3. An extra on-demand bolus facility is available in some designs. This allows boluses of 5 mL of solution with a lockout time of 60 minutes.
4. Some designs allow the simultaneous infusion of two surgical sites.
5. A silver-coated antimicrobial dressing is provided.

Problems in practice and safety features

1. Some of the local anaesthetic may get absorbed into the balloon.
2. The infusion rate profile can vary throughout the infusion. It is thought that the initial rate is higher than expected initially, especially if the pump is underfilled. The infusion rates tend to decrease over the infusion period. To reduce such potential risks, the Pajunk FuserPump, with a 350-mL capacity, has a hard shell, a flow rate selector and a locking key. Rates of 3, 5 and 8 mL/h can be delivered (Fig. 12.6).

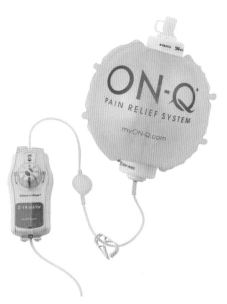

Fig. 12.5 The On-Q elastomeric pump. Note the flow restrictor, bacterial filter, antisyphon valve and attached catheter. (Used with permission from Avanos Medical, Inc.)

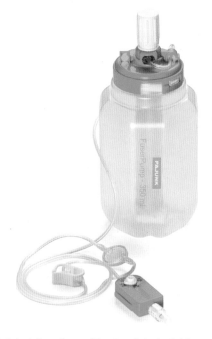

Fig. 12.6 Pajunk FuserPump. (Courtesy Pajunk, Geisingen, Germany.)

3. It is important to follow the manufacturer's instructions regarding positioning of the device in relation to the body and ambient temperature. Changes in temperature can affect the flow rate. A change of 10°C in the temperature of water-based fluids results in altered viscosity, which causes a 20%–30% change in flow rate.

Penthrox Inhaler 'Green Whistle' (Fig. 12.7)

Methoxyflurane is a volatile, halogenated inhalational agent. It was discontinued from routine anaesthetic usage due to concerns over nephrotoxicity at high dosage levels. However, self-administered in a controlled subanaesthetic dose from the Penthrox inhaler, it can provide an efficacious, safe, rapid (within 4–5 minutes) short-term pain relief following trauma in conscious adults. Methoxyflurane has minimal side effects, including negligible effects on the cardiovascular system and respiratory system, making it ideal for pain relief in the prehospital settings. In subanaesthetic doses, methoxyflurane does not carry a risk of nephrotoxicity.

Components (Fig. 12.8)
1. A cylindrical tube with the patient's mouthpiece.
2. A polypropylene wick within the tube to accommodate 3 mL of methoxyflurane.
3. An inlet chamber that allows the addition of methoxyflurane and fresh air.
4. An activated charcoal chamber.

Mechanism of action
1. The wick gradually vaporizes the 3 mL of methoxyflurane.
2. Patient inhales and exhales through the mouthpiece.
3. During inhalation, the patient gets vapour through the mouthpiece.
4. During exhalation, the expired methoxyflurane is captured by the activated charcoal, so reducing pollution.
5. 3-mL methoxyflurane provides 25–30 minutes of analgesia with continuous use. Longer durations can be achieved with intermittent use.
6. If stronger analgesia is needed, the inlet chamber is covered with a finger, allowing less dilution and higher concentration of methoxyflurane.

Problems in practice and safety features
A total dose of 6 mL (two vials) can be used in a day or 15 mL (five vials) in a week.

> **Penthrox inhaler**
> - Methoxyflurane vapour in subanaesthetic concentrations used to provide analgesia.
> - Rapid onset and effective analgesia for 25–30 minutes can be provided.
> - Activated charcoal is used to absorb exhaled methoxyflurane to reduce pollution.

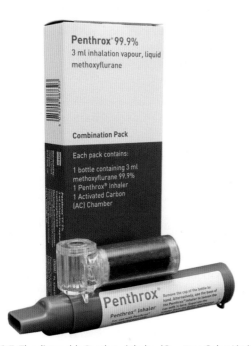

Fig. 12.7 The disposable Penthrox inhaler. (Courtesy Galen Limited, Distributor, UK.)

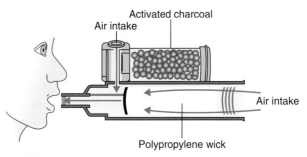

Fig. 12.8 Penthrox inhaler.

NRFit (ISO 80369-6:2016)

Luer connection presents the opportunity for a multitude of misconnection/wrong-route drug administration incidents. While not the unique cause, the Luer connection system has been identified as one of the root causes that enables such preventable events.

The development of safer small-bore connections, which are not compatible with Luer connectors, in medical care has been an ongoing patient safety initiative. In 2016, the International Organization for Standardization (ISO) developed a new standard for non-Luer devices and connectors used in neuroaxial/ regional blocks to avoid the accidental but potentially fatal connection of an intravenous infusion or injection. Making connections to the different devices incompatible will help minimize the risk of cross connection of devices intended for different clinical applications. This should minimize the risk of wrong route of administration drug errors.

NRFit (pronounced 'ner-fit') looks like a Luer connector but is 20% smaller and has unique design features that reduce cross-connections, especially with Luer connectors (Fig. 12.9). NRFit connectors have undergone a rigorous validation process and are considered to be functionally equivalent to conventional Luer connections. Adaptors to Luer connectors will not be manufactured, and syringes will need to have an application-specific connector.

In addition, manufacturers have incorporated yellow colouration into NRFit compatible equipment (Fig. 12.10).

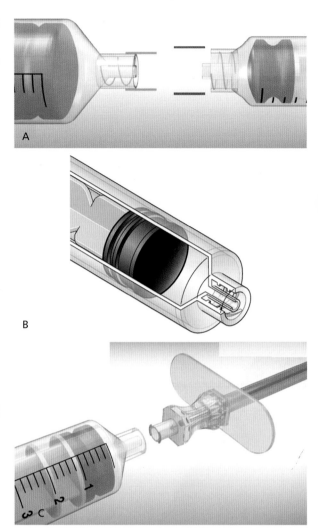

Fig. 12.9 NRFit devices. (A) Comparison of NRFit syringe *(left)* and standard Luer syringe *(right)*. (B) NRFit syringe cross-section. (C) NRFit epidural needle and syringe.

Epidural needles

Epidural needles are used to identify and cannulate the epidural space. The Tuohy needle is widely used in the United Kingdom (Fig. 12.11).

Components

1. The needle is 10 cm in length with a shaft of 8 cm (with 1-cm markings). A 15-cm version exists for obese patients.
2. The needle wall is thin in order to allow a catheter to be inserted through it.
3. The needle is provided with a stylet introducer to prevent occlusion of the lumen by a core of tissue as the needle is inserted.
4. The bevel (called a Huber point) is designed to be slightly oblique at 20 degrees to the shaft, with a rather blunt leading edge.
5. Some designs allow the wings at the hub to be added or removed.
6. The commonly used gauges are either 16 G or 18 G.

Mechanism of action

1. The markings on the needle enable the anaesthetist to determine the distance between the skin and the epidural space. Hence the length of the catheter left inside the epidural space can be estimated.
2. The shape and design of the bevel (Fig. 12.12) enable the anaesthetist to direct the catheter within the epidural space (either in a cephalic or caudal direction).

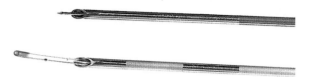

Fig. 12.12 Detail of a spinal needle introduced through a Tuohy needle *(top)*; an epidural catheter passing through a Tuohy needle *(bottom)*.

3. The bluntness of the bevel also minimizes the risk of accidental dural puncture.
4. Some anaesthetists prefer winged epidural needles for better control and handling of the needle during insertion.
5. A paediatric 19-G, 5-cm-long Tuohy needle (with 0.5-cm markings), allowing the passage of a 21-G nylon catheter, is available.
6. A combined spinal–epidural technique is possible using a 26-G spinal needle of about 12-cm length with a standard 16-G Tuohy needle. The Tuohy needle is first positioned in the epidural space, then the spinal needle is introduced through it into the subarachnoid space (see Fig. 12.12 and Fig. 12.13). A relatively high pressure is required to inject through the spinal needle because of its small bore. This might lead to accidental displacement of the tip of the needle from the subarachnoid space leading to a failed or partial block.
7. Echogenic epidural needles are available for ultrasound-guided use (Fig. 12.14).
8. An ultrasound spinal navigation system can be used to guide an epidural needle with real-time 3D navigation of lumbar and thoracic spines (Fig. 12.15). The portable, battery-operated ultrasound device is designed to visualize the bony landmarks, displaying the epidural space location and depth on a rotatable, touch screen display.

Problems in practice and safety features

1. During insertion of the catheter through the needle, if it is necessary to withdraw the catheter, the needle must be withdrawn simultaneously. This is because of the risk of the catheter being transected by the oblique bevel.
2. In accidental dural puncture, there is a high incidence of postdural headache due to the epidural needle's large bore (e.g. 16 G or 18 G).
3. NRFit design prevents wrong-route drug errors: in order to avoid administering drugs that were intended for intravenous administration, all epidural bolus doses are performed using syringes, needles and other devices with safety connectors that cannot connect with intravenous Luer connectors.

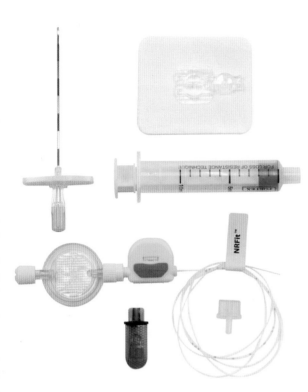

Fig. 12.10 Portex NRFit epidural set. (Courtesy Smiths Medical, Ashford, Kent, UK.)

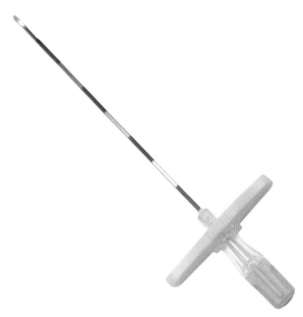

Fig. 12.11 Tuohy needle. Note the 1-cm markings along the shaft. (Courtesy Smiths Medical, Ashford, Kent, UK.)

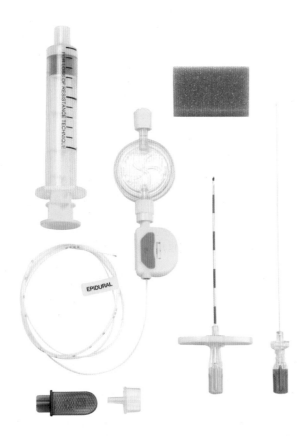

Fig. 12.13 Portex combined spinal–epidural set. (Courtesy Smiths Medical, Ashford, Kent, UK.)

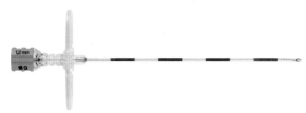

Fig. 12.14 Pajunk TuohySono echogenic epidural needle. Note the design of the distal part and tip to ensure good ultrasound visualization. (Courtesy Pajunk, Geisingen, Germany.)

Epidural needle

- The most popular needle is the 10-cm Tuohy needle with the oblique bevel (Huber point). 5- and 15-cm-long needles also exist.
- It has 1-cm markings to measure the depth of the epidural space.
- A stylet introducer is provided with the needle.
- A combined spinal–epidural technique is popular.
- NRFit design prevents wrong-route drug errors.

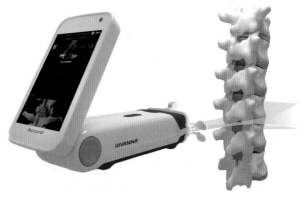

Fig. 12.15 The Accuro handheld ultrasound navigation system. (Courtesy Rivanna, Virginia, USA.)

Epidural catheter, filter and loss of resistance device (Fig. 12.10)

THE CATHETER

Components

1. The catheter is a 90-cm transparent, malleable tube made of either nylon or Teflon and is biologically inert. The 16-G version has an external diameter of about 1 mm and an internal diameter of 0.55 mm.
2. The distal end has two or three side ports with a closed and rounded tip in order to reduce the risk of vascular or dural puncture. Paediatric designs, 18 G or 19 G, have closer distal side ports.
3. Some designs have an open end.
4. The distal end of the catheter is marked clearly at 5-cm intervals, with additional 1-cm markings between 5 and 15 cm (Fig. 12.16).
5. The proximal end of the catheter is connected to a filter.
6. In order to prevent kinking, some designs incorporate a coil-reinforced catheter.
7. Some designs are radio-opaque. These catheters tend to be more rigid than the normal design. They can be used in patients with chronic pain to ensure correct placement of the catheter.

Mechanism of action

1. The catheters are designed to pass easily through their matched gauge epidural needles.
2. The markings enable the anaesthetist to place the desired length of catheter within the epidural space (usually 3–5 cm).

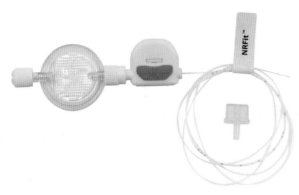

Fig. 12.16 Portex epidural catheter and filter. Note the markings up to 20 cm. (Courtesy Smiths Medical, Ashford, Kent, UK.)

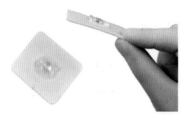

Fig. 12.17 Smiths Medical Portex LockIt Plus epidural catheter fixing device.

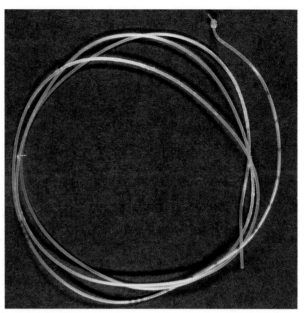

Fig. 12.18 An epidural catheter with a knot near its tip. (Courtesy Dr. M.S. Rao.)

3. There are catheters with a single port at the distal tip. These offer a rather sharp point and increase the incidence of catheter-induced vascular or dural puncture.
4. An epidural fixing device can be used to prevent the catheter falling out. The device clips on the catheter. It has an adhesive flange that secures it to the skin. The device does not occlude the catheter and does not increase the resistance to injection (Fig. 12.17).

Problems in practice and safety features

1. The patency of the catheter should be tested prior to insertion.
2. The catheter can puncture an epidural vessel or the dura at the time of insertion or even days later.
3. The catheter should not be withdrawn through the Tuohy needle once it has been threaded beyond the bevel as that can transect the catheter. Both needle and catheter should be removed in unison.
4. It is almost impossible to predict in which direction the epidural catheter is heading when it is advanced.
5. Once the catheter has been removed from the patient, it should be inspected for any signs of breakage. The side ports are points of catheter weakness where it is possible for the catheter to break. Usually, if a portion of the catheter was to remain in the patient

after removal, conservative management would be recommended.
6. Advancing the catheter too much can cause knotting (Fig. 12.18).

THE FILTER (see FIG. 12.16)

The hydrophilic filter is a 0.22-μm mesh that acts as a bacterial, viral and foreign body (e.g. glass) filter with a priming volume of about 0.7 mL. It is recommended that the filter should be changed every 24 hours if the catheter is going to stay in situ for long periods.

LOSS OF RESISTANCE DEVICE OR SYRINGE

The syringe has a special low-resistance plunger used to identify the epidural space by loss of resistance to either air or saline. Plastic and glass versions are available.

> **Epidural catheter, filter and syringe**
> - Marked 90-cm catheter with distal side or end ports.
> - It should not be advanced for more than 5 cm inside the epidural space.
> - The proximal end is connected to a 0.22-μm mesh bacterial, viral and foreign body filter.
> - A low-resistance plunger syringe is used to identify the epidural space.

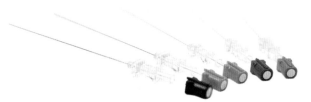

Fig. 12.19 Portex NRFit spinal needles. (Courtesy Smiths Medical, Ashford, Kent, UK.)

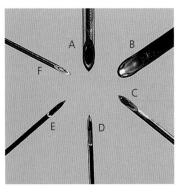

Fig. 12.20 Bevel design of (A) 18-G Quincke, (B) 16-G Tuohy, (C) 22-G Yale, (D) 24-G Sprotte, (E) 25-G Whitacre, (F) 25-G Yale needles.

Spinal needles

These needles are used to inject local anaesthetic(s) and/or opiates into the subarachnoid space. In addition, they are used to sample cerebrospinal fluid (CSF) or for intrathecal injections of antibiotics and cytotoxics (Fig. 12.19).

Components

1. The needle's length varies from 5 to 15 cm; the 10-cm version is most commonly used. They have a transparent hub in order to quickly identify the flow of CSF.
2. A stylet is used to prevent a core of tissue occluding the lumen of the needle during insertion. It also acts to strengthen the shaft. The stylet is withdrawn once the tip of the needle is (or is suspected to be) in the subarachnoid space.
3. Spinal needles are made in different sizes, from 18 G to 29 G in diameter. 32-G spinal needles have been described but are not widely used.
4. The 25-G and smaller needles are used with an introducer, which is usually an 18-G or 19-G needle.
5. The bevel has two designs. The cutting, traumatic bevel is seen in the Yale and Quincke needles. The noncutting, atraumatic pencil point, with a side hole just proximal to the tip, is seen in the Whitacre and Sprotte needles (Figs. 12.20 and 12.21).

Mechanism of action

1. The large 22-G needle is more rigid and easier to direct. It gives a better feedback feel as it passes through the different tissue layers.
2. The CSF is slower to emerge from the smaller-sized needles. Aspirating gently with a syringe can speed up the tracking back of CSF.
3. A 27-G 900-mm length microcatheter with a lateral orifice, very close to the atraumatic tip, can be inserted through a Sprotte spinal needle (23-G). A stylet inside the catheter is removed after the insertion. This allows continuous spinal anaesthesia and top-ups to be administered. The catheter can stay in situ for up to 7

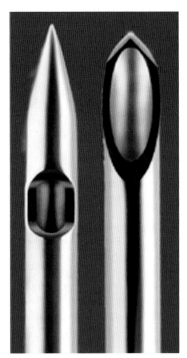

Fig. 12.21 Pencil-shaped Whitacre bevel *(left)* and cutting Quincke bevel *(right)*.

days. The maximum intrathecal catheter length should be less than 50 mm in order to avoid catheter knotting.

Problems in practice and safety features

1. Wrong-route errors: in order to avoid administering drugs that were intended for intravenous administration, NRFit system should be used with all spinal (intrathecal) needles, syringes and other devices with safer connectors that cannot connect with intravenous Luer connectors.

2. Dural headache:
   a. The incidence of dural headache is directly proportional to the gauge of the needle and the number of punctures made through the dura and indirectly proportional to the age of the patient. There is a 30% incidence of dural headache using a 20-G spinal needle, whereas the incidence is reduced to about 1% when a 26-G needle is used. For this reason, smaller-gauge spinal needles are preferred.
   b. The Whitacre and Sprotte atraumatic needles separate rather than cut the longitudinal fibres of the dura. The defect in the dura has a higher chance of sealing after the removal of the needles. This reduces the incidence of dural headache.
   c. Traumatic bevel needles cut the dural fibres, producing a ragged tear which allows leakage of CSF. Dural headache is thought to be caused by the leakage of CSF.
   d. The risk of dural headache is higher during pregnancy and labour, day-surgery patients and those who have experienced a dural headache in the past.
3. Spinal microcatheters
   a. They are difficult to advance.
   b. There is a risk of trauma to nerves.
   c. Cauda equina syndrome is thought to be due to the potential neurotoxicity from the anaesthetic solutions rather than the microcatheter.

Spinal needles
- They have a stylet and a transparent hub.
- Different gauges from 18 G to 32 G.
- The bevel can be cutting (Yale and Quincke) or pencil-like (Whitacre and Sprotte).
- Can cause dural headache.
- Continuous spinal block using a 27-G microcatheter is possible.

 Exam tip: Know the different designs of spinal needle tips and what influence these have on the incidence of spinal headache.

Nerve block needles

These needles are used in regional anaesthesia to identify a nerve plexus or peripheral nerve. To locate the nerve(s), these needles use either electrical nerve stimulation, ultrasound guidance or both.

The following describes the needles that use electrical stimulation. Needles that use ultrasound guidance are described later. It is important to emphasize the need for

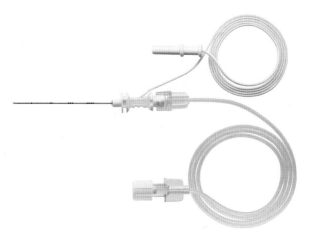
Fig. 12.22 Pajunk SonoPlex stimulating nerve needle, which also has echogenic properties. (Courtesy Pajunk, Geisingen, Germany.)

the World Health Organization checklist to be performed before starting any regional anaesthesia.

Components (Fig. 12.22)

1. They are made of steel with short, rather blunt bevels in order to cause minimal trauma to the nervous tissue. The bluntness makes skin insertion more difficult. This can be overcome by a small incision.
2. The needles have transparent hubs which allow earlier recognition of intravascular placement while performing blocks.
3. A port for injecting the local anaesthetic solution.
4. The needles are connected to a nerve stimulator to aid in localizing the nerve using an insulated cable to prevent leakage of current (see Chapter 15).
5. Although available in different sizes, 22-G size needles are optimal for the vast majority of blocks. There are different lengths depending on the depth of the nerve or plexus. Some suggested needle lengths for common blocks are:
   a. interscalene block: 25–50 mm
   b. axillary block: 35–50 mm
   c. psoas compartment block: 80–120 mm
   d. femoral nerve block: 50 mm
   e. sciatic nerve block (depending on the approach): 80–150 mm.
7. A pencil-shaped needle tip with a distal side hole for injecting local anaesthetic drugs is available.

Mechanism of action

1. The needle should first be introduced through the skin and subcutaneous tissues and then attached to the lead of the nerve stimulator.
2. An initial high output (e.g. 1–3 mA) from the nerve stimulator is selected. For superficial nerves, a

starting current of 1–2 mA should be sufficient in most cases. For deeper nerves, it may be necessary to increase the initial current to 3 mA or even more. The needle is advanced slowly towards the nerve until nerve stimulation is noticed. The output is then reduced until a maximal stimulation is obtained with minimal output. This current should be 0.2–0.4 mA. Contractions with such a low current mean that the tip of the needle is touching or very close to the nerve. Higher currents suggest that the needle is unlikely to be near the nerve. Contractions at a current less than 0.2 mA may indicate possible intraneural needle placement.

3. The blunt nerve block needle pushes the nerve ahead of itself as it is advanced, whereas a sharp needle is more likely to pierce the nerve. Blunt needles give better feedback as they pass through the different layers of tissues.

4. As the local anaesthetic solution is injected, the stimulation is markedly reduced after only a small volume (about 2 mL) is injected. This is due to displacement of the nerve from the needle tip. Failure of the twitching to disappear (or pain experienced by the awake patient) after injection may indicate intraneural needle placement.

5. The immobile needle technique is used for major nerve and plexus blocks when a large volume of local anaesthetic solution is used. One operator maintains the needle in position, while the second operator, after aspiration, injects the local anaesthetic solution through the injection port. This technique reduces the possibility of accidental misplacement and intravascular injection.

6. Catheters can be inserted and left in situ after localizing the nerve or plexus (Fig. 12.23). Repeat bolus or continuous infusion of local anaesthetic solution can then be administered. Catheter techniques can be used to enhance the spread (such as in the axillary block) or to prolong the duration of the block.

7. Stimulating catheters can also be inserted to provide a continuous block. The catheter body is made from insulating plastic material and usually contains a metallic wire inside, which conducts the current to its exposed tip electrode. Usually, such stimulating catheters are placed using a continuous nerve block needle, which is placed first using nerve stimulation. It acts as an introducer needle for the catheter. Once this needle is placed close to the nerve or plexus to be blocked, the stimulating catheter is introduced through it and the nerve stimulator is connected to the catheter. Stimulation through the catheter should reconfirm the catheter tip position in close proximity to the target nerve(s). However, it must be noted that the threshold currents with stimulating catheters may be considerably higher. Injection of local anaesthetic or saline (which is frequently used to widen the space for threading the catheter more easily) should be avoided as this may increase the threshold current considerably and may even prevent a motor response.

Problems in practice and safety features

It is essential to avoid injections of local anaesthetic into the nerve(s). This can lead to long-term or permanent damage to the nerve(s). The operator would notice an increase in injection pressure. This pressure can vary depending on the needle diameter and the specific nerve injected. However, it is prudent to avoid pressure >20 psi during the injection. The *NerveGuard* (Pajunk, Geisingen, Germany) (Fig. 12.24) stops the injection if the pressure exceeds 20 psi. Injection is reallowed when the injection pressure decreases after suitable manoeuvring of the needle.

Nerve block needles can be either insulated with an exposed tip or noninsulated.

INSULATED NEEDLES

These needles are Teflon coated with exposed tips. The current passes through the tip only (Fig. 12.25). The insulated needles have a slightly greater diameter than similar noninsulated needles, which may result in a higher risk of nerve injury. The plexus or nerve can be identified with a smaller current than that required using the noninsulated needles.

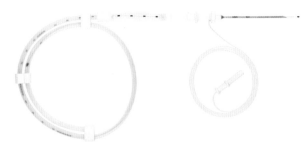

Fig. 12.23 Pajunk SonoLong-Echo needle and catheter set. Both the needle and catheter can be visualized by ultrasound. (Courtesy Pajunk, Geisingen, Germany.)

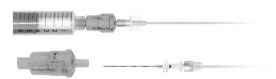

Fig. 12.24 Pajunk *NerveGuard* as part of the nerve blocking system. NerveGuard *(inset).* (Courtesy Pajunk, Geisingen, Germany.)

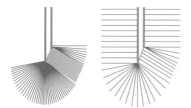

Fig. 12.25 Current density and flow from an insulated needle *(left)* and noninsulated needle *(right)*. Note the current leakage from the shaft in addition to the bevel of the latter.

NONINSULATED NEEDLES

These needles allow current to pass through the tip as well as the shaft (see Fig. 12.25). They are effective in regional anaesthesia because the maximum density of the current is being localized to the tip because of its lower resistance. However, a nerve may be stimulated via the shaft. In this situation, the local anaesthetic solution injected will be placed away from the nerve, resulting in an unsuccessful block.

> **Nerve block needles**
> - Made of steel with short blunt bevel to reduce trauma to nerves and improve feedback feel.
> - 22 G is optimal, with lengths of 50–150 mm available.
> - Can be insulated or noninsulated.
> - Immobile needle technique is commonly used.

Nerve stimulator for nerve blocks

This device is designed to produce visible muscular contractions at a predetermined current and voltage once a nerve plexus or peripheral nerve(s) has been located, without actually touching it, thereby providing a greater accuracy for local anaesthetic deposition (Fig. 12.26).

> **The ideal peripheral nerve stimulator**
> - Constant current output despite changes in resistance of the external circuit (tissues, needles, connectors, etc.).
> - Clear metre reading (digital) to 0.1 mA.
> - Variable output control.
> - Linear output.
> - Clearly marked polarity.
> - Short pulse width.
> - Pulse of 1–2 Hz.
> - Battery indicator.
> - High-quality clips of low resistance.

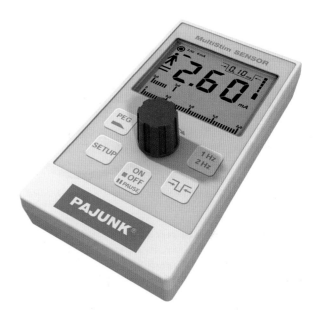

Fig. 12.26 Pajunk MultiStim Sensor nerve stimulator. (Courtesy Pajunk, Geisingen, Germany.)

Components

1. The nerve stimulator case has an on/off switch and a dial selecting the amplitude of the current.
2. Two leads complete the circuit. One is connected to an electrocardiogram (ECG) skin electrode and the other to the locating needle. The polarity of the leads should be clearly indicated and colour-coded with the negative lead being attached to the needle.

Mechanism of action

1. A small constant current (0.25–0.5 mA) is used to stimulate the nerve fibres, causing the motor fibres to contract. Less current is needed if the needle is connected to the negative lead rather than to the positive lead. When the negative (cathode) lead is used to locate the nerve, the current causes changes in the resting membrane potential of the cells, producing an area of depolarization and so causing an action potential. If the stimulating electrode is positive (anode), the current causes an area of hyperpolarization near the needle tip and a ring of depolarization distal to the tip. This requires a much higher current.
2. The frequency is set at 1–2 Hz. Tetanic stimuli are not used because of the discomfort caused. Using 2-Hz frequency allows more frequent feedback.
3. The duration of the stimulus should be short (50–100 ms) to generate painless motor contraction.
4. The nerve stimulator is battery operated to improve patient safety.

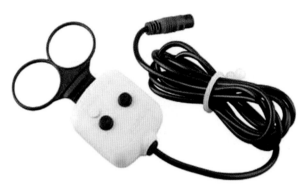

Fig. 12.27 Stimuplex remote control. (Courtesy B. Braun Medical Ltd.)

5. Nerve location can be very accurately defined, especially when low currents are used. The success rate of technically difficult nerve blocks can be increased by using a nerve stimulator. A sciatic nerve block with a success rate of over 90% can be achieved in experienced hands compared to about 50% without using a nerve stimulator.

6. Remote control of the nerve stimulator allows sterile one-hand operation (Fig. 12.27).

7. Percutaneous localization of nerves. This technique allows rapid, relatively painless and noninvasive localization of superficial nerves using a pen-like device (Fig. 12.28). This technique allows the identification of the optimal angle and needle entry point before introducing the needle into the patient. Such a device can be used to identify nerves up to 3 cm in depth. This system is ideal for teaching and training.

Problems in practice and safety features

1. Higher currents will stimulate nerve fibres even if the tip of the needle is not adjacent to the nerve. The muscle fibres themselves can also be directly stimulated when a high current is used. In both situations, the outcome will be an unsuccessful block once the local anaesthetic solution has been injected.

2. The positive ground electrode should have good contact with clear, dry skin. As the current flows between the two electrodes (needle and ground), it is preferable not to position the ground over a superficial nerve. The passage of the current through the myocardium should also be avoided.

3. Most stimulators have a connection/disconnection indicator to ensure that the operator is aware of the delivery or not of stimulus current.

4. It is not recommended to use nerve stimulators designed to monitor the extent of neuromuscular blockade for regional nerve blocks. These are high-output devices which can damage the nervous tissue.

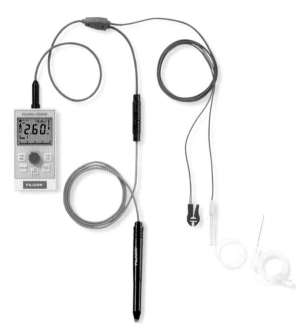

Fig. 12.28 Percutaneous localization of nerves. (Courtesy Pajunk, Geisingen, Germany.)

5. It should be remembered that using the nerve stimulator is no excuse for not having the sound knowledge of surface and neuroanatomy required to perform regional anaesthesia.

> **Peripheral nerve stimulator**
> - It has two leads, the positive one to the skin and the negative one to the needle.
> - A small current of 0.5 mA or less is used with a frequency of 1–2 Hz.
> - The stimulus is of short duration (1–2 ms).

 Exam tip: A good understanding of how the nerve stimulators and the insulated needles function is important.

Ultrasound guidance in regional anaesthesia

The use of ultrasound guidance and visualization to locate nerves/plexus has become a standard in regional anaesthesia. It is thought that a higher success rate can be achieved when it is used, together with lower complication rates.

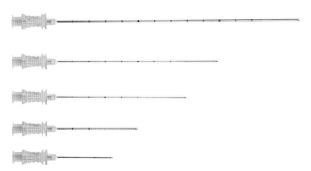

Fig. 12.29 Echogenic single-shot nerve block needles. (Courtesy Smiths Medical, Ashford, Kent, UK.)

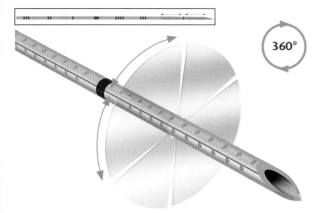

Fig. 12.30 *Cornerstone Reflectors* echogenic technology enhance needle ultrasound visualization. (Courtesy Pajunk, Geisingen, Germany.)

Specially designed needles for the use of ultrasound are available, allowing a better reflection of the ultrasound waves (Fig. 12.29). Special echogenic technology is used to facilitate better needle tip and its distal part visualization with minimal acoustic shadowing (see Fig. 12.28 and Fig. 12.30).

Most nerve blocks need ultrasound frequencies in the range of 10–14 MHz. Many broadband ultrasound transducers with a bandwidth of 5–12 MHz or 8–14 MHz can offer excellent resolution of superficial structures in the upper frequency range and good penetration depth in the lower frequency range.

The true echogenicity of a nerve is only captured if the sound beam is oriented perpendicularly to the nerve axis. This can be achieved best with *linear array transducers* with parallel sound beam emission rather than with *sector transducers*. The latter are characterized by diverging sound waves such that the echotexture of the nerves will only be displayed in the centre of the image.

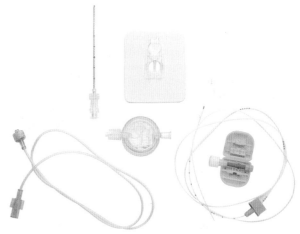

Fig. 12.31 Continuous ultrasound-guided nerve block set. (Courtesy Smiths Medical, Ashford, Kent, UK.)

The linear probes are most often used for the majority of peripheral blocks. The curved arrays are used for deep nerve structures (lower frequency is required). Smaller footprint probes are useful for smaller infants and children and for certain uses such as very superficial blocks (e.g. ankle blocks).

Continuous ultrasound-guided nerve(s) blocks can be achieved using catheter insertion (Fig. 12.23 and Fig. 12.31).

Portable ultrasound units are available.

Ultrasound is described in more detail in Chapter 13.

SUGGESTED FURTHER READING

Dalrymple, P., Chelliah, S., 2006. Electrical nerve locators. Cont. Educ. Anaesth. Crit. Care Pain 6 (1), 32–36.

Harrington. B.E., 2021. What Is ISO 80369-6:2016? The African Society for Regional Anesthesia (AFSRA). Available from: http://afsra.org/What_Is_ISO_80369_62016.html.

Keay, S., Callander, C., 2004. The safe use of infusion devices. Cont. Educ. Anaesth. Crit. Care Pain 4 (3), 81–85.

Marhofer, P., Greher, M., Kapral, S., 2005. Ultrasound guidance in regional anaesthesia. Br. J. Anaesth. 94 (1), 7–17.

Medicines and Healthcare products Regulatory Agency (MHRA), 2016. Total Intravenous Anaesthesia Sets (TIVA) – risk of leakage during use. Available from: https://www.gov.uk/drug-device-alerts/total-intravenous-anaesthesia-sets-tiva-risk-of-leakage-during-use.

MHRA, 2017. Alaris® syringe pumps (GH, CC, TIVA & PK models) – risk of uncontrolled bolus of medicine.

Available from: https://www.gov.uk/drug-device-alerts/alaris-syringe-pumps-gh-cc-tiva-pk-models-risk-of-uncontrolled-bolus-of-medicine.

The Royal College of Anaesthetists, 2010. Best practice in the management of epidural analgesia in the hospital setting. Available from: https://www.aagbi.org/sites/default/files/epidural_analgesia_2011.pdf.

US Food & Drug Administration, 2018. Infusion pumps. Available from: www.fda.gov/medical-devices/general-hospital-devices-and-supplies/infusion-pumps#:~:text=Many%20infusion%20pumps%20are%20equipped,delivers%20fluid%20to%20the%20patient.

SELF-ASSESSMENT QUESTIONS

Please check your eBook for additional self-assessment

MCQs

In the following lists, which of the statements (a) to (e) are true?

1. **Epidural catheters and filters**
   a. A minimum of 10 cm of the catheter should be inserted into the epidural space.
   b. The catheter should not be withdrawn through the Tuohy needle once it has been threaded beyond the bevel.
   c. Catheters with a single port at the distal tip reduce the incidence of vascular or dural puncture.
   d. The filter should be changed every 8 hours.
   e. Catheters can be radio-opaque.

2. **Regional anaesthesia using a nerve stimulator**
   a. The needles used have sharp tips to aid in localizing the nerves/plexuses.
   b. Alternating current (AC) is used to locate the nerve.
   c. A current of 1 A is usually used to locate a nerve.
   d. Paraesthesia is not required for successful blocks.
   e. 50-Hz frequency stimuli are used.

3. **Nerve stimulators in regional anaesthesia**
   a. They enable the block to be performed even without full knowledge of the anatomy.
   b. In the insulated nerve block needle, the current passes through the tip only.
   c. In the noninsulated nerve block needle, the current passes through the tip and the shaft.
   d. A catheter can be used for continuous nerve/plexus blockade.
   e. The immobile needle technique improves the success rate of the block.

4. **Incidence of spinal headache**
   a. Yale and Quincke needle designs have a lower incidence of spinal headache.
   b. It is inversely proportional to the size of the needle used.
   c. It is similar in young and elderly patients.
   d. It is proportional to the number of dural punctures.
   e. It is reduced using a pencil-shaped needle tip.

5. **Which of the following is/are true?**
   a. Using ultrasound guidance in regional anaesthesia, a frequency range of 10–14 kHz is adequate.
   b. It is important to prevent free flow from the syringe pump.
   c. There is no need to use antireflux valves in other infusion lines.
   d. Sector transducers can achieve better images when in regional anaesthesia.
   e. Syringe pumps should be positioned at the same level as the patient.

Single best answer (SBA)

6. **Spinal needles**
   a. Can be used to perform epidural block.
   b. Have an opaque hub to allow identification of cerebrospinal fluid (CSF).
   c. Dural puncture headache is eliminated with the cutting bevels.
   d. New guidelines make it impossible to administer drugs.
   e. Can be used as part of a combined spinal–epidural procedure.

Answers

1. Epidural catheters and filters
   a. *False. 3–5 cm of the catheter is left in the epidural space. This reduces the incidence of vascular or dural puncture, segmental or unilateral block (as the catheter can pass through an intervertebral foramina) and knotting.*
   b. *True. The withdrawal of the catheter through the Tuohy needle after it has been threaded beyond the bevel can lead to the transection of the catheter. This usually happens when the catheter punctures a vessel during insertion. The needle and the catheter should be removed together, and another attempt should be made to reinsert the needle and catheter.*
   c. *False. Catheters with a single port at the distal tip increase the incidence of vascular or dural puncture. This is due to the 'sharp' point at the end of the catheter. In contrast, catheters with side ports have a closed and rounded end, thus reducing the incidence of vascular or dural puncture.*
   d. *False. The filter can be used for up to 24 hours.*
   e. *True. Some catheters are designed to be radio-opaque. They are more rigid than the standard design. They are mainly used in patients with chronic pain to ensure the correct placement of the catheter.*

2. Regional anaesthesia using a nerve stimulator
   a. *False. There is a need for feedback from the needle as it goes through the different layers of tissue. A sharp needle will pass through the different layers of tissues easily with minimal feedback. A blunt needle will provide much better feedback.*
   b. *False. Direct current (DC) from a battery is used to operate nerve stimulators. By avoiding AC, patient safety is improved.*
   c. *False. This is a very high current. A current range of up to 5 mA is needed in locating the nerve. A current of 0.25–0.5 mA is used to stimulate the nerve fibres. Using a very high current, the tip of the needle might be far away from the nerve but might still lead to stimulation of the nerve fibres or the muscle fibres, directly leading to the failure of the block.*
   d. *True. There is no need for paraesthesia in order to achieve a successful block using a nerve stimulator. Paraesthesia implies that the needle is touching the nerve. With a nerve stimulator, the nerve can be stimulated electrically without being touched.*
   e. *False. Stimuli with a frequency of 1–2 Hz are used. Tetanic stimuli (e.g. 50-Hz frequency) are not used because of the discomfort caused.*

3. Nerve stimulators in regional anaesthesia
   a. *False. Full knowledge of the anatomical structure is essential for a successful block.*
   b. *True. As the tip is the only noninsulated part of the needle, the current passes only through it. Using a small current, the tip of the needle has to be very close to the nerve before stimulation is visible.*
   c. *True. In a noninsulated needle, the current passes through both the tip and the shaft. This might lead to nerve stimulation by current from the shaft even when the tip is far away from the nerve. This obviously leads to a failed block.*
   d. *True. After successful nerve stimulation, a catheter can be inserted. This allows a prolonged and continuous block using an infusion or boluses.*
   e. *True. The immobile needle technique allows one operator to maintain the needle in the correct position while the second operator injects the local anaesthetic. This also reduces the risk of accidental intravascular injection.*

4. Incidence of spinal headache
   a. *False. Yale and Quincke have a higher incidence of spinal headache. This is due to the traumatic bevel cutting the dural fibres, producing a ragged tear, which allows CSF leakage.*
   b. *False. The incidence is directly proportional to the size of the needle used. Using a 20-G spinal needle causes a 30% incidence of spinal headache, whereas a 26-G needle has a 1% incidence of headache.*
   c. *False. The incidence of spinal headache is much higher in young than in elderly patients.*
   d. *True. The incidence of spinal headache is increased with multiple dural punctures.*
   e. *True. The pencil-shaped needle tip separates rather than cuts the longitudinal dural fibres. After removal of the needle, the dura has a higher chance of sealing, reducing the incidence of spinal headache.*

5. Which of the following is/are true?
   a. *False. The frequencies needed for nerve blocks are in the range of 10–14 MHz. Most modern ultrasound devices can generate these frequencies.*
   b. *True. Antisiphon valves are used to prevent free flow from the syringe pump. In addition, the syringe should be securely clamped to the pump. Siphoning can also occur if there is a crack in the syringe, allowing air entry.*
   c. *False. An antireflux valve should be inserted in any other line that is connected to the infusion line. Antireflux valves prevent backflow up the secondary (usually with lower pressure) should a distal occlusion occur and avoid a subsequent inadvertent bolus.*

   d. *False. Sector transducers emit diverging sound waves such that the echotexture of the nerves will only be displayed in the centre of the image. The true echogenicity of a nerve is only captured if the sound beam is oriented perpendicularly to the nerve axis. This can best be achieved with linear array transducers with parallel sound beam emission.*
   e. *True. Gravitational pressure can be generated to overcome the friction between a nonsecured plunger and barrel, especially if the pump is positioned more than 100 cm above the patient.*

6. *e.*

Chapter 13

Additional equipment used in anaesthesia and intensive care

Continuous positive airway pressure (CPAP)

CPAP is a spontaneous breathing mode used in the intensive care unit during anaesthesia and for patients requiring respiratory support at home. It increases the functional residual capacity (FRC) and improves oxygenation. CPAP prevents alveolar collapse and possibly recruits already collapsed alveoli.

Components

1. A flow generator producing high flows of gas (Fig. 13.1) or a large reservoir bag may be needed.
2. It has a connecting tubing from the flow generator to the inspiratory port of the mask. An oxygen analyser is fitted along the tubing to determine the inspired oxygen concentration.
3. A tight-fitting mask or a hood has both inspiratory and expiratory ports. A CPAP valve is fitted to the expiratory port.
4. If the patient is intubated and spontaneously breathing, a T-piece with a CPAP valve fitted to the expiratory limb can be used.

Mechanism of action

1. Positive pressure within the lungs (and breathing system) is maintained throughout the whole of the breathing cycle.

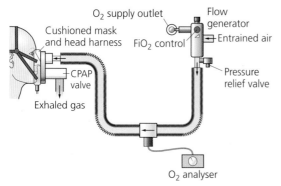

Fig. 13.1 A continuous positive airway pressure *(CPAP)* breathing system set-up. *FiO_2*, Fractional inspired oxygen concentration.

2. The patient's peak inspiratory flow rate can be met.
3. The level of CPAP varies depending on the patient's requirements. It is usually 5–15 cm H_2O.
4. CPAP is useful in weaning patients off ventilators, especially when positive end expiratory pressure (PEEP) is used. It is also useful in improving oxygenation in type 1 respiratory failure, where CO_2 elimination is not a problem.
5. Two levels of airway pressure support can be provided using *inspiratory positive airway pressure* (IPAP) and *expiratory positive airway pressure* (EPAP). IPAP is the pressure set to support the patient during inspiration. EPAP is the pressure set for the period of expiration. This is commonly used in reference to bilevel positive airway pressure (BiPAP). Using this mode, the airway pressure during inspiration is independent of expiratory airway pressure. This mode is useful in managing patients with type 2 respiratory failure as the work of breathing is reduced with improvements in tidal volume and CO_2 removal.

Problems in practice and safety features

1. CPAP has cardiovascular effects similar to PEEP but to a lesser extent. Although the arterial oxygenation may be improved, the cardiac output can be reduced. This may reduce the oxygen delivery to the tissues.
2. Barotrauma can occur.
3. A loose-fitting mask allows leakage of gas and loss of pressure.
4. A nasogastric tube is inserted in patients with depressed consciousness level to prevent gastric distension.
5. Skin erosion caused by the tight-fitting mask. This is minimized by the use of soft silicone masks or protective dressings or by using a CPAP hood. Rhinorrhoea and nasal dryness can also occur.
6. Nasal masks are better tolerated, but mouth breathing reduces the effects of CPAP.

> ### Continuous positive airway pressure
> - A tight-fitting mask or hood, CPAP valve and flow generator are used.
> - CPAP can be used in type 1 respiratory failure.
> - Two levels of airway pressure support (BiPAP) can also be used in type 2 respiratory failure.
> - Barotrauma, decrease in cardiac output and gastric distension are some of the complications.

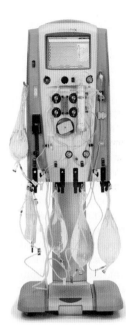

Fig. 13.2 The Prismaflex 1 haemofiltration system. (Courtesy Gambro Lundia AB.)

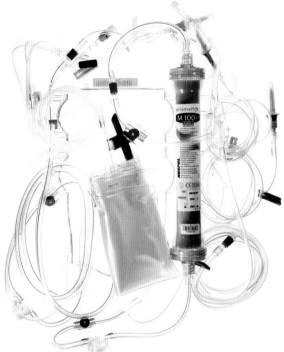

Fig. 13.3 The M100 Haemofilter set showing the filter, tubes and collecting bag. (Courtesy Gambro Lundia AB.)

Haemofiltration

Haemofiltration is a process of acute renal support used for critically ill patients. It is the ultrafiltration of blood.

Ultrafiltration is the passage of fluid under pressure across a semipermeable membrane where low molecular weight solutes (up to 20,000 Da) are carried along with the fluid by solvent drag (convection) rather than diffusion. This allows the larger molecules such as plasma proteins, albumin (62,000 Da) and cellular elements to be preserved.

The widespread use of haemofiltration has revolutionized the management of critically ill patients with acute renal failure within the intensive therapy environment (Fig. 13.2). Haemofiltration is popular because of its relative ease of use and higher tolerability in the cardiovascularly unstable patient.

In the critical care setting, haemofiltration can be delivered by:

1. *Continuous low flow therapy*, which is typically run 24 h/day for more than 1 day but may be stopped for procedures and filter or circuit changes. Continuous treatments are said to offer better cardiovascular stability and more efficient solute removal because of the steady biochemical correction and gradual fluid removal. Continuous therapy is also better suited to the frequently changing fluid balance situation in patients with multiorgan dysfunction in critical care.
2. *Intermittent high flow systems*, which is often a 4-hour session with a new filter and circuit for each session.

Components

1. Intravascular access lines can either be arteriovenous lines (such as femoral artery and vein or brachial artery and femoral vein) or venovenous lines (such as the femoral vein or the subclavian vein using a single double lumen catheter). The extracorporeal circuit is connected to the intravascular lines. The lines should be as short as possible to minimize resistance.
2. It has a filter or membrane (Fig. 13.3). Synthetic membranes are ideal for this process. They are made of polyacrylonitrile, polysulfone or polymethyl methacrylate. They have a large pore size to allow efficient diffusion (in contrast to the smaller size of dialysis filters).
3. Two roller pumps are positioned on the unit, one on each side of the circuit. Each pump peristaltically propels about 10 mL of blood per revolution and is positioned slightly below the level of the patient's heart.
4. The collection vessel for the ultrafiltrate is positioned below the level of the pump.

Mechanism of action

1. At its most basic form, the haemofiltration system consists of a circuit linking an artery to a vein with a filter positioned between the two.
2. The patient's blood pressure provides the hydrostatic pressure necessary for ultrafiltration of the plasma. This technique is suitable for fluid-overloaded patients who have a stable, normal blood pressure.
3. Blood pressure of less than a mean of 60 or 70 mmHg reduces the flow and the volume of filtrate and leads to clotting despite heparin.
4. In the venovenous system, a pump is added, making the cannulation of a large artery unnecessary (Fig. 13.4). The speed of the blood pump controls the maintenance of the transmembrane pressure. The risk of clotting is also reduced. This is the most common method used. Blood flows of 30–750 mL/min can be achieved, although flow rates of 150–300 mL/min are generally used. This gives an ultrafiltration rate of 25–40 mL/min.
5. The fluid balance is maintained by the simultaneous reinfusion of a sterile crystalloid fluid. The fluid contains most of the plasma electrolytes present in their normal values (sodium, potassium, calcium, magnesium, chloride, glucose and lactate or bicarbonate buffers) with an osmolality of 285–335 mOsmol/kg. Large amounts of fluid are needed such as 2–3 L/h.
6. Pressure transducers monitor the blood pressure in access and return lines. Air bubble detection facilities are also incorporated. Low inflow pressures can happen during line occlusion. High and low postpump pressures can happen in line occlusion or disconnection, respectively.

7. Some designs have the facility to weigh the filtrate and automatically supply the appropriate amount of reinfusion fluid.
8. Unfractionated heparin is added as the anticoagulant with a typical loading dose of 3000 IU followed by an infusion of 10 IU/kg body weight. Heparin activity is monitored by activated partial thromboplastin time or activated clotting time (ACT). Citrate or prostacyclin or low–molecular-weight heparin can be used as alternatives to heparin.
9. The filters are supplied in either a cylinder or a flat box casing. The packing of the filter material ensures a high surface area-to-volume ratio. The filter is usually manufactured as a parallel collection of hollow fibres packed within a plastic canister. Blood is passed, or pumped, from one end to the other through these tubules. One or more ports provided in the outer casing are used to collect the filtrate and/or pass dialysate fluid across the effluent side of the membrane tubules.
   a. They are highly biocompatible, causing minimal complement or leucocyte activation.
   b. They are also highly wettable, achieving high ultrafiltration rates.
   c. They have large pore size, allowing efficient diffusion.
   d. The optimal surface area of the membrane is 0.3–1.9 m^2.
   e. Both small molecules (e.g. urea, creatinine and potassium) and large molecules (e.g. myoglobin and some antibiotics) are cleared efficiently. Proteins do not pass through the membrane because of their larger molecular size.

Problems in practice and safety features

1. The extracorporeal circuit must be primed with 2 L of normal saline prior to use. This removes all the toxic ethylene oxide gas still present in the filter. (Ethylene oxide is used to sterilize the equipment after manufacture.)
2. Haemolysis of blood components by the roller pump.
3. The risk of cracks to the tubing after long-term use.
4. The risk of bleeding must be controlled by optimizing the dose of anticoagulant.

> **Haemofiltration**
> * An effective method of renal support in critically ill patients using ultrafiltration of the blood.
> * Usually, venovenous lines are connected to the extracorporeal circuit (filter and a pump).
> * Synthetic filters with a surface area of 0.5–1.5 m^2 are used.
> * Citrate can be used as an alternative to heparin for anticoagulation during haemofiltration. It is usually delivered as an infusion prefilter.

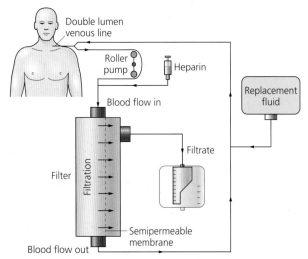

Fig. 13.4 Diagrammatic representation of venovenous haemofiltration.

Arterial blood gas analyser (Fig. 13.5)

In order to measure arterial blood gases, a sample of heparinized, anaerobic and fresh arterial blood is needed.

1. Heparin should be added to the sample to prevent clotting during the analysis. The heparin should only fill the dead space of the syringe and form a thin film on its interior. Excess heparin, which is acidic, lowers the pH of the sample.
2. The presence of air bubbles in the sample increases the oxygen partial pressure and decreases carbon dioxide partial pressure.
3. An old blood sample has a lower pH and oxygen partial pressure and a higher carbon dioxide partial pressure. If there is a need to delay the analysis (e.g. machine self-calibration), the sample should be kept on ice.

The measured parameters are:

1. arterial blood oxygen partial pressure
2. arterial carbon dioxide partial pressure
3. the pH of the arterial blood.

From these measurements, other parameters can be calculated, e.g. actual bicarbonate, standard bicarbonate, base excess and oxygen saturation.

Polarographic (Clark) oxygen electrode

This measures the oxygen partial pressure in a blood (or gas) sample (Fig. 13.6).

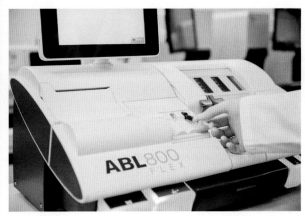

Fig. 13.5 The ABL800 Flex blood gas analyser. (Courtesy Radiometer Medical ApS, Brønshøj, Denmark. All rights reserved. Used with permission.)

Components

1. A platinum cathode is sealed in a glass body.
2. A silver/silver chloride anode is present.
3. It has a sodium chloride electrolyte solution.
4. An oxygen-permeable Teflon membrane separates the solution from the sample.
5. It has a power source of 700 mV.

Mechanism of action

1. Oxygen molecules cross the membrane into the electrolyte solution at a rate proportional to their partial pressure in the sample.
2. A very small electric current flows when the polarization potential is applied across the electrode in the presence of oxygen molecules in the electrolyte solution. Electrons are donated by the *anode* and accepted by the *cathode*, producing an electric current within the solution. The circuit is completed by the input terminal of the amplifier.

Cathode reaction:

$$O_2 + 2H_2O + 4e^- = 4OH^-$$

Electrolyte reaction:

$$NaCl + OH^- = NaOH + Cl^-$$

Anode reaction:

$$Ag + Cl^- = AgCl + e^-$$

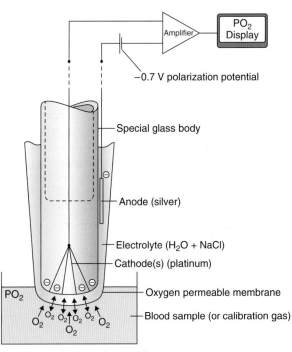

Fig. 13.6 Mechanism of action of the oxygen electrode.

The oxygen partial pressure in the sample can be measured since the amount of current is linearly proportional to the oxygen partial pressure in the sample.

3. The electrode is kept at a constant temperature of 37°C.

Problems in practice and safety features

1. The membrane can deteriorate and perforate, affecting the performance of the electrode. Regular maintenance is essential.
2. Protein particles can precipitate on the membrane affecting the performance.

Polarographic oxygen electrode
- Consists of a platinum cathode, silver/silver chloride anode, electrolyte solution, membrane and polarization potential of 700 mV.
- The flow of the electrical current is proportional to the oxygen partial pressure in the sample.
- Requires regular maintenance.

---

pH Electrode

This measures the activity of the hydrogen ions in a sample. Described mathematically, it is:

$$pH = -\log[H^+]$$

It is a versatile electrode which can measure samples of blood, urine or cerebrospinal fluid (CSF) (Fig. 13.7).

Components

1. A glass electrode (silver/silver chloride) incorporates a bulb made of pH-sensitive glass holding a buffer solution.
2. A calomel reference electrode (mercury/mercury chloride) is in contact with a potassium chloride solution via a cotton plug. The arterial blood sample is in contact with the potassium chloride solution via a membrane.
3. A meter displays the potential difference across the two electrodes.

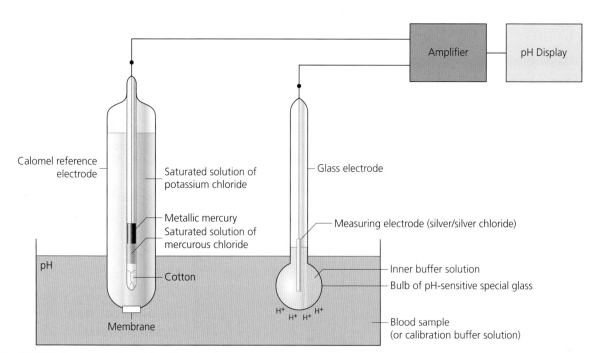

Fig. 13.7 Mechanism of action of the pH electrode.

Mechanism of action

1. The reference electrode maintains a constant potential.
2. The pH within the glass remains constant due to the action of the buffer solution. However, a pH gradient exists between the sample and the buffer solution. This gradient results in an electrical potential.
3. Using the two electrodes to create an electrical circuit, the potential can be measured. One electrode is in contact with the buffer, and the other is in contact with the blood sample.
4. A linear electrical output of about 60 mV per unit pH is produced.
5. The two electrodes are kept at a constant temperature of 37°C.

Problems in practice and safety features

1. It should be calibrated before use with two buffer solutions.
2. The electrodes must be kept clean.

> **pH Electrode**
> - Two half cells linked via the sample.
> - The electrical potential produced is proportional to the pH of the sample.

Carbon dioxide electrode (Severinghaus electrode)

A modified pH electrode is used to measure carbon dioxide partial pressure, as a result of change in the pH of an electrolyte solution (Fig. 13.8).

Components

1. A pH-sensitive glass electrode with a silver/silver chloride reference electrode forms its outer part.
2. The electrodes are surrounded by a thin film of an electrolyte solution (sodium bicarbonate).
3. It has a carbon dioxide permeable rubber or Teflon membrane.

Mechanism of action

1. Carbon dioxide (not hydrogen ions) diffuses in both directions until equilibrium exists across the membrane between the sample and the electrolyte solution.

2. Carbon dioxide reacts with the water present in the electrolyte solution, producing hydrogen ions resulting in a change in pH:

$$CO_2 + H_2O \rightarrow H^+ + HCO_3^-$$

3. The change in pH is measured by the glass electrode.
4. The electrode should be maintained at a temperature of 37°C. Regular calibration is required.

Problems in practice and safety features

1. The integrity of the membrane is vital for accuracy.
2. Slow response time because diffusion of carbon dioxide takes 2–3 minutes.

> **Carbon dioxide electrode**
> - A modified pH electrode measures changes in pH due to carbon dioxide diffusion across a membrane.
> - Maintained at 37°C.
> - Slow response time.

👍 **Exam tip:** Know how the various electrodes in a blood gas analyser work. Knowledge of the factors that can affect the accuracy of the measurements is important.

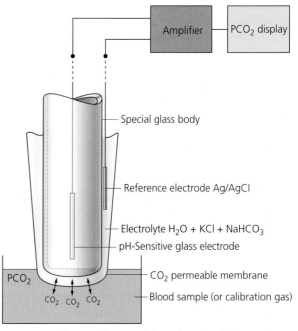

Fig. 13.8 Mechanism of action of the carbon dioxide electrode.

Intra-aortic balloon pump (IABP)

This is a catheter incorporating a balloon which is inserted into the aorta to support patients with severe cardiac failure. Its core principle is synchronized counterpulsation. It is usually inserted using a percutaneous femoral approach, over a guidewire, under fluoroscopic or transoesophageal echo guidance. The correct position of the pump is in the descending aorta, just distal to the left subclavian artery (Fig. 13.9).

Components

1. The unit contains from a 7-FG up to an 8-FG catheter with a balloon.
2. The catheter has two coaxial lumens: an outer lumen for helium gas exchange to and from the balloon and a fluid-filled central lumen for continuous aortic pressure monitoring via a transducer. The most modern versions use fibreoptics instead to monitor aortic pressure, which is faster and more sensitive, generating faster response times.
3. The usual volume of the balloon is 40 mL. A smaller, 34-mL balloon is available for small individuals. The size of the balloon should be 80%–90% of the diameter of the aorta. The pump is attached to a console (Fig. 13.10) which controls the flow of helium in and out of the balloon and monitors the patient's blood pressure and electrocardiogram (ECG). The console allows the adjustment of the various parameters in order to optimize counterpulsation.

Mechanism of action

1. The balloon is inflated in early diastole, immediately after the closure of the aortic valve.

This leads to an increase in peak diastolic blood pressure (diastolic augmentation) and an increase in coronary artery perfusion pressure. This increases myocardial oxygen supply. Inflation should be at the dicrotic notch on the arterial pressure waveform (Fig. 13.11) and corresponding to the peak of T-wave on ECG.

2. The balloon is deflated at the end of diastole just before the aortic valve opens and remains deflated during systole. This leads to a decrease in aortic end-diastolic pressure, causing a decrease in left ventricular afterload and decreased myocardial oxygen demand. This will lead to an increase in left ventricular performance, stroke work and ejection fraction. Deflation should be at the lowest point of the arterial diastolic pressure.
3. During myocardial ischaemia, the main benefits of the IABP are the reduction of myocardial oxygen demand (by lowering of the left ventricular pressure) and the increase in myocardial oxygen supply (by increasing the coronary artery perfusion).
4. The effectiveness of the balloon depends on the ratio of the balloon to aorta size, heart rate and rhythm, compliance of the aorta and peripheral vessels and the precise timing of the counterpulsation. Correctly timed IABP should be able to increase the augmented

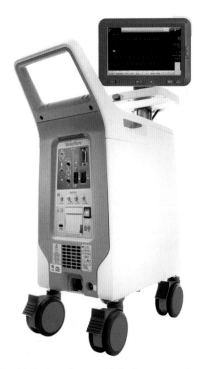

Fig. 13.10 AC3 Optimus intra-aortic balloon pump. (Image courtesy Teleflex Incorporated. © [2021] Teleflex Incorporated. All rights reserved.)

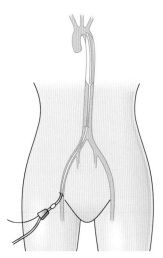

Fig. 13.9 The intra-aortic balloon pump in situ.

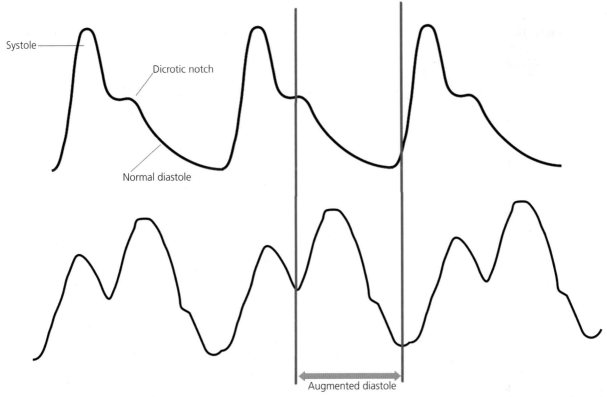

Systole

Dicrotic notch

Normal diastole

Augmented diastole

Fig. 13.11 Effect of intra-aortic balloon pump on the arterial blood waveform; (above) a sinus rhythm arterial blood pressure trace; (below) an intra-aortic balloon pump with a 1:1 sequence. Note the augmentation occurring after the aortic valve closure (dicrotic notch).

diastolic pressure to higher than the systolic pressure. IABP is expected to increase diastolic pressure by 30%, decrease the systolic pressure by 20% and improve cardiac output by 20%.

5. Helium is used due to its low density, hence promoting a laminar flow and reducing a turbulent flow (decreasing Reynold's number) so improving the flow rate.

In laminar flow: Flow rate $\propto$ driving pressure

In turbulent flow: flow rate $\propto \sqrt{}$ driving pressure

Indications for use of IABP

- Refractory ventricular failure.
- Acute myocardial infarction complicated with cardiogenic shock, mitral regurgitation, ventricular septal defect.
- Impending myocardial infarction.
- Unstable angina refractory to medical treatment.
- High-risk angioplasty.
- Ischaemia-related ventricular arrhythmias.
- Pre- and post-coronary bypass surgery, including weaning from cardiopulmonary bypass.

Contraindications for use of IABP

- Severe aortic regurgitation.
- Aortic dissection.
- Major coagulopathy.
- Severe bilateral peripheral arterial disease.
- Bilateral femoral–popliteal bypass graft.
- Sepsis.

Problems in practice and safety features

1. If the balloon is too large, it may damage the aorta. If it is too small, counterpulsation will be ineffective.
2. Dyssynchrony
3. Limb ischaemia.
4. Thrombosis and embolism. Low-dose heparinization is often used to counteract this.
5. Arterial dissection or perforation.
6. Bleeding.
7. Balloon rupture causing gas embolism as helium is not readily absorbed.
8. Infection.

Intra-aortic balloon pump

- 7-FG to 8-FG catheter with a balloon positioned in the descending aorta.
- Two lumens: a central one to monitor blood pressure and an outer one for inflation and deflation of the balloon with helium.
- Balloon inflation occurs at the dicrotic notch of the arterial pressure waveform.
- Balloon deflation occurs at the lowest point of the arterial diastolic pressure.

Intravenous giving sets

These are designed to administer intravenous fluids, blood and blood products (Fig. 13.12).

Components

1. Adult giving set includes the following:
   a. A clear plastic tube of about 175 cm in length and 4 mm in internal diameter. One end is designed for insertion into the fluid bag, whereas the other end is attached to an intravascular cannula with a Luer-Lok connection.

b. Blood giving sets have a filter with a mesh of about 150–200 μm and a fluid chamber (Fig. 13.12B). Giving sets with finer mesh filter of about 40 μm are available (Fig. 13.12C).
c. Some designs have a one-way valve and a three-way tap attachment or a rubber injection site at the patient's end. The maximum size needle used for injection should be 23G.
d. A flow controller determines the drip rate (20 drops of clear fluid is 1 mL and 15 drops of blood is 1 mL).

2. Paediatric set (Fig. 13.12D) includes the following:
   a. In order to attain accuracy, a burette (30–200 mL) in 1-mL divisions is used to measure the volume of fluid to be infused. The burette has a filter, an air inlet and an injection site on its top. At the bottom, a flap/ball valve prevents air entry when the burette is empty.
   b. There are two flow controllers: one is between the fluid bag and the burette and is used to fill the burette; the second is between the burette and the patient and controls the drip rate. An injection site should be close to the patient to reduce the dead space.
   c. Drop size is 60 drops/mL of clear fluid. A burette with a drop size similar to the adult's version (15 drops/mL) is used for blood transfusion.

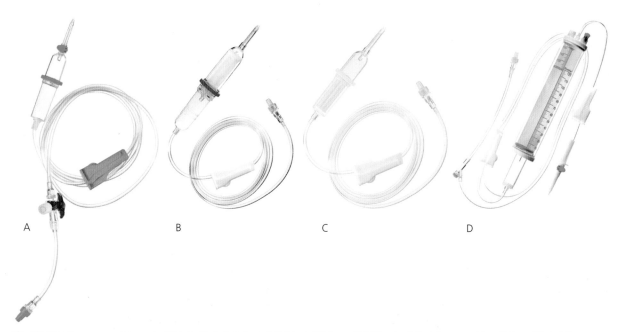

Fig. 13.12 Intravenous giving sets: (A) Intrafix Safe Set adult fluid set; (B) SangofixB blood adult giving set with a 200-μm filter; (C) Sangopur adult blood set with a 40-μm filter; (D) Dosifix paediatric fluid set with a burette. (Courtesy B. Braun Medical Ltd.)

d. 0.2-µm filters can be added in line to filter out air and foreign bodies, e.g. glass or plastic particles. Infusion-related thrombophlebitis can be reduced by the use of these filters.

Intravenous cannulae

Intravenous cannulae are made of plastic. They are made by different manufacturers with different characteristics (Fig. 13.13).

Intravenous cannulae can be either with or without a port. Some designs offer protection against the risk of needlestick injuries (Fig. 13.14), covering the sharp needle tip with a blunt end.

More recent designs are the 'closed and integrated' cannulae (Fig. 13.15). A 'closed' system may offer better protection against bacterial exposure than conventional 'open' ports. As the blood does not naturally escape from the catheter hub, these devices further minimize the risk of exposing the clinician to blood during the insertion procedure.

Using distilled water at a temperature of 22°C and under a pressure of 10 kPa, the flow through a 110-cm tubing with an internal diameter of 4 mm is as follows:
20G: 40–80 mL/min.
18G: 75–120 mL/min.
16G: 130–220 mL/min.
14G: 250–360 mL/min.

Blood and fluid warmers

These are used to warm blood (and other fluids) before administering them to the patient. The aim is to deliver blood/fluids to the patient at 37°C. At this temperature, there is no significant haemolysis or increase in osmotic fragility of the red blood cells (RBCs). Various designs with the coaxial fluid/blood warmer devices are most popular (Fig. 13.16). A coaxial tubing is used to heat and deliver the fluids to the patient. The outside tubing carries heated sterile water. The inside tubing carries the intravenous fluid. The sterile water is heated to 40°C and stored in the heating case. The water is circulated through the outside tubing. The intravenous fluid does not come in contact with the circulating water. The coaxial tubing extends to the intravenous cannula, reducing the loss of heat as fluid is exposed to room temperature.

For patients requiring large and rapid intravenous therapy, special devices are used to deliver warm fluids (Fig. 13.17). Fluids are pressurized to 300 mmHg and warmed with a countercurrent recirculation fluid at a temperature of 42°C.

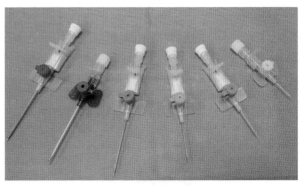

Fig. 13.13 A range of intravenous cannulae.

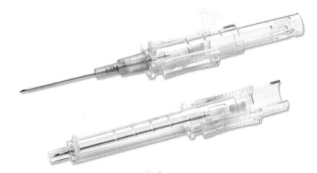

Fig. 13.14 ProtectIV safety cannula. (Courtesy Smiths Medical, Ashford, Kent, UK.)

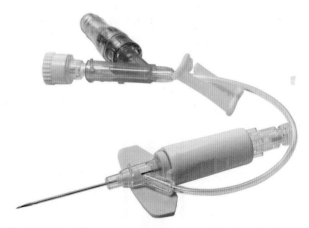

Fig. 13.15 DeltaVen closed system IV cannula. (Courtesy Smiths Medical, Ashford, Kent, UK.)

Forced-air warmers (Fig. 13.18)

These devices are used to maintain the temperature of patients during surgery. They have been found to be effective even when applied to a limited surface body

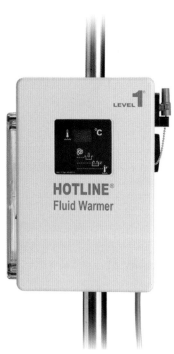

Fig. 13.16 The Hotline fluid warmer. (Courtesy Smiths Medical, Ashford, Kent, UK.)

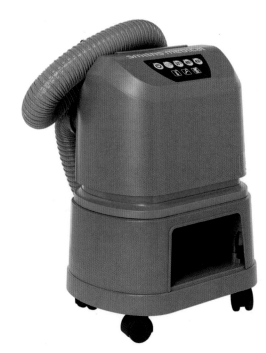

Fig. 13.18 Level 1 forced-air warmer. The ambient air passes through a HEPA air filter. (Courtesy Smiths Medical, Ashford, Kent, UK.)

area. They consist of a case where warm ambient air is pumped at variable temperatures between 32°C and 37°C. The warm air is delivered via a hose to a thin-walled, channelled bag/blanket positioned on the patient's body. Different bags are available depending on which part of the body is covered (e.g. upper or lower body). A thermostat to prevent overheating controls the temperature of the warm air. The ambient air passes through a HEPA air filter before being delivered to the patient. Cooling versions also exist for surgery where body temperature <37°C is desirable, e.g. neurosurgery.

Defibrillator

This is a device that delivers electrical energy to the heart, causing simultaneous depolarization of an adequate number of myocardial cells to allow a stable rhythm to be established. Defibrillators can be divided into the automated external defibrillators (AEDs) (Fig. 13.19) and manual defibrillators (Fig. 13.20). AEDs offer interaction with the rescuer through voice and visual prompts.

Components

1. The device has an on/off switch, Joules setting control, charge and discharge buttons.

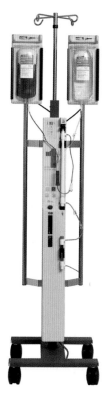

Fig. 13.17 Level 1 fast fluid warmer. (Courtesy Smiths Medical, Ashford, Kent, UK.)

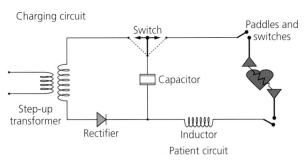

Charging circuit

Switch

Paddles and switches

Capacitor

Step-up transformer

Rectifier

Inductor

Patient circuit

Fig. 13.21 Defibrillator electric circuit.

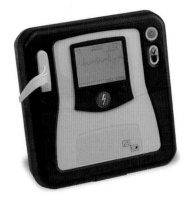

Fig. 13.19 The Zoll Pro automated external defibrillator. (Courtesy Zoll Medical.)

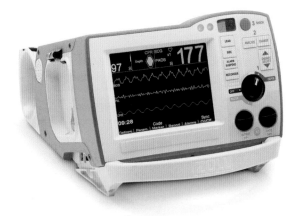

Fig. 13.20 The Zoll R manual defibrillator. (Courtesy Zoll Medical.)

2. Paddles can be either external (applied to the chest wall) or internal (applied directly to the heart). The external paddles/pads are usually 8–8.5 cm in size.

Mechanism of action

1. Direct current (DC) energy rather than alternating current (AC) energy is used. DC energy is more effective, causing less myocardial damage and being less arrhythmogenic than AC energy. The lower the energy used, the less the damage to the heart.
2. Transformers are used to step up mains voltage from 240 V AC to 5000–9000 V AC. A rectifier converts it to 5000 V DC. A variable voltage step-up transformer is used so that different amounts of charge may be selected. Most defibrillators have internal rechargeable batteries that supply DC in the absence of mains supply. This is then converted to AC by means of an inverter and then amplified to 5000 V DC by a step-up transformer and rectifier (Fig. 13.21).
3. The DC shock is of brief duration and produced by discharge from a capacitor. The capacitor stores energy

in the form of an electrical charge and then releases it over a short period of time. The current delivered is maintained for several milliseconds in order to achieve successful defibrillation. As the current and charge delivered by a discharging capacitor decay rapidly and exponentially, inductors are used to prolong the duration of current flow.

4. The external paddles/pads are positioned on the sternum and on the left midaxillary line (at the fifth–sixth rib). An alternative placement is one paddle positioned anteriorly over the left precordium and the other positioned posteriorly behind the heart. Firm pressure on the paddles is required in order to reduce the transthoracic impedance and achieve a higher peak current flow. Using conductive gel pads helps in reducing the transthoracic impedance. Disposable adhesive defibrillator electrode pads are currently used instead of paddles, offering hands-free defibrillation.
5. Most of the current is dissipated through the resistance of the skin, and the rest of the tissues and only a small part of the total current (about 35 A) flows through the heart. The impedance to the flow of current is about 50–150 Ohms; however, repeated administration of shocks in quick succession reduces impedance.
6. Waveform:
   a. *Monophasic defibrillators* deliver current that is unipolar (i.e. one direction of current flow) (Fig. 13.22A). They are not used in modern practice as they were likely to have waveform modification depending on transthoracic impedance (e.g. larger patients with high transthoracic impedance received considerably less transmyocardial current than smaller patients).
   b. *Biphasic defibrillators* deliver a two-phased current flow in which electrical current flows in one direction for a specified duration, then reverses and flows in the opposite direction for the remaining milliseconds of the electrical discharge. Biphasic defibrillators can either be *biphasic truncated exponential* (Fig. 13.22B)

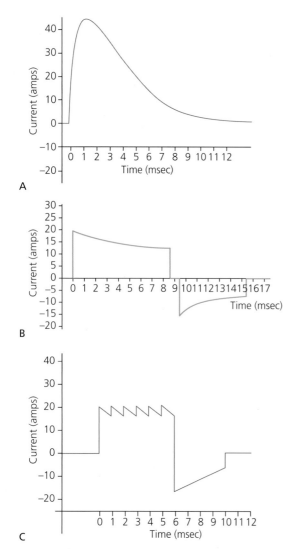

Fig. 13.22 Defibrillator waveforms. (A) Monophasic defibrillator waveform. (B) Biphasic truncated exponential defibrillator waveform. (C) Biphasic rectilinear defibrillator waveform.

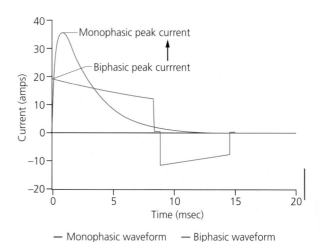

Fig. 13.23 Performance of monophasic versus biphasic defibrillator currents.

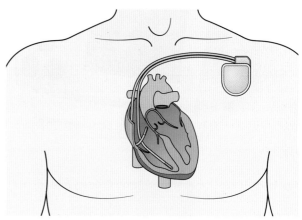

Fig. 13.24 Implantable cardiac defibrillator. (Courtesy Medtronic Ltd.)

or *rectilinear biphasic* (Fig. 13.22C). Biphasic defibrillators compensate for the wide variations in transthoracic impedance by electronically adjusting the waveform magnitude and duration to ensure optimal current delivery to the myocardium, irrespective of the patient's size.

c. *Monophasic versus biphasic performance*: as can be seen in Fig. 13.23, the highest part of the current waveform is known as the 'peak current' when the most current is flowing. Note the difference in height (amps) between the monophasic peak current and the biphasic peak current. Too much peak current during the shock can injure the heart. The peak current, not energy, can injure the heart. The goal of defibrillation is to deliver enough current to

the heart to stop the lethal rhythm but with a low enough peak current to decrease the risk of injury to the heart muscle.

7. For internal defibrillation, the shock delivered to the heart depends on the size of the heart and the paddles.

8. Some designs have an ECG oscilloscope and paper recording facilities. DC defibrillation can be synchronized with the top of the R-wave in the treatment of certain arrhythmias such as atrial fibrillation.

9. The implantable automatic internal defibrillator (Fig. 13.24) is a self-contained, diagnostic and therapeutic device placed next to the heart. It consists of a battery and electrical circuitry (pulse generator) connected to one or more insulated wires. The pulse generator and batteries are sealed together and implanted under the skin, usually near the shoulder. The

wires are threaded through blood vessels from the implantable cardiac defibrillator (ICD) to the heart muscle. It continuously monitors the rhythm, and, when malignant tachyarrhythmias are detected, a defibrillation shock is automatically delivered. ICDs are subject to malfunction due to internal short circuit when attempting to deliver an electrical shock to the heart or due to a memory error. Newer devices also provide overdrive pacing to electrically convert a sustained ventricular tachycardia and 'back-up' pacing if bradycardia occurs. They also offer a host of other sophisticated functions (such as storage of detected arrhythmic events and the ability to do 'non-invasive' electrophysiologic testing).

Problems in practice and safety features

1. Skin burns.
2. Further arrhythmias.

Defibrillators
- AEDs and manual versions are available.
- A step-up transformer increases mains voltage then a rectifier converts it to DC. DC energy is discharged from a capacitor.
- Modern defibrillators use a biphasic current flow.
- Implanted automatic internal defibrillators are becoming more popular with pacemaker capabilities.

 Exam tip: Knowing the physical principles of the devices used in cardioversion is important.

Chest drain

Used for the drainage of air, blood and fluids from the pleural space.

Components

1. A drainage tubing that has distal ports (Fig. 13.25).
2. An underwater seal and a collection chamber that measures approximately 20 cm in diameter.

Mechanism of action

1. An air-tight system is required to maintain a subatmospheric intrapleural pressure. The underwater seal acts as a one-way valve through which air is expelled from the pleural space and prevented from reentering during the next inspiration. This allows reexpansion of the lung after a pneumothorax and restores haemodynamic stability by minimizing mediastinal shift.

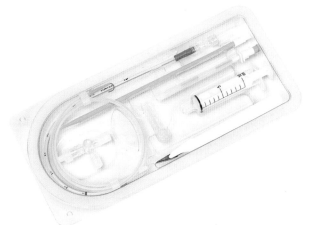
Fig. 13.25 Seldinger chest drainage kit. (Courtesy Smiths Medical, Ashford, Kent, UK.)

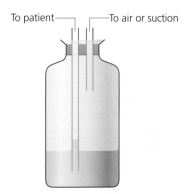
Fig. 13.26 Chest drain underwater seal.

2. Under asepsis, skin and subcutaneous tissues are infiltrated with local anaesthetic at the level of the fourth–fifth intercostal space in the midaxillary line. The chest wall is incised, and blunt dissection using artery forceps through to the pleural cavity is performed. Using the tip of the finger, adherent lung is swept away from the insertion site.
3. The drain is inserted into the pleural cavity and slid into position (usually towards the apex). The drain is then connected to an underwater seal device.
4. Some designs have a flexible trocar to reduce the risk of trauma.
5. The drainage tube is submerged to a depth of 1–2 cm in the collection chamber (Fig. 13.26). This ensures minimum resistance to drainage of air and maintains the underwater seal even in the face of a large inspiratory effort.
6. The collection chamber should be about 100 cm below the chest as subatmospheric pressures up to −80 cm H_2O may be produced during obstructed inspiration.
7. A Heimlich flutter one-way valve can be used instead of an underwater seal, allowing better patient mobility.

8. Drainage can be allowed to occur under gravity, or suction of about –15–20 mmHg may be applied.

Problems in practice and safety features

1. Retrograde flow of fluid may occur if the collection chamber is raised above the level of the patient. The collection chamber should be kept below the level of the patient at all times to prevent fluid being siphoned into the pleural space.
2. Absence of oscillations may indicate obstruction of the drainage system by clots or kinks, loss of subatmospheric pressure or complete reexpansion of the lung.
3. Persistent bubbling indicates a continuing bronchopleural air leak.
4. Clamping a pleural drain in the presence of a continuing air leak may result in a tension pneumothorax.

Chest drain

- An air-tight system to drain the pleural cavity usually inserted at the fourth–fifth intercostal space in the midaxillary line.
- The underwater seal chamber should be about 100 cm below the level of the patient.
- Absence of oscillation is seen with complete lung expansion, obstruction of the system or loss of negative pressure.
- Persistent bubbling is seen with a continuing bronchopleural air leak.

The ultrasound machine (Fig. 13.27)

Ultrasound (US) is a longitudinal high-frequency wave. It travels through a medium by causing local displacement of particles. This particle movement causes changes in pressures with no overall movement of the medium. A US machine consists of a probe connected to a control unit that displays the US image.

Components

1. A beamformer applies high-amplitude voltage to energize the crystals.
2. The transducer converts electrical energy to mechanical (US) energy and vice versa.
3. The receiver detects and amplifies weak signals.
4. Memory stores video display.

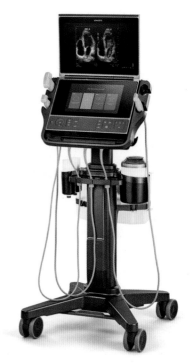

Fig. 13.27 Sonosite PX ultrasound machine. (Courtesy FUJIFILM Sonosite, Bothell, WA, USA.)

Mechanism of action

1. The probe transmits and receives the US beam once placed in contact with the skin via 'acoustic coupling' jelly.
2. US is created by converting electrical energy into mechanical vibration utilizing the piezoelectric (PE) effect. The PE materials vibrate when a varying voltage is applied. The frequency of the voltage applied determines the frequency of the sound waves produced. The thickness of the PE element determines the frequency at which the element will vibrate most efficiently, i.e. its resonant frequency (RF). RF occurs when the thickness of the element is half the wavelength of the sound wave generated.
3. An image is generated when the pulse wave emitted from the transducer is transmitted into the body, reflected off the tissue interface and returned to the transducer. Returning US waves cause PE crystals (elements) within the transducer to vibrate. This causes the generation of a voltage. Therefore the same crystals can be used to send and receive sound waves.

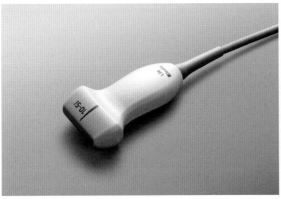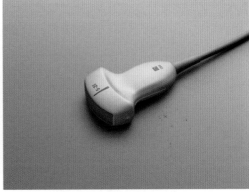

Fig. 13.28 Different ultrasound probes. The probe on the *left*, '*L38 xi*', can be used for superficial nerve blocks, down to 9-cm depth; whereas the curved probe on the *right*, '*rC60 xi*', can be used for deeper nerve blocks, down to 30-cm depth. (Courtesy FUJIFILM Sonosite, Bothell, WA, USA.)

4. Two-dimensional (2D) images of structures are displayed. Procedures requiring precise needle placement such as venous cannulation or nerve
   blocks can be performed under direct US control.
   This helps to minimize the possible risks of the procedure.
5. The image can be displayed in a number of modes:
   a. A-mode (amplitude): not used any more
   b. B-mode (brightness): most commonly used for regional anaesthesia
   c. M-mode (motion): most commonly for cardiac and foetal imaging
   d. 2D-real time.
6. Structures can then be identified via their US characteristics and anatomical relationships.
7. Increasing the depth allows visualization of deeper structures. The depth of the image should be optimized so that the target is centred in the display image.
8. Transducer probes come in many shapes and sizes (Fig. 13.28). The shape of the probe determines its field of view, and the frequency of emitted sound waves determines how deep the sound waves penetrate and the resolution of the image.

Problems in practice and safety features

1. One of the commonest mistakes in US imaging is the use of incorrect gain settings. Insufficient gain can result in missed structures of low reflectivity, such as thrombus. Excessive gain can result in artefacts.
2. The characteristics differentiating vein from artery are listed in Table 13.1.

Table 13.1 Differentiating veins from arteries

	Vein	**Artery**
Appearance	Black	Black
Movement	None	Pulsatile
Compressible	Yes	No
Colour flow	Constant flow	Pulsatile

Ultrasound machine
- US is longitudinal high-frequency waves.
- Created by converting electrical energy into mechanical vibration using piezoelectric effect.
- Same crystals can be used to send and receive sound wave.
- Shape of probe determines its field of view, whereas frequency of emitted sounds determines the depth of penetration and resolution of image.

Red blood cell salvage; cell saver (Figs. 13.29 and 13.30)

This is a device that allows autologous transfusion of RBCs of lost blood during surgery or trauma. Due to the risk of complications and cost associated with allogenic

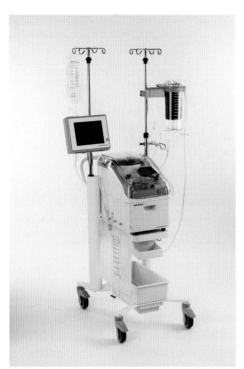

Fig. 13.29 Cell Saver Elite. (Courtesy Haemonetics, Glasgow, UK. Images of the TEG® 6s hemostasis analyzer and Cell Saver® Elite®+ autologous blood recovery device used by permission of Haemonetics Corporation. TEG®, Cell Saver ® and Elite® are registered trademarks of Haemonetics Corporation in the US, other countries or both.)

blood transfusion, its use has increased significantly in the operating theatre. Used in a wide range of surgery such as cardiac; major vascular; major hepatobiliary; major spinal surgery; arthroplasty surgery, particularly revision hip replacement; major urological surgery; surgery for thoracic, abdominal and pelvic trauma; and obstetric procedures and major obstetric haemorrhage.

Components

1. Suction tube with a wide-bore tip (>4 mm).
2. Anticoagulant citate dextrose (ACDA) or heparinized saline to anticoagulate blood on collection.
3. Reservoir to collect the salvaged blood with a filter a mesh of 40–150-μm mesh.
4. Bowl and centrifuge.
5. Blood collection bag to store the salvaged RBCs.
6. Waste bag.

Mechanism of action

1. Blood is sucked using a wide-bore tip tube with the minimal negative suction pressure possible to reduce haemolysis. A pressure of –100 to –150 mmHg is usually used and is autoregulated by the device to maximize red cell recovery.
2. An anticoagulant is added in the collection reservoir. This could be heparin using 1:5 ratio (20 mL of anticoagulant to 100 mL blood) or citrate using 1:7 ratio (15 mL of anticoagulant to 100 mL blood). Heparin saline is usually prepared with 30,000 units

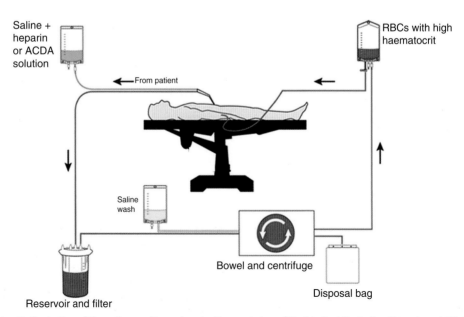

Fig. 13.30 Schematic illustration of the cell saver. (Reproduced with permission of the Medical Illustration Department, Wythenshawe Hospital, Manchester University NHS Foundation Trust.) *ACDA,* Anticoagulant citate dextrose; *RBCs,* Red blood cells.

of heparin in 1 L of normal saline. A rate of 60–80 drops per minute if heparin saline is used and 40–60 drops if premixed citrate-based anticoagulant is used.

3. The contents of the reservoir are filtered to remove large clots and debris.

4. After filtration, the blood enters a centrifuge where sterile isotonic saline is pumped into the bowl. The size of the bowl varies according to the volume of collected blood. The RBCs (being denser) are held against the outer wall of the bowl by the forces of the centrifuge. Plasma, being less dense, moves towards the centre of the bowl, spilling into the waste bag. Some RBCs could be lost in this process.

5. Using photo-optics, the maximum cell density can be measured to start the process of washing of the packed suspension with saline.

6. Packed RBCs are collected and salvaged in a separate preprepared blood collection bag.

7. The collected red cells can be reinfused immediately or for up to 4 hours after processing and kept at room temperature. A standard blood infusion IV giving set is used. The transfused blood has a haematocrit of 60%–70%. Compared with stored allogenic RBCs, salvaged RBCs have higher concentrations of 2,3 DPG and ATP.

8. The waste products (plasma, platelets, clotting factors, WBCs and fat) are channelled into a disposal bag as clinical waste.

9. It is recommended to use 'collect-only' mode for potential cell salvage where blood loss exceeds 10% of calculated total blood volume.

Problems in practice and safety features

1. There are no absolute contraindications to the cell saver; however, potential contamination of the aspirated blood with bowel contents, infection or tumour cells should be regarded as a relative contraindication, depending on the likelihood/degree of contamination.

2. In cancer or infected field surgery, it is recommended to use leucodepletion filters during reinfusion.

3. It is important to remember that the retransfused blood lacks platelets or clotting factors.

4. Certain drugs/chemicals should not be aspirated during the collection such as iodine skin preparations, chlorhexidine, antibiotics not licensed for IV use, fibrin-based glues, topical clotting agents and unset orthopaedic cement.

Cell saver
- Used in intraoperative blood salvage.
- RBCs are retransfused back to the patient.
- Platelets, white blood cells and clotting factors are lost.
- Has a wide range of indications with no absolute con-traindications.

Extracorporeal membrane oxygenation (ECMO)

The technology that already existed to allow oxygenation and removal of carbon dioxide using cardiopulmonary bypass (CBP) during heart operations has been modified and miniaturized to allow bedside insertion and continuous use for moderate periods of time (days to weeks).

Indications have grown as the ease of use and safety profile has improved.

Since the H1N1 influenza 2009 pandemic and the more recent COVID 19 pandemic caused by SARS CoV 2, ECMO can be used to replace lung-damaging mechanical ventilation. ECMO has been a valuable addition to the management options for viral pneumonias.

Commonly accepted indications for ECMO:

- Hypoxia, especially due to potentially recoverable viral pneumonias (e.g. SARS CoV 1 and 2 infection).
- Cardiogenic shock or cardiac arrest.
- Failure to wean from CPB following heart surgery.
- Bridge to transplantation or long-term mechanical support (e.g. ventricular assist device (VAD)).

ECMO exists as two modalities: veno-veno (VV)-ECMO and veno arterial (VA)-ECMO.

1. VV-ECMO is used to oxygenate and remove carbon dioxide. This technique is used to support only the lungs.
   - Adequate systemic circulation is provided by the patient's own cardiac output.
   - Deoxygenated blood is drained from the venous circulation into the ECMO circuit.
   - Blood is oxygenated via the oxygenator and is returned to the right atrium.
   - Cannula position: drains from major vein and returns to a major vein.

2. VA-ECMO is used to pump blood around the body as well as oxygenate and remove carbon dioxide. This technique supports both the heart and lungs.
   - Deoxygenated blood is drained from the venous circulation into the ECMO circuit.
   - Passes through the oxygenator and is pumped directly to the arterial circulation.
   - Cannula position: drains from major vein and returns to major artery.

Components

1. Large-bore cannulae that allow large flows of blood to be pumped through the ECMO circuit.
2. A polycarbonate semipermeable membrane (oxygenator) that allows oxygenation and removal of carbon dioxide.

3. An electric centrifugal pump capable of pumping up to 12 L/min of blood through the circuit.

Mechanism of action

1. The oxygenator provides oxygenation to the drained venous blood. This supplements the lung-protective conventional ventilation.
2. The removal of carbon dioxide is dependent on the gas flow across the membrane oxygenator. Clearance of carbon dioxide needs adjustment. Usually, 3 L/min of oxygen delivered to the membrane oxygenator is a reasonable starting flow. By increasing the flow, more carbon dioxide is removed.
3. The ECMO circuit usually has a prime volume of approximately 1 L of crystalloid such as Hartman's solution.
4. Heparinization is essential. This is achieved usually through a continuous heparin infusion. An ACT machine and TEG machine are used to provide guidance.

Problems in practice and safety features

1. Localized bleeding: Cannulation of vessels is fundamental and, although VV-ECMO only cannulates low-pressure venous vessels, VA-ECMO cannulates the higher pressure arterial vessel(s) also. So correct identification of the vessel to be cannulated and meticulous insertion technique are important to avoid bleeding.
2. Bleeding in other parts of the body: The most common serious areas of bleeding are cerebral (10%) and gastrointestinal.
3. Femoral artery cannulation can often lead to blockage of the distal femoral arterial flow, rendering the leg ischaemic. A small bypass cannula into the distal femoral artery can reestablish perfusion.
4. Flow and pressure alarms exist on the centrifugal pump.
5. A hand crank is used as a backup power source if the centrifugal pump fails.
6. There is a battery backup if the mains electricity supply fails.
7. Transmembrane pressure of >50 mmHg suggests clot formation within the oxygenator.

SUGGESTED FURTHER READING

Carroll, C., Young, F., 2021. Intraoperative cell salvage. BJA Education 21 (3), 95–101.

Limbert, V.M., Amiri, A.M., 2019. Intra-aortic balloon pump for patients with cardiac conditions: an update on available techniques and clinical applications. MDPI, Reports. Available from: https://www.mdpi.com/2571-841X/2/3/19/htm.

Medicines and Healthcare products Regulatory Agency (MHRA), 2010. Medical device alert: intravenous (IV) extension sets with multiple ports: all brands. (MDA/2010/073). Available from: http://www.mhra.gov.uk/Publications/Safetywarnings/MedicalDeviceAlerts/CON093966.

Medicines and Healthcare Products Regulatory Agency, 2017. All LIFEPAK 1000 automatic external defibrillators (AEDs) - risk of device shutting down unexpectedly during patient treatment and possible failure to deliver therapy. Available from: https://www.gov.uk/drug-device-alerts/all-lifepak-1000-automatic-external-defibrillators-aeds-risk-of-device-shutting-down-unexpectedly-during-patient-treatment-and-possible-failure-to-deliver-therapy.

NHS, 2020. Guidance for the role and use of non-invasive respiratory support in adult patients with coronavirus (confirmed or suspected). Available from: https://amhp.org.uk/app/uploads/2020/03/Guidance-Respiratory-Support.pdf.

Oxford Medical Education, Oxford Medical Education. Intercostal drain (chest drain/pleural drain) insertion. Available from: http://www.oxfordmedicaleducation.com/clinical-skills/procedures/intercostal-drain/.

SELF-ASSESSMENT QUESTIONS

Please check your eBook for additional self-assessment

MCQs

In the following lists, which of the statements (a) to (e) are true?

1. Concerning defibrillators

a. Alternating current (AC) is commonly used instead of direct current (DC).
b. The electric current released is measured in watts.
c. Consists of an inductor that releases the electric current.
d. Can cause skin burns.
e. The same amount of electrical energy is used for external and internal
f. Defibrillation.

2. Concerning arterial blood gases analysis

a. Excess heparin in the sample increases the hydrogen ion concentration.
b. Blood samples with air bubbles have a lower oxygen partial pressure.
c. If there is a delay in the analysis, the blood sample can be kept at room temperature.
d. Normal H^+ ion concentration is 40 mmol/L.
e. CO_2 partial pressure can be measured by measuring the pH.

3. Concerning the CO_2 electrode

a. KCl and $NaHCO_3$ are used as electrolyte solutions.
b. A carbon dioxide-sensitive glass electrode is used.
c. The electrical signal generated is directly proportional to the log of CO_2 tension in the sample.
d. It has a response time of 10 seconds.
e. It should be kept at room temperature.

4. Continuous positive airway pressure (CPAP)

a. CPAP is a controlled ventilation mode.
b. It can improve oxygenation by increasing the functional residual capacity (FRC).
c. Pressures of up to 15 kPa are commonly used.
d. It has no effect on the cardiovascular system.
e. A nasogastric tube can be used during CPAP.

5. Haemofiltration

a. Solutes of molecular weight up to 20,000 Da can pass through the filter.
b. It should not be used in the cardiovascularly unstable patient.
c. Blood flows of 150–300 mL/min are generally used.
d. Warfarin is routinely used to prevent the filter clotting.
e. The optimal membrane surface area is 0.5–1.5 cm^2.

6. Intra-aortic balloons

a. The usual volume of the balloon is 40 mL.
b. The inflation of the balloon occurs at the upstroke of the arterial waveform.
c. The deflation of the balloon occurs at the end of diastole just before the aortic valve opens.
d. It is safe to use in aortic dissection.
e. Helium is used to inflate the balloon.

7. Chest drains

a. The underwater seal chamber can be positioned at any level convenient to the patient.
b. Persistent air bubbling may be a sign of a continuing bronchopleural air leak.
c. They function by expelling intrapleural fluids during deep inspiration.
d. Negative pressure of about –15–20 mmHg may be applied to help in the drainage.
e. Clamping a pleural drain in the presence of a continuing air leak may result in a tension pneumothorax.

Single best answers

8. CPAP respiratory support
  a. Should be administered by a loose-fitting mask.
  b. Can only be used in type 2 respiratory failure.
  c. Can be used with high inspired oxygen concentrations.
  d. Typically uses an expiratory valve between 20 and 30 cm H_2O.
  e. Has no effects on the cardiovascular system.

9. The blood gas analyser
  a. Can use either heparinized or unheparinized samples.
  b. All the results are individually measured by the machine.
  c. The pH is related to the $[H^+]$.
  d. Its results are unaffected by temperature.
  e. Only blood samples can be analysed.

Answers

1. Concerning defibrillators
  a. *False. DC used as the energy generated is more effective and causes less myocardial damage. Also DC energy is less arrhythmogenic than AC energy.*
  b. *False. Joules, not watts, are used to measure the electric energy released.*
  c. *False. The defibrillator consists of a capacitor that stores then discharges the electric energy in a controlled manner. Step-up transformers are used to change mains voltage to a much higher AC voltage. A rectifier converts that to a DC voltage. Inductors are used to prolong the duration of current flow as the current and charge delivered by a discharging capacitor decay rapidly and exponentially.*
  d. *True. Because of the high energy release, skin burns can be caused by defibrillators, especially if gel pads are not used.*
  e. *False. The amount of electrical energy used in internal defibrillation is a very small fraction of that used in external defibrillation. In internal defibrillation, the energy is delivered directly to the heart. In external defibrillation, a large proportion of the energy is lost in the tissues before reaching the heart.*

2. Concerning arterial blood gases analysis
  a. *True. Heparin is added to the blood sample to prevent clotting during the analysis. Heparin should only fill the dead space of the syringe and form a thin layer on its interior. Heparin is*

  acidic and in excess will increase the hydrogen ion concentration (lowering the pH) of the sample.
  b. *False. As air consists of about 21% oxygen in nitrogen, the addition of an air bubble(s) to the blood sample will increase the oxygen partial pressure in the sample.*
  c. *False. At room temperature, the metabolism of the cells in the blood sample will continue. This leads to a low oxygen partial pressure and a high H^+ concentration and CO_2 partial pressure. If there is a delay in the analysis, the sample should be kept on ice.*
  d. *False. The normal H^+ concentration is 40 nmol/L, which is equivalent to a pH of 7.4.*
  e. *True. CO_2 partial pressure in a sample can be measured by measuring the changes in pH of an electrolyte solution using a modified pH electrode. The CO_2 diffuses across a membrane, separating the sample and the electrolyte solution. The CO_2 reacts with the water present, producing H^+ ions resulting in changes in pH.*

3. Concerning the carbon dioxide electrode
  a. *True. KCl, $NaHCO_3$ and water are the electrolyte solutions used. The CO_2 reacts with the water, producing hydrogen ions.*
  b. *False. A pH-sensitive glass electrode is used to measure the changes in pH caused by the formation of H^+ ions resulting from the reaction between water and CO_2.*

c. **True.** The electrical signal generated at the electrode is directly proportional to the pH of the sample or the –log of H^+ concentration. The latter is related to the CO_2 tension in the sample.

d. **False.** The CO_2 electrode has a slow response time as the CO_2 takes 2–3 minutes to diffuse across the membrane.

e. **False.** The CO_2 electrode, like the pH electrode, should be kept at 37°C. Dissociation of acids or bases changes when temperature changes.

4. CPAP

a. **False.** CPAP is continuous positive airway pressure used in spontaneously breathing patients via a face mask or a tracheal tube.

b. **True.** Oxygenation can be improved by CPAP as the alveoli are held open throughout the ventilatory cycle, preventing airway closure thus increasing the FRC.

c. **False.** Pressures of up to 15 cm H_2O are commonly used during CPAP.

d. **False.** CPAP reduces the cardiac output (similar to PEEP, although to a lesser extent). The arterial oxygenation might improve with the application of CPAP, but oxygen delivery might be reduced because of the reduced cardiac output.

e. **True.** A nasogastric tube is inserted in patients with a depressed consciousness level to prevent gastric distension.

5. Haemofiltration

a. **True.** Solutes of up to 20,000 Da molecular weight are carried along the semipermeable membrane with the fluid by solvent drag (convection).

b. **False.** One of the reasons for the popularity of haemofiltration in the intensive care unit setup is that it has a higher tolerability in cardiovascularly unstable patients.

c. **True.** Although blood flows of 30–750 mL/min can be achieved during haemofiltration, blood flows of 150–300 mL/min are commonly used. This gives a filtration rate of 25–40 mL/min.

d. **False.** Heparin is the anticoagulant of choice during haemofiltration. If there is a contraindication for its use, prostacyclin can be used instead.

e. **False.** The filters have a large surface area with large pore size and are packed in such a way as to ensure a high surface area to volume ratio. The optimal surface area is 0.5–1.5 m^2.

6. Intra-aortic balloons

a. **True.** The usual volume of the balloon is 40 mL. A smaller version, 34 mL, can be used in small patients. The size of the balloon should be 80%–90% of the diameter of the aorta.

b. **False.** The balloon should be inflated in early diastole immediately after the closure of the aortic valve at the dicrotic notch of the arterial waveform. This leads to an increase in coronary artery perfusion pressure.

c. **True.** This leads to a decrease in aortic end-diastolic pressure, so reducing the left ventricular afterload and myocardial oxygen demand.

d. **False.** Aortic dissection is one of the absolute contraindications to intra-aortic balloon pump.

e. **True.** Helium is used to inflate the balloon. Because of its physical properties (low density), it allows rapid and complete balloon inflation and deflation.

7. Chest drains

a. **False.** The collection chamber should be about 100 cm below the chest as subatmospheric pressures up to –80 cm H_2O may be produced during obstructed inspiration. Retrograde flow of fluid may occur if the collection chamber is raised above the level of the patient.

b. **True.**

c. **False.** Deep inspiration helps in expanding the lung, whereas deep expiration helps in the drainage of fluids from the pleural space.

d. **True.** Drainage can be allowed to occur under gravity, or suction of about –15–20 mmHg may be applied.

e. **True.**

8. c.

9. c.

Chapter 14

Point-of-care testing

Introduction

Point-of-care (POC) testing is an ever-expanding area of biomedical science and is now essential to efficient patient care. As the name implies, the goal is to collect the specimen to be tested and obtain the results in a short period of time (Fig. 14.1). This ideally should be done at, or at least near, the location of the patient. All processes are integrated and automated.

Historically, blood gas analysis was the forerunner of POC testing, with blood glucose analysis revolutionized diabetic care.

Now tests as diverse as human immunodeficiency virus, C-reactive protein, haemoglobin A1C and cardiac markers can be rapidly obtained at the POC. Use of polymerase chain reaction technology has allowed the detection and measurement of the specific genetic material of bacteria, viruses, etc.

This chapter considers only a few of the available POC tests and goes into detail on some of the more common machines seen in healthcare theatres.

HemoCue, haemoglobin measurement (Fig. 14.2)

A reliable compact device that measures haemoglobin concentration.

Components

1. A handheld and portable device houses a photometer.
2. It has a disposable microcuvette into which a drop of capillary, venous or arterial blood is placed.

Mechanism of action

1. The microcuvette contains a dried reagent mixture. Sodium deoxycholate haemolyses red blood cells, releasing the haemoglobin. Sodium nitrite converts haemoglobin to methaemoglobin, which, together with sodium azide, gives azide methaemoglobin.

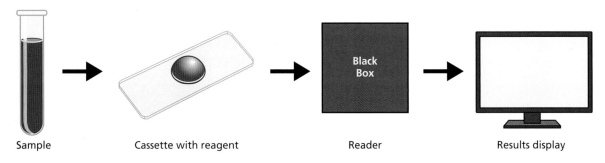

| Sample | Cassette with reagent | Reader | Results display |

Fig. 14.1 Point-of-care testing concepts.

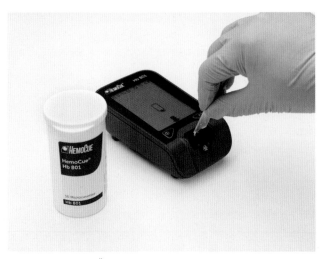

Fig. 14.2 HemoCue Hb 801. (Courtesy HemoCue AB, Ängelholm, Sweden.)

2. A specific photometer is housed in the device and measures the absorbance at 570 nm and 880 nm.
3. Results are displayed digitally almost immediately.

Problems in practice and safety features

1. Quality control is necessary to ensure accuracy is maintained.
2. The microcuvettes need to be stored in a dry environment.

Hemochron Junior, activated clotting time measurement

This is a compact, mains or battery-powered device that measures activated clotting time (ACT) (Fig. 14.3). The ACT is used to monitor unfractionated heparin therapy.

Each different version of an ACT machine has its own baseline reference value. The normal range for the Hemochron Junior is usually between 90 and 140 seconds.

After a dose of unfractionated heparin, the measured ACT value should rise. The two versions of cuvette commonly used are low range and high range.

Components

1. A handheld device contains the test chamber.
2. A 'Keypad' and 'Results' display panel.
3. The test cuvette contains the following activation reagents:
   a. low range: celite, potato dextrin, stabilizers and buffers
   b. high range: silica, kaolin, phospholipid, stabilizers and buffers.

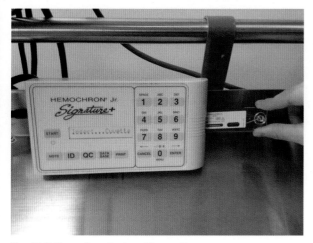

Fig. 14.3 Hemochron Junior with cassette.

Mechanism of action

1. The cuvette is warmed to 37°C.
2. A single drop of blood is needed to be added to the warmed cuvette.
3. The result is available in minutes.

Problems in practice and safety features

1. Memory function to store results.
2. Printer option available.
3. Quality control testing is necessary at regular intervals.
4. The ACT reading is prolonged by heparin, hypothermia, haemodilution, low platelet count, warfarin, clotting factor deficiencies, hypofibrinogenaemia, qualitative platelet abnormalities, aprotinin.

Original TEG/ROTEM

BACKGROUND

Speed to clot formation and the firmness (quality) of the clot formed at the POC can be assessed by two similar technologies. They differ in essence via the simple principles of testing the firmness of a clot as it forms. One spins a cup around a fixed pin (thromboelastography [TEG]). The other spins a pin in a fixed cup (rotational thromboelastometry [ROTEM]).

Prothrombin time, activated partial thromboplastin time and thrombin time are traditional coagulation laboratory-based tests, with the associated time delay to results being available.

Because of the speed of access to results with TEG/ROTEM, these POC machines are rapidly becoming the gold standard for the treatment of bleeding in major trauma, cardiac and liver transplantation surgery and massive haemorrhage resulting from other causes.

A small volume of whole blood is added to a cup containing a clot activator assay. Other cups that contain heparinase (an enzyme that neutralizes heparin) with the clot activator and other reagents are also available.

How it works

The cup is placed on the machine, and a sensor pin is inserted into the blood. Rotational movement occurs between the pin and the cup in one direction, followed by a short pause. Rotation then occurs in the opposite direction. This back and forth rotation continues throughout the analysis and is intended to represent sluggish venous blood flow. The whole system is kept

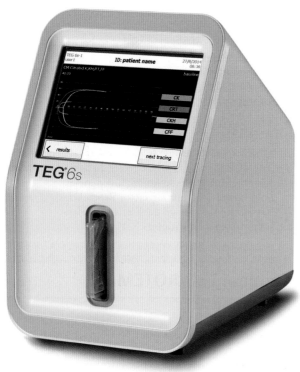

Fig. 14.4 TEG 6s with cartridge. (Courtesy Haemonetics, Glasgow, UK. Images of the TEG® 6s hemostasis analyzer and Cell Saver® Elite®+ autologous blood recovery device used by permission of Haemonetics Corporation. TEG®, Cell Saver ® and Elite® are registered trademarks of Haemonetics Corporation in the US, other countries or both.)

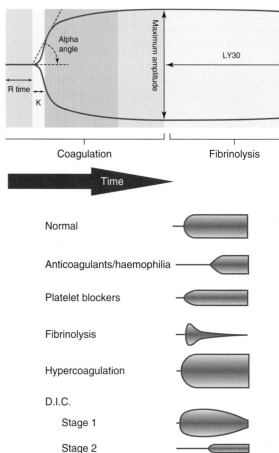

Fig. 14.5 TEG patterns.

at 37°C. As the clot begins to form, the blood becomes more viscous and exerts more resistance to rotation. This resistance is detected and plotted on a graph of clot strength against time.

TEG 6s

This is one of the most modern and truly portable POC devices at the time of publication (Fig. 14.4). This device uses a resonance method instead of a cup and pin (as discussed previously) to produce the clot formation measurements.

Components

1. A compact, portable unit that has an interactive screen to display and control the functions of the TEG 6s.
2. The unit accepts a single microfluidic cartridge that is primed with fresh whole blood from the patient. Each cartridge can have an array of tests depending on preference.

Mechanism of action

1. To measure clot strength with the resonance method, the sample is exposed to a fixed vibration frequency range (20–500 Hz). With light-emitting diode illumination, a detector measures up/down motion of the blood meniscus. A fast Fourier transform is used to identify frequency leading to resonance, and this is converted to a TEG trace via a mapping function (Fig. 14.5). Stiffer (stronger) clots have higher resonant frequencies and higher TEG traces.
2. Up to four assays can be run simultaneously on the TEG 6s.
3. From the global haemostasis cartridge, the following parameters are rapidly available, giving a complete picture and allowing therapy to be targeted (Table 14.1).

Choices of cartridges include:

1. **Global haemostasis cartridge (citrated multi-channel):** The standard TEG assay uses kaolin for activation of coagulation. This provides a measure of the time it takes for the first measurable clot to be formed, the

Table 14.1 Thromboelastometry

Component	Definition	Normal values	Problem with	Treatment
R Time	Time to start forming clot	5–10 minutes	Coagulation factors	FFP
K Time	Time clot reaches 20-mm amplitude	1–3 minutes	Fibrinogen	Cryoprecipitate
Alpha angle	Speed of fibrin accumulation	53–72 degrees	Fibrinogen	Cryoprecipitate
Maximum amplitude	Highest vertical amplitude of the TEG	50–70 mm	Platelets	Platelets +/or DDAVP
Lysis at 30 minutes (LY30)	Percent of MA reduction at 30 minutes	0%–8%	Excess fibrinolysis	TXA

DDAVP, Desmopressin (1-desamino-8-d-arginine vasopressin) is a synthetic analogue of vasopressin; *FFP,* Fresh frozen plasma; *K time,* From end of R until clot reaches 20-mm so represents speed of clot formation; *MA,* Maximal amplitude-a measurement of maximal clot strength; equals the maximal width of TEG. Normal value is 45–55 mm); *R time,* From start of test till start of clot or fibrin formation; *TXA,* Tranexaminic acid.

kinetics of clot formation, the strength of the clot and the breakdown of the clot, or fibrinolysis.

2. **Kaolin TEG with heparinase (CKH):**
   The addition of heparinase (an enzyme that removes the anticoagulant effects of heparin) eliminates the effect of heparin in the test sample. In conjunction with a kaolin TEG, this assesses the presence of systemic heparin (e.g. during or after cardiac surgery).
3. **RapidTEG (CRT):**
   An accelerated assay with tissue factor and kaolin for activation, offering a more rapid assessment of coagulation properties and enabling appropriate haemostatic therapy to be administered with minimal time delay.
4. **TEG functional fibrinogen (CFF):**
   1. Tissue factor is used for coagulation activation with platelet function inhibited by a GPIIb/IIIa inhibitor. The functional fibrinogen contribution to the clot strength is examined. Also, by subtracting this functional fibrinogen contribution from the overall clot strength, the specific contribution of platelet function is extrapolated.
   2. By using both the information from the RapidTEG and TEG functional fibrinogen, information is provided on a fibrinogen or platelet deficiency.

Problems in practice and safety features

1. The machine needs regular quality control checks.
2. Results are not instantaneous and require interpretation.
3. The sample blood needs to be citrated by adding it to a citrated blood test bottle.

ABL90 Flex Plus (Fig. 14.6)

This is a portable and automated, POC and battery-operated blood gas analyser. It can also be used in the laboratory. Up to 39 critical care parameters (plus up to 40 derived

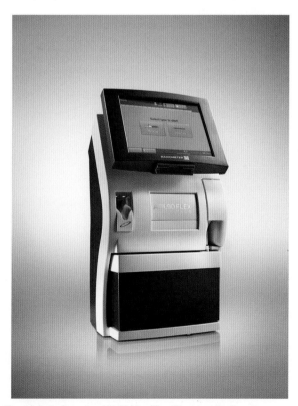

Fig. 14.6 Radiometer ABL90 Flex Plus. (Courtesy Radiometer Medical ApS, Brønshøj, Denmark. All rights reserved. Used with permission.)

parameters) including pH, pCO_2 and pO_2 are measured using a very small sample, 0.065 mL (0.045 mL in micromode) of blood from a syringe or capillary tube via an automatic inlet. Results are displayed within 35 seconds. An automatic quality management system including but not limited to performing calibrations, quality controls, clot detection and removal makes the analyser very easy to operate in POC settings.

Although the device uses pH and CO_2 electrodes with technology similar to the traditional blood gases analyser (see Chapter 13), it uses an optical technology, phosphorescence quenching spectroscopy, for oxygen measurements. Optical technology makes O_2 measurement very stable, reducing the need for the self-calibrations to once every 24 hours. As a result, the analyser is practically always ready for blood sample measurements with more than 23 hours uptime. There are only two consumables, sensor cassette and solution pack, requiring replacements every 14 or 30 days depending on the parameter panel.

Using the same sample, other parameters such as glucose, creatinine, urea, lactate, bilirubin, sodium, potassium, calcium and chloride levels can be measured and calculated. Oximetry parameters include oxygen saturation, total haemoglobin, oxyhaemoglobin, reduced haemoglobin, carboxyhaemoglobin, methaemoglobin and foetal haemoglobin.

For the arterial blood samples, the analyser can display Acid-Base Chart—a nomogram combining pH, pCO_2 and extracellular base excess results—facilitating the interpretation of the patient's acid–base status.

The measurements are displayed on an 8-inch touch screen, printed on inbuild printing and could be sent to the hospital laboratory information system.

SUGGESTED FURTHER READING

Haas, T., Spielmann, N., Mauch, J., Speer, O., Schmugge, M., Weiss, M., 2012. Reproducibility of thrombelastometry (ROTEM): point-of-care versus hospital laboratory performance. Scand. J. Clin. Lab. Invest. 72 (4), 313–317.

Perry, D.J., Fitzmaurice, D.A., Kitchen, S., Mackie, I.J., Mallett, S., 2010. Point–of–care testing in haemostasis. Br. J. Haematol. Available from: https://onlinelibrary.wiley.com/doi/full/10.1111/j.1365-2141.2010.08223.x.

St John, A., Price, C.P., 2014. Existing and emerging technologies for point-of-care testing. Clin. Biochem. Rev. 35 (3), 155–167. Available from: https://www.ncbi.nlm.nih.gov/pmc/articles/PMC4204237/.

SELF-ASSESSMENT QUESTIONS

Please check your eBook for additional self-assessment

MCQs

In the following lists, which of the following statements (a) to (e) are true?

1. Concerning thromboelastography (TEG)
a. Heparin will always cause an abnormal reading.
b. An elevated LY 30 indicates good clot stability.
c. TEG has an important role in cardiac anaesthesia.
d. TEG and HemoCue are similar technologies.
e. TEG/rotational thromboelastometry (ROTEM) are laboratory-based tests.

2. The activated clotting time (ACT)
a. Can be measured at any temperature.
b. Is prolonged by haemodilution.
c. Is not affected by unfractionated heparin.
d. Is commonly used in cardiac surgery.
e. Is useful to monitor the effect of protamine on heparinized blood.

Answers

1. Concerning TEG
   a. *False. A heparinase cartridge can be used that neutralises the effect of heparin.*
   b. *False. LY 30 is a measure of clot lysis, not stability.*
   c. *True. Due to the TEG's speed of delivery of results.*
   d. *False. The TEG and HemoCue are very different machines.*
   e. *False. The TEG 6s is very portable.*

2. Concerning TEG
   a. *False. The cuvette and the blood are warmed to 37°C.*
   b. *True. Coagulation is hindered by dilution as clotting factor concentration decreases.*
   c. *False. ACT is used as a measure of how well a patient is heparinized after dosing with unfractionated heparin.*
   d. *True. Heparinization is used in almost all cardiac surgery.*
   e. *True. Heparin is reversed by protamine. This can be quantified by the change in the ACT value returning to baseline after appropriate protamine dosing.*

Chapter 15

Electrical safety

The electrical equipment used in the operating theatre and intensive care unit is designed to improve patient care and safety. At the same time, however, there is the potential of exposing both the patient and staff to an increased risk of electric shock. It is essential for the anaesthetist to have a thorough understanding of the basic principles of electricity, even though these devices include specific safety features.

In the United Kingdom, mains power source of electricity is supplied as an alternating current (AC) with a frequency of 50 Hz. The current travels from the power station to the substation where it is converted to main power voltage by a transformer. From the substation, the current travels in two conductors: the live and neutral wires. The live wire is at a potential of 240 V (or more accurately 240 root mean square [RMS]). The neutral is connected to the earth at the substation, so keeping its potential approximately the same as earth. The live wire carries the potential to the equipment, whereas the neutral wire returns the current back to the source, so completing the circuit.

Principles of electricity (Fig. 15.1)

ELECTRIC CURRENT (I)

An electric current is the flow of electrons through a conductor past a given point per unit of time, propelled by the driving force, i.e. the voltage (potential difference). The current is measured in amperes (A). One ampere represents a flow of 6.24×10^{18} electrons (one coulomb of charge) past a specific point in 1 second.

1. *Direct current (DC):* the current flows in one direction (e.g. flow from a battery).
2. *Alternating current (AC):* the flow of electrons reverses direction at regular intervals (e.g. main power supply);

in the United Kingdom, the frequency of AC is 50 cycles per second (Hz).

POTENTIAL DIFFERENCE OR VOLTAGE (V)

It is the electrical force that drives the electrical current. When a current of 1 A is carried along a conductor, such that 1 watt (W) of power is dissipated between two points, the potential difference between those points is 1 volt (V).

ELECTRICAL RESISTANCE (R)

Electrical resistance is the resistance along a conductor to the flow of electrical current. It is not dependent on the frequency of the current. Electrical resistance is measured in ohms (Ω).

IMPEDANCE (Z)

Impedance is the sum of the forces that oppose the movement of electrons in an AC circuit. The unit for impedance is the ohm (Ω). The term *impedance* covers resistors, capacitors and inductors and is dependent on the frequency of the current. Substances with high impedance are known as insulators. Substances with low impedance are known as conductors. The impedance through capacitors and inductors is related to the frequency (Hz) at which AC reverses direction. Such an impedance, i.e. frequency related, is known as reactance (X).

1. Capacitor: impedance $\propto$ 1/frequency.
2. Inductor: impedance $\propto$ frequency.

OHM'S LAW

Electric potential (volts) = current (amperes) × resistance (ohms) [E = I × R]

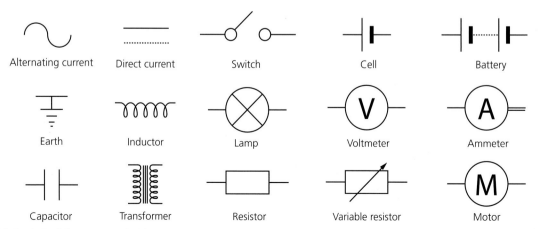

Fig. 15.1 Symbols of the common electric components.

CAPACITANCE

Capacitance is a measure of the ability of a conductor or system to store an electrical charge. A capacitor consists of two parallel conducting plates separated by an insulator (dielectric). The unit for capacitance is the farad.

With AC, the plates change polarity at the same current frequency (e.g. 50/s). This will cause the electrons to move back and forth between the plates, so allowing the current to flow.

The impedance of a capacitor = distance between the plates/current frequency × plate area.

INDUCTANCE

Inductance occurs when electrons flow in a wire resulting in a magnetic field being induced around the wire. If the wire is coiled repeatedly around an iron core, as in a transformer, the magnetic field can be very powerful.

Identification of medical electrical equipment

A *single-fault condition* is a condition when a single means for protection against hazard in equipment is defective or a single external abnormal condition is present, e.g. short circuit between the live parts and the applied part.

The following classes of equipment describe the method used to protect against electrocution according to an International Standard (IEC 60601).

Class I equipment

This type of equipment offers basic protection whereby the live, neutral and earth wires do not come into contact with each other. There is a secondary protection whereby parts that can be touched by the user, such as the metal case, are insulated from the live electricity and connected to an earth wire via the plug to the main power supply. Fuses are positioned on the live and neutral supply in the equipment. In addition, in the United Kingdom, a third fuse is positioned on the live wire in the main power source plug. This fuse melts and disconnects the electrical circuit in the event of a fault, protecting the user from electrical shock. The fault can be due to deteriorating insulation or a short circuit, making the metal case 'live'. Current will pass to earth, causing the fuse to blow (this current is called 'leakage current'). Some tiny nonfault leakage currents are always present as insulation is never 100% perfect. A faultless earth connection is required for this protection to function.

Class II equipment

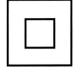

This type of equipment, also called double-insulated equipment, has double or reinforced insulation protecting the accessible parts. There is no need to earth this type of equipment. The power cable has only 'live' and 'neutral' conductors with only one fuse.

Class III equipment

This type of equipment does not need electrical supply exceeding 24 V AC or 50 V DC. The voltage used is called safety extra low voltage (SELV). Although this does not cause an electrical shock, there is still a risk of a microshock. This equipment may contain an internal power source or be connected to the main power supply by an adaptor or a SELV transformer. The power input port is designed to prevent accidental connection with another cable.

The following types of equipment define the degree of protection according to the maximum permissible leakage current.

Type B equipment

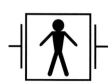

This may be class I, II or III main source-powered equipment or equipment with an internal power source. This equipment is designed to have low leakage currents, even in fault conditions, such as 0.5 mA for class I and 0.1 mA for class II. It may be connected to the patient externally or internally but is not considered safe for direct connection to the heart.

The equipment may be provided with defibrillator protection.

Type BF equipment

This is similar to type B equipment, but the part applied to the patient is isolated from all other parts of the equipment using an isolated (or floating) circuit. This isolation means that allowable leakage current under single-fault conditions is not exceeded even when 1.1 times the rated main power source voltage is applied between the attachment to the patient and the earth. The maximum AC leakage current is 0.1 mA under normal conditions and 0.5 mA under a single-fault condition. It is safer than type B but still not safe enough for direct connection to the heart.

The equipment may be provided with defibrillator protection.

Type CF equipment

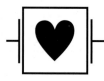

This can be class I or II equipment powered by mains power source with an internal electrical power source but considered safe for direct connection to the heart. Isolated circuits are used. There is no risk of electrocution by leakage currents (allows 0.05 mA per electrode for class I and 0.01 mA per electrode for class II). This provides a high degree of protection against electrical shock. This is used in electrocardiogram (ECG) leads, pressure transducers and thermodilution computers.

The equipment may be provided with defibrillator protection.

Attention!

DANGER

The user must consult the accompanying documents for any equipment. A black triangle on a yellow background with an exclamation mark means that there is no standardized symbol for the hazard:

High voltage and risk of electrocution!

Protective earth

The equipment itself has its own earth connection via the green-and-yellow lead in the conventional three-pin plug. The earth lead is connected to the external case of the equipment, so reducing it to zero potential. Although this provides some protection, it does not guarantee it.

Functional earth

This is part of the main circuit. The current is returned via the neutral wire back to the substation and so to earth. In effect, all conventional electrical circuits have functional earth. It is necessary for proper functioning of electrical equipment and is not a safety feature. On older equipment, the same symbol may have been used to denote protective earth.

Additional protective earth

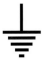

This equipment carries an additional protective earth. This protects against electric shock in cases of a single-fault condition.

Equipotentiality

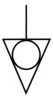

This is used to ensure that all metalwork is normally at or near zero voltage. Therefore under fault conditions, all the metalwork will increase to the same potential. Simultaneous contact between two such metal appliances would not cause a flow of current because they are both at the same potential, therefore no shock results. This provides some protection against electric shock by joining together all the metal appliances and connecting to earth.

Drip proof, splash proof, water tight

Depending on the nature and use of the equipment, some are drip proof, splash proof or water proof.

Anaesthetic-proof equipment

Anaesthetic-proof (AP) equipment standards are based on the ignition energy required to ignite the most flammable mixture of ether and air. They can be used within 5–25 cm of gas escaping from a breathing system. The temperature should not exceed 200°C. It is a less stringent requirement.

Anaesthetic-proof equipment category G

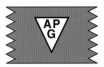

AP equipment category G standards are based on the ignition energy required to ignite the most flammable mixture of ether and oxygen. They can be used within 5 cm of gas escaping from a breathing system. The temperature should not exceed 90°C. This is a more stringent requirement as the energy level should be less than 1 mJ.

This is the UK conformity mark that supersedes the European CE mark.

CE

It means conformity has been met according to the Council of Europe Directive 93/42/EEC concerning medical devices.

Isolated or floating circuit

This is a safety feature whereby current is not allowed to flow between the electrical source and earth. These circuits are used to isolate individual equipment. An isolating transformer is used with two coils insulated from each other. The main power source circuit is earthed, whereas the patient's circuit is not earthed, so floating. As current flows through the main power source coil (producing an electromagnetic field), a current is induced in the patient's coil. To complete the patient's circuit, wires A and B should be connected. Contact with wire A or B alone will not complete a circuit, even if the subject is earthed.

Current-operated earth leakage circuit breakers (COELCB)

These safety features are also known as an earth trip or residual circuit breakers. They consist of a transformer with a core that has an equal number of windings of a live and a neutral wire around it. These are connected via a third winding to the coil of a relay that operates the circuit breaker. Under normal conditions, the magnetic fluxes cancel themselves out, as the current in the live and neutral wires is the same. In the case of a fault (e.g. excessive leakage current), the current in the live and neutral wires will be different, so resulting in a magnetic field. This induces a current in the third winding, causing the relay to break circuit. The COELCB is designed to be very sensitive. A very small current is needed to trip the COELCB (e.g. 30 mA) for a very short period of time, reducing the risk of electrocution.

Maintenance of equipment

Two factors should be checked during the maintenance of equipment (details of the tests are beyond the scope of this book):
1. *Earth leakage*: the maximum current allowed is less than 0.5 mA. Devices that are connected directly to the patient's heart should have a leakage current of less than 10 mA.

2. *Earth continuity*: the maximum resistance allowed is less than 0.1 Ω.

Hazards of electrical shock

An electric shock can occur whenever an individual becomes part of the electric circuit. The person has to be in contact with the circuit at two points with a potential difference between them for the electrons to flow. This can happen either with a faulty high-leakage current or by a direct connection to the main power source. Main power source frequency is very dangerous as it can cause muscle spasm or tetany. As the frequency increases, the stimulation effect decreases but with an increase in heating effect. With a frequency of over 100 kHz, heating is the only effect. Electric shock can happen with both AC and DC. The DC required to cause ventricular fibrillation is very much higher than the AC.

If a connection is made between the live wire and earth, electricity will flow through that connection to earth. This connection can be to a patient or to a member of staff. Main power source supplies are maintained at a constant voltage (240 V in the United Kingdom). According to Ohm's law, current flow is $\propto$ 1/impedance. A high impedance will reduce the current flow and vice versa. The main impedance is the skin resistance, which can vary from a few hundred thousand ohms to one million ohms. Skin impedance can be reduced in inflamed areas or when skin is covered with sweat.

Current density is the amount of current per unit area of tissues. In the body, the current diffusion tends to be in all directions. The larger the current or the smaller the area over which it is applied, the higher the current density.

Regarding the heart, a current of 100 mA (100,000 μA) is required to cause ventricular fibrillation when the current is applied to the surface of the body. However, only 0.05–0.1 mA (50–100 μA) is required to cause ventricular fibrillation when the current is applied directly to the myocardium. This is known as *microshock*.

Methods to reduce the risk of electrocution

- General measures: adequate maintenance and testing of electrical equipment at regular intervals, wearing antistatic shoes and having antistatic flooring in theatres.
- Ensuring that the patient is not in contact with earthed objects.
- Equipment design: all medical equipment used in theatres must comply with British Standard 5724 and *International Electro-technical Committee* (IEC) 60601-1 describing the various methods used for protection and the degree of protection (see earlier).
- Equipotentiality (see earlier).
- Isolated circuits (see earlier).
- Circuit breakers (COELCB) (see earlier).

Electricity can cause electrocution, burns or ignition of a flammable material, so causing fire or explosion. Burns can be caused as heat is generated due to the flow of the current. This is typically seen in the skin. Fires and explosions can occur through sparks caused by switches or plugs being removed from wall sockets and igniting inflammable vapours.

Damage caused by electrical shock can occur in two ways:

1. Disruption of the normal electrical function of cells. This can cause contraction of muscles, alteration of the cerebral function, paralysis of respiration, and disruption of normal cardiac function, resulting in ventricular fibrillation.
2. Dissipation of electrical energy throughout all the tissues of the body. This leads to a rise in temperature due to the flow of electrons and can result in burns.

The severity of the shock depends on:

1. The size of current (number of amperes) per unit of area.
2. Current pathway (where it flows). A current passing through the chest may cause ventricular fibrillation or tetany of the respiratory muscles, leading to asphyxia. A current passing vertically through the body may cause loss of consciousness and spinal cord damage.
3. The duration of contact. The shorter the contact, the less damage caused.
4. The type of current (AC or DC) and its frequency. The higher the frequency, the less risk to the patient. A 50-Hz current is almost the most lethal frequency. The myocardium is most susceptible to the arrhythmogenic effects of electric currents at this frequency, and muscle spasm prevents the victim letting go of the source. As the frequencies increase to >1 kHz, the risks decrease dramatically.

THE EFFECTS OF ELECTROCUTION

As a general guide to the effects of electrocution, the following might occur:

1. 1 mA: tingling pain.
2. 5 mA: pain.
3. 15 mA: tonic muscle contraction and pain.
4. 50 mA: tonic contraction of respiratory muscles and respiratory arrest.
5. 75–100 mA: ventricular fibrillation.
6. 1000 mA: extensive burns and charring.

The body can form part of an electrical circuit either by acting as the plate of a capacitor (capacitance coupling) without being in direct contact with a conductor or as an electrical resistance (resistive coupling).

Resistive coupling

This can be caused by:

1. faulty equipment allowing a contact with a live wire if it touches the casing of the equipment
2. leakage current. As there is no perfect insulation or infinite resistance, some small currents will flow to earth because the equipment is at a higher potential than earth.

Diathermy

Diathermy is frequently used to coagulate a bleeding vessel or to cut tissues. Unipolar diathermy is commonly used. As the current frequency increases above 100 kHz (i.e. radiofrequency), the entire effect is heat generating.

Components

1. Diathermy is achieved with an active or live electrode.
2. Patient's neutral or passive plate is used.
3. Diathermy case where the frequency and voltage of the current used can be adjusted. An isolating capacitor is situated between the patient's plate and earth.

Mechanism of action (Fig.15.2)

1. Heat is generated when a current passes through a resistor, depending on the current density (current per unit area). The amount of heat generated (H) is proportional to the square of current (I^2) divided by the area (A) ($H = I^2/A$). So the smaller the area, the greater the heat generated. The current density around the active electrode can be as much as 10 A/cm², generating a heating power of about 200 W.
2. A large amount of heat is produced at the tip of the diathermy forceps because of its small size (high current density). Whereas at the site of the patient's plate, because of its large surface area, no heat or burning is produced (low current density).
3. A high-frequency current (in the radiofrequency range) of 500,000 to more than 1,000,000 Hz is used. This high-frequency current behaves differently from the standard 50-Hz current. It passes directly across the precordium without causing ventricular fibrillation. This is because high-frequency currents have a low tissue penetration without exciting the contractile cells.
4. The isolating capacitor has low impedance to a high-frequency current, i.e. diathermy current. The capacitor has a high impedance to 50-Hz current, thus protecting the patient against electrical shock.

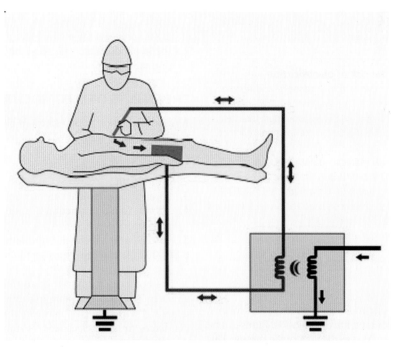

Fig. 15.2 Surgical diathermy. Note the isolating capacitor between the patient's plate and earth. (Source: Boyd, D.E., MacG Palmer, J.H., 2013. Surgical diathermy. Anaesthesia & Intensive Care Medicine, 14(10), pp.431–433.)

5. Earth-free circuit diathermy can be used. The patient, the tip of the diathermy forceps and the patient plate are not connected to earth. This reduces the risk of burns to the patient. This type of circuit is known as a floating patient circuit.

6. Cutting diathermy uses a continuous sine waveform at a voltage of 250–3000 V. Coagulation diathermy uses a modulated waveform. Coagulation can be achieved by fulguration or desiccation. Blended modes (cutting and coagulation) can be used with a variable mixture of both cutting and coagulation.

7. Bipolar diathermy does not require a patient plate. The current flows through one side of the forceps, through the patient and then back through the other side of the forceps. The current density and heating effect are the same at both electrodes. Usually low power can be achieved from a bipolar diathermy with a good coagulation effect but less cutting ability. Bipolar diathermy is frequently used during neurosurgery or ophthalmic surgery.

Problems in practice and safety features

1. If the area of contact between the plate and the patient is reduced, the patient is at risk of being burned at the site of the plate. If the plate is completely detached, current might flow through any point of contact between patient and earth, for example earthed ECG electrodes or temperature probes. Modern diathermy machines do not function with any of the above.

2. Electrical interference with other electrical monitoring devices. The use of electrical filters can solve this problem.

3. Interference with the function of cardiac pacemakers. Damage to the electrical circuits or changes in the programming can occur. This is more of a hazard with cutting diathermy than with coagulation diathermy. Modern pacemakers are protected against diathermy.

4. Fires and explosions may be caused by sparks igniting flammable material such as skin cleansing solutions or bowel gas.

Static electricity

Measures to stop the build-up of static electricity in the operating theatre are necessary to prevent the risk of sparks, fire and explosions. The electrical impedance of equipment should allow the leakage of charge to earth but should not be so low that there is a risk of electrocution and electrical burns.

Some of the measures used to prevent the build-up of static electricity are:

1. Tubings, reservoir bags and face masks are made of carbon-containing rubber; they are black with yellow labels.
2. Staff wear antistatic footwear.
3. Trolleys have conducting wheels.
4. The relative humidity in the operating theatre is kept at more than 50% with a room temperature of more than 20°C.

With modern anaesthesia, the significance of these measures is questionable as the flammable inhalational agents (e.g. ether and cyclopropane) are not used any more.

Lasers

Lasers are being used more frequently, both inside and outside the operating theatre. Lasers have the ability to cut tissue with precision with almost perfect haemostasis. They are used in thoracic surgery (excision of central airway tumours such as bronchial carcinoma); ear, nose and throat surgery (e.g. excision of vocal cord tumours), gynaecology (excision of endometriosis), urology (benign prostatic hyperplasia), skin lesion and myopia. Basic knowledge of laser principles is essential for both patient and staff safety.

Laser stands for *l*ight *a*mplification by the *s*timulated *e*mission of *r*adiation. Laser produces a nondivergent light beam of a single colour or frequency (monochromatic) with a high-energy intensity and has a very small cross-sectional area. The energy of the beam depends on the frequency.

Diathermy
- High-frequency current is used.
- An isolating capacitor is used to protect the patient against mains power frequency current.
- Floating patient circuit (earth-free circuit) is used.
- There is a high current density at the tip of the diathermy forceps generating heat.

Types of laser
- Solid-state laser such as the Nd–YAG laser that emits light at 1064 nm (infrared).
- Semiconductor laser such as the gallium arsenide (GaAs) laser. The power output tends to be low.
- Liquid laser.
- Gas laser such as the helium–neon laser (emits red light), carbon dioxide laser (emits infrared light) and argon laser (emits green light).

Problems in practice and safety features

Increasing the distance from the laser offers little increase in safety as the laser is a high-energy nondivergent beam.

1. Permanent damage to the eye retina or the head of the optic nerve can be caused by laser beams in the visible portion. Infrared light can cause damage to cornea, lens and aqueous and vitreous humours. All staff should wear eye protection appropriate for the type of laser and within the laser-controlled area. This should offer adequate protection against accidental exposure to the main beam. Spectacles do not give reliable peripheral visual field protection.
2. Burning can be caused if the laser hits the skin.
3. A non–water-based fire extinguisher should be used immediately.
4. All doors should be locked and all windows covered in order to protect those outside the operating theatre.

Table 15.1 shows the different classes of laser products.

AIRWAY LASER SURGERY

There is a high risk of fire due to the combination of an oxygen-enriched environment and the very high thermal energy generated by the laser. The risk can be reduced by avoiding the use of nitrous oxide, the use of lower oxygen concentrations (25% or less), the use of the laser-resistant tracheal tubes, protecting other tissues with wet swabs and using nonreflective matt-black surgical instruments, so reducing reflection of the main laser beam.

If fire occurs, the laser should be switched off and the site of surgery flooded with saline. The breathing system should be disconnected and the tracheal tube removed. The patient can then be ventilated with air using a bag–valve–mask system.

SUGGESTED FURTHER READING

Alkatout, I., Schollmeyer, T., Hawaldar, N.A., Sharma, N., Mettler, L., 2012. Principles and safety measures of electrosurgery in laparoscopy. J. Laparoendosc. Surg. 16 (1), 130–139.

Boumphrey, S., Langton, J.A., 2003. Electrical safety in the operating theatre. BJA CPED Rev. 3 (1), 10–14.
Electrical Safety. Available from: https://www.ebme.co.uk/articles/electrical-safety.
Kitching, A.J., Edge, C.J., 2003. Laser and surgery. BJA CPED Rev. 8 (5), 143–146.

Table 15.1 Classification of laser products

Class 1	Power not to exceed maximum permissible exposure for the eye or safe because of engineering design
Class 2	Visible laser beam only (400–700 nm), powers up to 1 mW, eye protected by blink-reflex time of 0.25 second
Class 2 m	As class 2, but not safe when viewed with visual aids such as eye loupes
Class 3a	Relaxation of class 2–5 mW for radiation in the visible spectrum (400–700 nm) provided the beam is expanded so that the eye is still protected by the blink reflex Maximum irradiance must not exceed 25 W/m for intrabeam viewing For other wavelengths, hazard is no greater than class 1
Class 3b	Powers up to 0.5 W Direct viewing hazardous Can be of any wavelength from 180 nm to 1 mm
Class 4	Powers over 0.5 W Any wavelength from 180 nm to 1 mm Capable of igniting inflammable materials, extremely hazardous

SELF-ASSESSMENT QUESTIONS

Please check your eBook for additional self-assessment

MCQs

In the following lists, which of the statements (a) to (e) are true?

1. Concerning electric current
   a. Inductance is a measure of the ability to store a charge.
   b. Main power source current in the United Kingdom is at a frequency of 50 Hz.
   c. The leakage current of a central venous pressure monitoring device should be less than 10 mA.
   d. Current density is the current flow per unit of area.
   e. In alternating current (AC), the flow of electrons is in one direction.

2. Electrical impedance
   a. When current flow depends on the frequency, impedance is used in preference to resistance.
   b. The impedance of an inductor to low-frequency current is high.
   c. Isolating capacitors in surgical diathermy are used because of their low impedance to high-frequency current.
   d. With electrocardiogram (ECG), skin electrodes need a good contact to reduce impedance.
   e. Ohms are the units used to measure impedance.

3. Which of the following statements are correct?
   a. With equipotentiality, all metal work is normally at or near zero voltage.
   b. Functional earth found on medical devices acts as a safety feature.
   c. Ohm's law states that electric resistance = current × potential difference.
   d. Type CF equipment can be safely used with direct connection to the heart.
   e. Defibrillators cannot be used with type B equipment.

4. Electrical shock
   a. It does not happen with DC.
   b. The main impedance is in the muscles.
   c. A current of 50 Hz is lethal.
   d. A current of 100 mA applied to the surface of the body can cause ventricular fibrillation.
   e. It can result in burns.

5. Diathermy
   a. The current density at the patient's plate should be high to protect the patient.
   b. An isolating capacitor is incorporated to protect the patient against low-frequency electrical shock.
   c. A floating patient circuit can be used.
   d. Filters can reduce interference with ECG.
   e. A current of 50 Hz is used to cut tissues.

Answers

1. Concerning electric current
   a. *False. Inductance occurs when a magnetic field is induced as electrons flow in a wire. The ability to store a charge is known as capacitance. In an inductor, the impedance is proportional to the frequency of the current. In a capacitor, impedance is inversely proportional to the current frequency.*
   b. *True. The frequency of the main power source supply in the United Kingdom is 50 Hz. At this relatively low frequency, the danger of electric shock is high.*
   c. *True. A central venous pressure monitoring device can be in direct contact with the heart. Ventricular fibrillation can occur with very small current, between 50 and 100 mA, as the current is applied directly to the myocardium (microshock). Such devices should have a leakage current of less than 10 mA to prevent microshock.*
   d. *True. The amount of current flow per unit of area is known as the current density. This is important in the function of diathermy. At the tip of the diathermy forceps, the current density is high, so heat is generated. At the patient plate, the current density is low, so no heat is generated.*
   e. *False. In AC, the flow of electrons reverses direction at regular intervals. In the United Kingdom, the AC is 50 cycles per second (Hz). In DC, the flow of electrons is in one direction only.*

2. Electrical impedance
   a. *True. Impedance is the sum of the forces that oppose the movement of electrons in an AC circuit. In capacitors, the impedance is low- to high-frequency current and vice versa. The opposite is correct in inductors.*
   b. *False. Inductors have low impedance to low-frequency current and vice versa.*
   c. *True. Capacitors have low impedance to high-frequency current and high impedance to low-frequency current. The latter is of most importance in protecting the patient from low-frequency current. High-frequency currents have low tissue penetration without exciting the contractile cells, allowing the current to pass directly across the heart without causing ventricular fibrillation.*
   d. *True. The skin forms the main impedance against the conduction of the ECG signal. In order to reduce the skin impedance, there should be good contact between the skin and the electrodes.*
   e. *True. Ohms are used to measure both impedance and electrical resistance. Ohm = volt/ampere.*

3. Which of the following statements are correct?
   a. *True. Equipotentiality is a safety feature when, under fault conditions, all metalwork increases to the same potential. Current will not flow during simultaneous contact between two such metal appliances as they are both at the same potential and no shock results.*
   b. *False. Functional earth is not a safety feature. It is necessary for the proper functioning of the device. It is part of the main circuit where the current, via the neutral wire, is returned to the substation and so to earth.*
   c. *False. Ohm's law states that the potential difference (volts) = current (ampere) × resistance (ohms).*
   d. *True. Type CF equipment can be used safely in direct contact with the heart. The leakage current is less than 50 μA in class I and less than 10 μA in class II, providing a high degree of protection against electrical shock.*
   e. *False. Type B equipment can be provided with defibrillator protection. The same applies to type BF and type CF equipment.*

4. Electrical shock
   a. *False. Electric shock can happen with DC, although the amount of current required to cause ventricular fibrillation is much higher than that of AC.*
   b. *False. The main impedance is in the skin and not in the muscles. Skin impedance is variable and can be from 100,000 to 1,000,000 Ω depending on the area of contact and whether or not the skin is wet.*
   c. *True. The severity of the electric shock depends on the frequency of the current. The lower the frequency, the higher the risk. A current of 50 Hz is almost the most lethal frequency.*
   d. *True. A current of 100 mA, when applied to the surface of the body, can cause ventricular fibrillation. Most of the current is lost as the current travels through the body, and only 50–100 μA are required to cause ventricular fibrillation.*
   e. *True. The electrical energy is dissipated throughout the tissues of the body, leading to a rise in temperature and resulting in burns.*

5. Diathermy
   a. **False.** In order to protect the patient from burns, the current density at the plate should be low. The same current is passed through the tip of the diathermy forceps where the current density is high, thus producing heat. The current density at the plate is low because of its large surface area.
   b. **True.** The isolating capacitor protects the patient from low-frequency current (50 Hz) shock because of its high impedance to low-frequency currents. It has low impedance to high-frequency (diathermy) currents.
   c. **True.** A floating patient circuit can be used to reduce the risk of burns. The diathermy circuit is earth free. The patient, the tip of the diathermy forceps and the patient's plate are not connected to earth.
   d. **True.** Diathermy can cause electrical interference with ECG and other monitoring devices. The use of electrical filters can solve this.
   e. **False.** Very-high–frequency current (in the radiofrequency range) of 500,000 to 1,000,000 Hz is used. This high-frequency current behaves differently from the standard 50-Hz current; because of its low tissue penetration, it passes directly through the heart without causing ventricular fibrillation.

Appendices

APPENDIX A

CHECKING ANAESTHETIC EQUIPMENT

Checking Anaesthetic Equipment 2012, AAGBI Safety Guidelines. Available from: https://www.aagbi.org/sites/default/files/checking_anaesthetic_equipment_2012.pdf.

Checklist for Anaesthetic Equipment 2012 sheet- AAGBI. Available from: https://www.aagbi.org/sites/default/files/checklist_for_anaesthetic_equipment_2012.pdf.

Recommendations for standards of monitoring during anaesthesia and recovery.

RECOMMENDATIONS FOR STANDARDS OF MONITORING DURING ANAESTHESIA AND RECOVERY

AAGBI, 2021. Recommendations for standards of monitoring during anaesthesia and recovery. Available from: https://anaesthetists.org/Home/Resources-publications/Guidelines/Recommendations-for-standards-of-monitoring-during-anaesthesia-and-recovery-2021.

APPENDIX B

Graphical symbols for use in labelling medical devices

LOT

Batch code.

134°C

Can be autoclaved.

Cannot be autoclaved.

REF

Catalogue number.

Certified to British Standards.

Date of manufacture.

Expiry date.

SN

Serial number.

Do not reuse (single use only).

STERILE

Sterile.

STERILE EO

Method of sterilization using
ethylene oxide.

STERILE R

Method of sterilization using
irradiation.

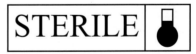

STERILE

Method of sterilization using
dry heat or steam.

Do not use if package is opened or damaged. Do not use if the product sterilization barrier or its packaging is compromised.

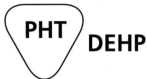

Contains phthalate – DEHP – The potential effects of phthalates on pregnant/nursing women or children have not been fully characterized and there may be concern for reproductive and developmental effects.

MR safe. This means the item poses no known hazards in *all* magnetic resonance imaging (MRI) environments.

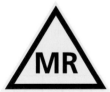

MR conditional. This means an item has been demonstrated to pose no known hazards in a *specified* MRI environment with *specified* conditions of use.

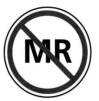

MR unsafe. This means an item is known to pose hazards in all MRI environments.

Manufacturer. This symbol is accompanied by the name and address of the manufacturer.

Order Number = Reference Number = Catalogue Number

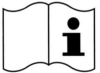

Consult instructions for use.

APPENDIX C

Decontamination of medical equipment

Healthcare-associated infections are the leading cause of preventable disease. In the United Kingdom, they are responsible for more than 5000 deaths per year and cost the National Health Service over £1 billion every year. Failure to adequately decontaminate equipment carries not only the risk associated with breach of the host barriers but the additional risk of person-to-person transmission (e.g. hepatitis B virus) and transmission of environmental pathogens. *Decontamination* is a term encompassing all the processes necessary to enable a reusable device to be reused. This includes cleaning, disinfecting, inspecting, packaging, sterilizing, transporting, storing and using (Table AppC.1). The decontamination process is required to make medical devices:

1. safe for users to handle and
2. safe for use on the patient.

Clean, disinfect or sterilize instruments?

As there is no need to sterilize all clinical items and some items cannot be sterilized, healthcare policies must identify whether cleaning, disinfecting or sterilizating is indicated based primarily on the items' intended use.

Earle H. Spaulding devised a classification system where instruments and items used for patient care are divided into three categories based on the degree of risk of infection involved in the use of the items (Table AppC.2).

Table AppC.1 Cleaning, disinfection and sterilization

Cleaning	Disinfection	Sterilization

Cleaning is the removal of visible soil (e.g. organic and inorganic material) from objects and surfaces.
    It is normally accomplished by manual or mechanical means using water with detergents or enzymatic products.
    Cleaning does much to reduce risk of vCJD.
	Disinfection describes a process that eliminates many or all pathogenic microorganisms on inanimate objects with the exception of bacterial spores.
	    It is usually accomplished by the use of liquid chemical and heat (washer disinfector).
		Sterilization is the complete elimination or destruction of all forms of microbial life. This is accomplished in healthcare facilities by either physical or chemical processes.

vCJD, Variant Creutzfeldt-Jakob disease.

Table AppC.2 Spaulding classification

Critical	Semicritical	Noncritical

Items which enter normally sterile tissue or the vascular system or through which blood flows.
    They have a high risk of infection. These items should be sterile.
    Examples: surgical instruments and needles.
	Items that touch the mucous membranes or skin that is not intact.
	    They require a high-level disinfection process, i.e. mycobactericidal.
	    As intact mucous membranes are generally resistant to infection, such items pose an intermediate risk.
	    Such devices should ideally be sterilized, but chemical disinfection is usually reserved for those that are intolerant of heat sterilization.
	    Example: laryngoscopes.
		Items that touch only intact skin require low-level disinfection.
		    As skin is an effective barrier to microorganisms, such items pose a low risk of infection.
		    Examples: bedpans and blood pressure cuffs.

???? Prions ????
- Bacterial spores
- Mycobacteria
- Non-lipid or small viruses
- Fungi
- Vegetative bacteria
- Lipid or medium-size viruses

Fig. AppC.1 Descending order of resistance of microorganisms against inactivation.

This classification has been successfully used by infection control professionals and others when planning methods for disinfection or sterilization.

The ease of inactivation differs according to the microorganisms involved (Fig. AppC.1).

Cleaning

Involves physical removal of the infectious material or organic matter on which microorganisms thrive. The critical parameters for cleaning are the following:

1. Temperature: initial wash temperatures must be below 45°C to prevent coagulation of tissue/blood residues.
2. Chemicals: detergents used are a complex formulation of chemicals designed to remove soil (proteins, carbohydrates, lipids, etc.) from instruments. Detergents have an optimal concentration and pH to work effectively.
3. Energy: may take the form of manual washing, ultrasonic energy or water jets/sprays in automated washer disinfectors.
4. Time: cleaning cycle requires a suitable time period to achieve its desired effect.
   Cleaning can be achieved either by:

Manual cleaning

1. Immersion in a diluted detergent at 35°C: Nonimmersion techniques involve a cloth soaked in cleaning solution and used to wipe the items. This can be used for electrical equipment.
2. Mechanical cleaning: This uses thermal disinfection, chemical disinfection (see later) or ultrasonic cleaners. Ultrasonic cleaning is used in areas that are difficult to access. The ultrasonic waves create small bubbles on the surfaces of the instruments. These bubbles expand until they cavitate and collapse, producing areas of vacuum that dislodge the contaminants.

Disinfection

Involves reduction of microorganisms on devices.
1. Thermal washer disinfectors combine cleaning and disinfection. Powerful water and detergent jets heated to about 80°C are used. Most organisms are inactivated except for bacterial spores, some heat-resistant viruses and cryptosporidia.
2. Chemical disinfection is the destruction of microorganisms by chemical or physiochemical means. This process is difficult to control and validate. It is frequently used for devices that are heat sensitive in the semicritical category such as endoscopes. Examples are glutaraldehyde 2% for 20 minutes, hydrogen peroxide 6%–7.5% for 20–30 minutes, peracetic acid 0.2%–0.35% for 5 minutes and orthophthalaldehyde (OPA) for 5–12 minutes.
3. Pasteurization (heat disinfection): heating to 60°C–100°C for approximately 30 minutes to reduce the number of pathogens by killing a significant number of them. The higher the temperature, the shorter the time needed.

Sterilization

The complete destruction of all microorganisms. Sterility is the probability of complete sterilization. This probability is known as the *sterility assurance level* (SAL). A sterile device has a SAL of 10^{-6}, which means that the probability of an organism surviving on that device is one in a million, using a validated process.

The methods used to achieve sterility include the following:

1. *Steam sterilization* is currently the gold standard method (Table AppC.3). It is reliable, easy to monitor, nontoxic, inexpensive, sporicidal and has high lethality, rapid heating and good penetration of fabrics. The temperature and pressure reached determine the time to sterilization. Usually a temperature of 134°C maintained for a period of 3 minutes under a pressure of 2.25 bars is used.
2. *Ionizing radiation* using γ rays to produce sterility. It is ideal for prepacked, heat-labile, single-use items such as IV cannulae and syringes. This technique of sterilization is widely used in industry.

Table AppC.3 Steam sterilization

Advantages	Disadvantages
Highly effective Rapid heating and penetration of instruments Nontoxic Inexpensive Can be used to sterilize liquids	Items must be heat and moisture resistant Does not sterilize powders, ointments or oils Needs good maintenance

Table AppC.4 Indicators used to monitor sterilization

Physical indicators	Chemical indicators	Biological indicators
These indicators are part of the steam sterilizer itself: They record and allow the observation of time, temperature and pressure readings during the sterilization cycle.	There are different chemical indicators: There are tapes with heat- or chemical-sensitive inks that change colour when the intended temperature, time and pressure are reached (Fig. AppC.2). Such a tape does not assure sterility. It merely states that the pack has been through a heating process. Bowie Dick test uses heat-sensitive inks to ensure that the steam sterilizer is functioning appropriately (Fig. AppC.3).	These are rarely used in UK hospitals: Bacillus spores that are heat sensitive can directly measure sterilization. They are inherently unreliable but can be used as an additional method of validation for some forms of sterilization such as ethylene oxide.

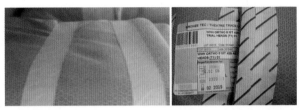

Fig. AppC.2 Heat- or chemical-sensitive inks that change colour. *Right*: presterilization. *Left*: poststerilization with the sterilization trace label. Note the date of sterilization that is valid for 1 year and details to track any object.

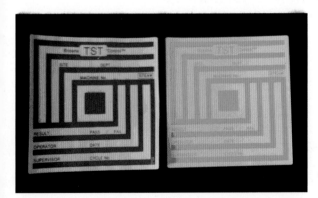

Fig. AppC.3 Bowie Dick test. This is a daily test to ensure that the steam sterilizer is functioning appropriately. Paper patches with heat-sensitive inks are used. The blue patch *(left)* is a PASS, the yellow patch *(right)* is FAILED.

3. *Dry heat sterilization* (hot air oven): a constant supply of electricity is needed. Used for reusable glass, metal instruments, oil, ointments and powders.
4. *Ethylene oxide* can effectively sterilize most equipment that can withstand temperatures of 50°C–60°C. However, it is used under carefully controlled conditions because it is extremely toxic, carcinogenic, flammable and an explosion risk. Although it is very versatile and can be used for heat-sensitive equipment, fluids and rubber, a long period of aeration is necessary to remove all traces of gas before the equipment can be distributed. The processing time ranges from 2 to 24 hours and is a very costly process.

Sterilization monitoring

The sterilization process should demonstrate a spore kill to achieve a SAL of 1×10^{-6}. To ensure that sterilization has been successful, indicators are used (Table AppC.4). For steam sterilization, for example, this requires the direct contact of saturated steam with the device in question in the absence of air at the required pressure/temperature and time.

SINGLE-USE ITEMS

The use of single-use items should be encouraged when possible. This practice ensures the sterility of the equipment and prevents cross-infection. The quality of such devices must be the same as the reusable ones. As a large proportion of these devices are made from polyvinyl chloride (PVC) plastic materials, a balance should be struck between the reduction in infection risk and effect on the environment. Incinerating PVC has no or very small effect on the levels of dioxin produced. The operating conditions of an incineration plant are the key factor in determining dioxin production and emissions rather than the quantity or source of the chlorine entering the incinerator. It must be emphasized that any equipment that is designated 'single-use' must be used for one patient only and for a single treatment episode and not reused even for the same patient during subsequent visits.

SUGGESTED FURTHER READING

Association of Anaesthetists in Great Britain and Ireland, 2008. Infection Control in Anaesthesia. AAGBI, London. Available from: http://www.aagbi.org/sites/def ault/files/infection_control_08.pdf.

MHRA, 2010. Sterilization, Disinfection and Cleaning of Medical Equipment: Guidance on Decontamination from the Microbiology Advisory Committee (the MAC manual). Available from: http://www.mhra.gov .uk/Publications/Safetyguidance/Otherdevicesafetygui dance/CON007438.

TSE Working Group, 2008. Transmissible Spongiform Encephalopathy Agents: Safe Working and the Prevention of Infection. Guidance from the Advisory Committee on Dangerous Pathogens. Available from: http://www.advisorybodies.doh.gov.uk/acdp/tseguidan ce/Index.htm.

APPENDIX D

Directory of manufacturers

AMBU

Ambu Ltd
Alconbury Weald
Cambridgeshire PE28 4XA
UK
Tel: 01480 498 403
www.ambu.co.uk

ANAEQUIP UK

2 Millstream Bank
Worthen
Shrewsbury SY5 9EY
UK
Tel: 01743 891140
www.anaequip.com

BAXTER

Wallingford Road
Compton
Newbury
Berkshire RG20 7QW
UK
Tel: 01635 206000
www.baxterhealthcare.co.uk

BD

1030 Eskdale Road
Winnersh Triangle Wokingham
Berkshire RG41 5TS
UK
Tel: 0800 917 8776
www.bd.com

BLUE BOX MEDICAL LTD

Unit 29 New Forest Enterprise Centre
Chapel Lane
Totton
Southampton
Hants SO40 9LA
UK
Tel: 0238 066 9000
www.blueboxmedical.co.uk

BOC

The Priestley Centre
10 Priestley Road
The Surrey Research Park
Guildford
Surrey GU2 7XY
UK
Tel: 01483 579 857
https://www.boconline.co.uk/en/index.html

B BRAUN MEDICAL LTD

Brookdale Road
Thorncliffe Park
Sheffield S35 2PW
UK
Tel: 0114 225 9000
www.bbraun.co.uk

COOK MEDICAL

O'Halloran Road
National Technology Park
Limerick
Ireland
Tel: 00353 61 334440
www.cookmedical.com

DELTEX MEDICAL LTD

Terminus Road
Chichester
West Sussex PO19 8TX
UK
Tel: 01243 774837
www.deltexmedical.com

DIAMEDICA (UK) LTD

Grange Hill Industrial Estate
Bratton Fleming
Barnstaple EX31 4UH
UK
Tel: 01598 710066
www.diamedica.co.uk

DYNASTHETICS

Pentland Medical Ltd.
48 Craighall Road
Edinburgh EH6 4RU
UK
Tel: 0131 467 5764
www.pentlandmedical.co.uk/

DRÄGER MEDICAL UK LTD

The Willows
Mark Road
Hemel Hempstead
Hertfordshire HP2 7BW
UK
Tel: 01442 213542
www.draeger.com

EDWARDS LIFESCIENCES LTD

The Sector 3 Newbury Business Park
London Road
Newbury RG14 2PZ
UK
Tel: 0870 606 2040
www.edwards.com

GE DATEX-OHMEDA MEDICAL EQUIPMENT SUPPLIES LTD

61 Great North Road
Hatfield
Herts AL9 5EN
UK
Tel: 01707 263570
www.gehealthcare.com

GETINGE AB

14–15 Burford Way
Boldon Business Park
Sunderland
Tyne & Wear NE35 9PZ
UK
Tel: 0191 519 6200
www.getinge.com

HEMOCUE AB

Manor Court
Manor Royal
Crawley
West Sussex RH10 9FY
UK
Tel: 01293 517599
www.radiometer.co.uk

INTERSURGICAL

Dray House
Molly Millars Lane
Wokingham
Berkshire RG41 2PX
UK
Tel: 0118 965 6300
www.intersurgical.com

MASIMO EUROPE LIMITED

Matrix House,
Basing View
Basingstoke
Hampshire RG21 4DZ
UK
Tel: 01256 479988
www.masimo.co.uk

MEDTRONIC LTD

Building 9
Croxley Green Business Park
Hatters Lane
Watford, Hertfordshire WD18 8WW
UK
Tel: 01923 212213
www.covidien.com

OLYMPUS KEYMED (MEDICAL & INDUSTRIAL EQUIPMENT) LTD

Keymed House
Stock Road
Southend-on-Sea SS2 5QH
UK
Tel: 01702 616333
www.keymed.co.uk

PAJUNK

The Waterfront Goldcrest Way
Newcastle upon Tyne NE15 8NY
UK
Tel: 0191 264 7333
www.pajunk.com

PENLON LTD

Abingdon Science Park
Barton Lane
Abingdon
Oxon OX14 3PH
UK
Tel: 01235 547000
www.penlon.com

PHILIPS HEALTH CARE

Philips Centre
Guildford Business Park
Guildford
Surrey GU2 8XH
UK
Tel: 01483 792004
www.healthcare.philips.com

PROACT MEDICAL

9-13 Oakley Hay Lodge
Great Folds Road
Corby NN18 9AS
UK
Tel: 01536 461981
www.proactmedical.co.uk

RADIOMETER LTD

Manor Court
Manor Royal
Crawley
West Sussex RH10 9FY
UK
Tel: 01293 517599
www.radiometer.co.uk

RIMER ALCO LTD

2-4 Kelvin Place
Thetford
Norfolk IP24 3RR
UK
Tel: 01842 766441
https://www.camdenboss.com/

SIEMENS HEALTHCARE

Newton House
Sir William Siemens Square
Frimley
Camberley
Surrey GU16 8QD
UK
Tel: 01276 696000
www.medical.siemens.com

SMITHS MEDICAL

1500 Eureka Park
Lower Pemberton
Ashford
Kent TN25 4BF
UK
Tel: 0845 850 0445
www.smiths-medical.com

SPACELABS HEALTHCARE LTD

John Tate Road
Unit B, Foxholes Centre
Hertford SG13 7DT
UK
Tel: 01992 507700
www.spacelabshealthcare.com

TELEFLEX

Grosvenor House
Horseshoe Crescent
Old Town
Beaconsfield HP9 1LJ
UK
Tel: 01494 53 27 61
www.teleflex.com

TRITON ELECTRONIC SYSTEMS LTD

620100 Ekaterinburg
Russia
Sibirsky Tract 12/5
www.treat-on.com

VERATHON MEDICAL UNITED KINGDOM LTD

Rutland House
148 Edmund Street
Birmingham B3 2JRUK
Tel: 01494 682650
www.verathon.com

VYGON (UK) LTD

The Pierre Simonet Building
V Park
Gateway North
Latham Road
Swindon
Wiltshire SN25 4DL
UK
Tel: 01793 748800
www.vygon.co.uk

ZOLL MEDICAL UK

16 Seymour Court
Tudor Road
Manor Park
Runcorn
Cheshire WA7 1SY
UK
Tel: 01928 595160
www.zollaed.co.uk

Index